DIALYSIS HANDBOOK 2026

A Clinical Textbook Covering Kidney Replacement Therapy, Vascular Access, and Bedside Complication Response for Nephrology Fellows

Ramon C. Henson, MD

This textbook is intended solely for educational and informational purposes and is designed to support the continuing professional development of licensed healthcare providers. The clinical content presented herein reflects information believed to be accurate and current at the time of publication; however, medicine evolves rapidly, and readers are advised that new research findings, updated clinical practice guidelines, and revised regulatory approvals may alter or supersede information contained in this work after its publication date.

Nothing in this publication constitutes medical advice, clinical guidance specific to any individual patient, or a substitute for the independent professional judgment of a licensed and qualified healthcare provider. No clinician-patient relationship is established, implied, or intended by the use of this textbook or any portion thereof. All clinical decisions, including but not limited to diagnosis, therapeutic selection, drug dosing, and patient monitoring, must be individualized based on thorough and direct assessment of the patient, the totality of current published evidence, applicable clinical practice guidelines, institutional protocols, and the informed professional judgment of the responsible clinician.

Drug information, dosages, treatment protocols, and therapeutic recommendations presented in this publication are offered for educational reference only and must be independently verified against current prescribing information, pharmacopeial references, and applicable regulatory approvals prior to clinical application. The author and publisher have made every reasonable effort to ensure the accuracy and completeness of the information presented; nevertheless, they expressly disclaim all liability for any adverse outcomes, clinical errors, patient harm, loss, or injury alleged to arise, directly or indirectly, from the use, misuse, or application of any information, recommendation, protocol, or clinical guidance contained in this publication.

TABLE OF CONTENTS

DIALYSIS RECOGNITION & RESPONSE SYSTEM — Special Population Arcs 359

DIALYSIS RECOGNITION & RESPONSE SYSTEM — Transplant Transition Arcs 369

PREFACE

Dialysis medicine is practiced against a clock. A patient's blood pressure begins to fall twenty minutes into a hemodialysis run; a fistula that thrilled normally last week now feels different under the fingers; a peritoneal dialysis effluent turns cloudy overnight. In each case, the clinician at the bedside has minutes, not hours, to recognize the pattern, weigh the alternatives that mimic it, and act. Most nephrology references are built to answer a different question — what is the complete pathophysiology of this condition — and answer it exceptionally well. This handbook is built to answer the question the reader actually has in the moment: what is happening, what does it rule in or out, and what happens next.

This textbook covers the full clinical territory of kidney replacement therapy: the physiology and prescription of hemodialysis, peritoneal dialysis, and continuous renal replacement therapy; the creation, surveillance, and troubleshooting of vascular and peritoneal access; the recognition and management of intradialytic emergencies; and the systemic complications — anemia, mineral and bone disorder, cardiovascular disease, nutrition, and infection — that accompany long-term dialysis dependence. Special populations and the transitions surrounding transplantation and conservative kidney management receive dedicated treatment, reflecting how much of dialysis practice is about matching therapy to the individual patient's trajectory rather than applying a single protocol uniformly.

Threaded through every chapter is the Dialysis Recognition & Response System, this book's integrated approach to bedside decision-making. At each major clinical decision point, a named pattern is presented alongside its recognizable bedside signature, the decision it should trigger, the look-alike presentation most likely to be confused with it, and a single anchoring fact meant to be recalled instantly under pressure. Every chapter closes by consolidating its patterns into a scannable recap, and the book closes with a comprehensive, cross-referenced index of every pattern introduced — organized so that a reader standing at a dialysis station can find the relevant entry in seconds.

This is a reference text, not an examination-preparation tool. It contains no practice questions, review items, or self-assessment exercises of any kind; its purpose is to be read, consulted, and trusted as an authoritative clinical companion. It is written for nephrology fellows building clinical judgment during training, for dialysis nurses and technicians managing patients at the bedside, for nephrology nurse practitioners and physician assistants, and for practicing nephrologists who want a fast, reliable point-of-care reference that has not sacrificed clinical depth for brevity.

Kidney replacement therapy has grown more individualized over the past decade — incremental prescriptions, home and intensive modalities, and patient-centered adequacy targets have all displaced older, one-size-fits-all conventions. This handbook reflects that shift throughout, teaching the reasoning behind each decision rather than a single fixed algorithm, so that the clinician using it is prepared not only for the textbook presentation but for the patient in front of them.

CHAPTER 1: CHRONIC KIDNEY DISEASE PROGRESSION AND THE DECISION TO INITIATE KIDNEY REPLACEMENT THERAPY

Learning Objectives

Stage chronic kidney disease by glomerular filtration rate and albuminuria category and relate that staging to expected trajectory.

Distinguish uremic signs and symptoms that mandate urgent initiation of kidney replacement therapy from those that permit continued conservative management.

Weigh the evidence on early versus late initiation of dialysis against an individual patient's trajectory and symptom burden.

Sequence the practical steps of patient preparation, including vein preservation and access referral, ahead of anticipated kidney failure.

Apply the Dialysis Recognition & Response System to the initiation decision, distinguishing true indications for urgent start from look-alike presentations that do not require it.

Chapter Overview

The decision to begin kidney replacement therapy is rarely made at a single moment. It is the endpoint of a trajectory that a clinician has usually been tracking for months or years, punctuated by an inflection point at which the kidneys' remaining function can no longer keep the internal environment within a range the body tolerates. Because that inflection point can arrive gradually, as a slow accumulation of fatigue and appetite loss, or abruptly, as pulmonary edema or a seizure, the clinician's task is twofold: to recognize where a given patient sits on the trajectory of chronic kidney disease, and to recognize, in real time, whether the current presentation has crossed the threshold that makes further delay dangerous. This chapter builds both skills before the book turns, in later chapters, to the mechanics of the therapies themselves.

Staging and Trajectory of Chronic Kidney Disease

Confirming Chronicity Before Staging

Staging by GFR and albuminuria category presumes that the kidney impairment being staged is genuinely chronic, and this presumption is only valid once abnormalities have been documented for at least three months, per the conventional definition of chronic kidney disease. A single abnormal GFR or albuminuria measurement, however low, describes kidney impairment of undetermined duration and should prompt repeat testing rather than immediate staging and the trajectory-based planning that staging is meant to support, because a substantial fraction of single abnormal values reflect an acute process — dehydration, an acute illness, or a transient hemodynamic insult — that resolves rather than persists.

Supporting evidence for chronicity beyond the three-month criterion includes a compatible history of long-standing diabetes, hypertension, or other known chronic kidney disease etiology; imaging findings such as reduced kidney size or increased echogenicity, discussed later in this chapter; and, where available, prior laboratory values establishing that the impairment substantially predates the current presentation. When chronicity cannot be confirmed and the clinical context does not otherwise suggest a chronic process, the more accurate framing is unexplained kidney impairment of undetermined duration, with staging and trajectory planning deferred until repeat testing clarifies the picture, rather than a chronic kidney disease stage assigned prematurely on a single value.

CKD Staging by GFR and Albuminuria Categories

Chronic kidney disease is staged along two independent axes rather than one, because glomerular filtration rate alone understates risk in patients whose filtration barrier is already leaking protein. The estimated glomerular filtration rate, staged from G1 through G5, describes how much filtering capacity remains; the albuminuria category, staged from A1 through A3, describes how much of the filtration barrier's selectivity has already been lost. A patient with preserved filtration but heavy albuminuria carries a materially higher risk of progression to kidney failure than a patient with the same filtration rate and normal albumin excretion, because albuminuria is not merely a marker of glomerular injury but a mediator of it: filtered protein is reabsorbed by proximal tubular cells, which triggers an inflammatory and profibrotic response that accelerates nephron loss. The two-axis staging system is therefore not an administrative convenience but a reflection of two separable, additive mechanisms of decline.

Because G-category and A-category interact multiplicatively rather than additively in their effect on prognosis, the two axes are conventionally displayed together as a heat map, allowing a clinician to locate a patient's overall risk of progression to kidney failure, cardiovascular events, and mortality at a glance. The heat map is reproduced below in its conventional form.

GFR Category (mL/min/1.73m^2)	A1: Normal-to-Mildly Increased (<30 mg/g)	A2: Moderately Increased (30–300 mg/g)	A3: Severely Increased (>300 mg/g)
G1 (≥90, Normal or High)	Low Risk	Moderately Increased Risk	High Risk
G2 (60–89, Mildly Decreased)	Low Risk	Moderately Increased Risk	High Risk
G3a (45–59, Mild-to-Moderate)	Moderately Increased Risk	High Risk	Very High Risk

G3b (30–44, Moderate-to-Severe)	High Risk	Very High Risk	Very High Risk
G4 (15–29, Severely Decreased)	Very High Risk	Very High Risk	Very High Risk
G5 (<15, Kidney Failure)	Very High Risk	Very High Risk	Very High Risk

This handbook's focus begins in earnest at the G4-to-G5 boundary, where the clinical question shifts from slowing progression to preparing for and timing replacement therapy. A patient entering G5 has not necessarily reached the point at which dialysis must start; G5 describes filtration below fifteen milliliters per minute, a threshold chosen because it is where uremic complications become common, not because it is where they become universal. Some patients tolerate a GFR of ten or eleven for an extended period with adequate residual clearance of potassium, acid, and volume; others become symptomatic well before reaching that number because comorbid heart failure or diabetes narrows their physiologic reserve. Staging identifies who to watch closely; it does not by itself answer when to start.

Trajectories of Decline and Their Clinical Significance

Two patients arriving at the same GFR by different routes are not equivalent patients. A patient whose filtration has declined by two milliliters per minute per year for a decade is approaching kidney failure along a trajectory that allows deliberate, unhurried preparation: modality education, vascular access referral, and a Life-Plan discussion can all proceed on a timeline measured in months. A patient whose filtration has fallen by ten milliliters per minute in the last three months, by contrast, is on a trajectory that compresses all of that preparation into weeks, and it is the rate of decline, not the absolute number, that should trigger urgency in referral and access planning. Because slope is more informative than any single value, this handbook treats a trend line of at least three GFR measurements over six to twelve months as the minimum dataset needed to characterize a patient's trajectory, rather than anchoring management decisions to a single laboratory value.

Rapid decline should also prompt a search for a reversible or partially reversible contributor before the trajectory is accepted as the patient's new baseline. Superimposed acute kidney injury from volume depletion, nephrotoxic medication exposure, urinary obstruction, or an intercurrent illness can masquerade as accelerated chronic progression, and distinguishing the two matters enormously: a patient whose apparent rapid decline is substantially acute-on-chronic injury may recover meaningful function once the precipitant is removed, while a patient whose decline reflects true, sustained loss of nephron mass will not. This distinction is the first Recognition & Response pattern of the chapter, developed below.

DIALYSIS RECOGNITION & RESPONSE SYSTEM — Initiation Decision Arcs

The Pattern: A patient with known chronic kidney disease presents with a creatinine substantially higher than their established trend.

Stem Signature: Rapid rise in creatinine over days to a few weeks, often accompanied by a clear precipitant such as a new nephrotoxic medication, a diarrheal illness, contrast exposure, or a change in diuretic dosing; urine output may be preserved or reduced.

The Decision: Evaluate for and remove reversible contributors — hold nephrotoxins, correct volume depletion, rule out obstruction with renal ultrasound — before accepting the new creatinine as the patient's chronic baseline or accelerating the initiation timeline on the basis of it.

Trap Logic: True accelerated chronic progression looks similar on a single lab draw, but it lacks an identifiable precipitant, shows a smoother multi-month rather than an abrupt multi-day rise, and does not improve after volume repletion and nephrotoxin removal.

Response Anchor: Do not stage a new baseline off a single creatinine value obtained during an acute illness; recheck after the precipitant has resolved.

Estimating GFR at the Threshold of Kidney Failure

Creatinine-based estimating equations become progressively less reliable as filtration falls toward the threshold for kidney failure, because at very low clearance a growing fraction of creatinine elimination occurs through tubular secretion rather than filtration, which the estimating equations do not account for. This tends to make estimated GFR overstate true filtration in advanced disease, particularly in patients with low muscle mass, in whom creatinine generation is reduced independently of kidney function and can produce a falsely reassuring estimate. Cystatin C–based or combined creatinine-cystatin C equations partially correct for this muscle-mass dependence and are preferred when the clinical picture and the estimated GFR disagree, such as a frail, sarcopenic patient whose creatinine-based GFR seems inconsistent with visible uremic symptoms.

When precision at the threshold genuinely matters — for example, when timing a vascular access referral or planning a dialysis start date — a measured creatinine clearance from a timed urine collection, imperfect as it is, still provides information that estimating equations cannot: an approximation of residual kidney function grounded in the patient's actual urine output rather than a population-derived formula. This is used selectively rather than routinely, reserved for cases where the estimating equations are suspected to mislead.

A twenty-four-hour urine collection for creatinine clearance carries its own sources of error, chiefly incomplete collection, which is common enough that most laboratories report the total urine creatinine alongside the calculated clearance so the clinician can sanity-check the collection against expected daily creatinine excretion for the patient's age, sex, and muscle mass; a total urine creatinine well below the expected range signals a likely incomplete collection rather than an unusually low clearance. Because creatinine clearance overestimates true GFR at low filtration rates, owing to the same tubular secretion that undermines estimating equations, some centers average measured creatinine and urea clearances from the same collection to arrive at a value that splits the difference between creatinine's overestimation and urea's underestimation of true filtration. Regardless of which correction is used, the measured clearance is best treated as one additional data point weighed against the clinical trajectory rather than as a definitive replacement for the estimating equation, since both approaches share the underlying limitation that no single number fully captures a patient's physiologic reserve.

Figure 1.1: Nephron Loss and Compensatory Hyperfiltration in Progressive Chronic Kidney Disease

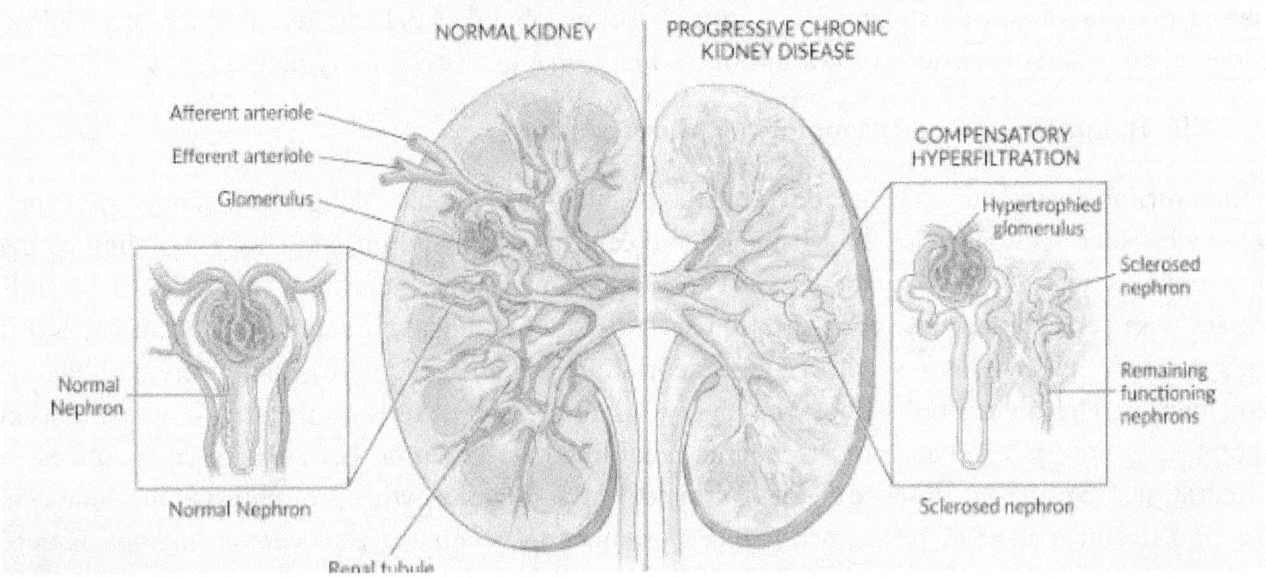

Uremic Signs and Symptoms Prompting Initiation

Constitutional and Neurologic Uremic Manifestations

The earliest uremic symptoms are often the least specific, which is precisely what makes them easy to under-recognize. Fatigue, anorexia, a metallic or diminished sense of taste, and mild cognitive slowing accumulate gradually enough that patients and families frequently attribute them to aging, depression, or unrelated illness rather than to declining kidney function, because no single symptom among these points unambiguously to uremia. Clustered together and trending in parallel with a falling GFR, however, they form a recognizable constellation, and part of this chapter's purpose is to train the reader to see that constellation as one pattern rather than as several unrelated complaints.

As filtration falls further, the neurologic manifestations become more specific and more dangerous. Asterixis, a coarse, irregular flapping tremor elicited by asking the patient to extend the wrists and fingers, reflects the diffuse metabolic encephalopathy of accumulating uremic toxins and is a reliable bedside sign that uremia has progressed beyond the mild, nonspecific stage. Its appearance, together with lethargy progressing toward frank confusion, marks the transition into uremic encephalopathy, a syndrome that in its most severe form can progress to seizure and coma, and its presence should be treated as an indication that further delay in initiating replacement therapy carries real risk rather than as a symptom to be managed conservatively while awaiting a more convenient start date.

Because the early cognitive slowing of uremia can be subtle enough to escape casual observation, particularly in patients who already have a mild baseline cognitive impairment from unrelated causes, a brief, structured cognitive screen repeated at intervals as GFR approaches the kidney-failure range can detect a meaningful decline that neither the patient nor family has spontaneously reported. This is particularly relevant in the differential between uremic encephalopathy and other causes of confusion common in this population — medication accumulation from reduced renal clearance, an intercurrent infection, or an unrelated primary neurologic process — each of which requires a different response than initiating dialysis, and a documented cognitive baseline obtained before advanced uremia makes that differential considerably easier to work through when a change is eventually noted.

Metabolic, Hematologic, and Dermatologic Manifestations

Uremic pruritus, historically attributed to cutaneous calcium-phosphate deposition, is now understood to involve a broader disturbance of the peripheral and central opioid and inflammatory signaling pathways, which explains why it often responds poorly to topical measures alone and why it does not reliably correlate with serum phosphate concentration in individual patients. Clinically it presents as a diffuse, often symmetric itch, sometimes with visible excoriations, and its severity tracks loosely with the overall uremic burden. Uremic frost, the fine, whitish crystalline deposit of urea on the skin left behind as sweat evaporates, is now rare because most patients reach medical attention before urea accumulates to the concentrations required to produce it, but its historical association with pre-dialysis-era kidney failure makes it a useful marker of just how advanced uremia can become if replacement therapy is deferred indefinitely.

Hematologic manifestations compound the constitutional symptoms rather than standing apart from them. Anemia of chronic kidney disease, discussed in full in a later chapter, contributes independently to the fatigue that patients often attribute solely to uremia itself, and a platelet dysfunction specific to the uremic milieu — impaired platelet aggregation and adhesion despite a normal platelet count — produces a bleeding tendency that becomes clinically relevant around the time of vascular or peritoneal access placement. Recognizing this platelet dysfunction preoperatively, rather than only after a bleeding complication, is one of the practical reasons access planning benefits from occurring well before the anticipated start of dialysis.

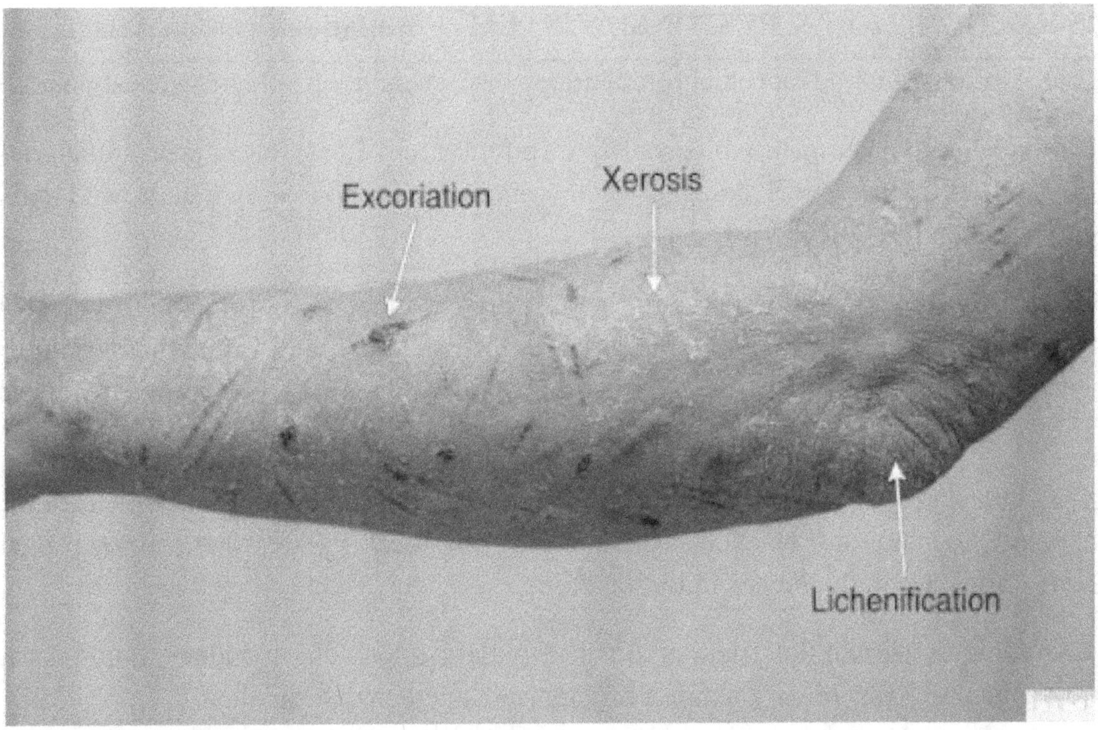

CLINICAL PEARL: Asterixis is elicited by asking the patient to extend both arms with wrists dorsiflexed and fingers spread; a positive result is a coarse, irregular flap, not a fine tremor, and its presence should prompt reassessment of the initiation timeline the same day it is found.

Fluid Overload and Cardiopulmonary Signs

As residual kidney function falls, sodium and water excretion become progressively less flexible, narrowing the margin between euvolemia and overt fluid overload. Early volume overload presents as lower extremity edema and modest weight gain that may be attributed to dietary indiscretion; more advanced overload produces elevated jugular venous pressure, pulmonary crackles, and, in its most severe form, frank pulmonary edema with hypoxemic respiratory distress. Because diuretic responsiveness itself declines as GFR falls — there is simply less filtered sodium delivered to the diuretic's site of action — a patient who previously controlled volume status comfortably on an established diuretic regimen may become refractory to escalating doses, and this diuretic resistance is itself a signal that the kidneys' capacity to manage volume independently is running out.

Uremic pericarditis, an inflammatory pericardial process driven by accumulated uremic toxins rather than infection, presents with pleuritic chest pain, a pericardial friction rub, and, in advanced cases, signs of tamponade physiology such as pulsus paradoxus and a narrowed pulse pressure. It is one of the few uremic complications considered an absolute indication for urgent initiation of dialysis regardless of the numeric GFR, because the pericardial inflammation itself is a direct consequence of uremic toxin accumulation and because tamponade from uremic pericardial effusion is immediately life-threatening. Recognizing pericarditis as a dialysis-urgent finding, rather than treating it symptomatically while continuing conservative management, is the second Recognition & Response pattern in this chapter.

The Pattern: A patient with advanced chronic kidney disease develops pleuritic chest pain.

Stem Signature: Sharp chest pain worsened by inspiration and lying flat, a pericardial friction rub on auscultation, and, in more severe cases, jugular venous distension with a narrowed pulse pressure suggesting tamponade physiology.

The Decision: Treat this as uremic pericarditis until proven otherwise in a patient with this degree of kidney impairment, obtain an echocardiogram to assess effusion size and hemodynamic significance, and initiate urgent dialysis — uremic pericarditis is an absolute indication for urgent start regardless of the numeric GFR.

Trap Logic: Acute coronary syndrome and pulmonary embolism can both produce pleuritic-quality chest pain in this population and must be excluded, but neither produces a pericardial friction rub, and both are far less likely to improve with dialysis initiation alone.

Response Anchor: A pericardial friction rub in a patient approaching kidney failure is an absolute indication for urgent dialysis initiation, not a finding to manage symptomatically.

Timing of Initiation: Early Versus Late Start

Evidence on Early Versus Late Initiation

For much of the modern dialysis era, prevailing practice favored initiating dialysis at higher residual GFR values on the theoretical assumption that starting earlier would spare patients the cumulative burden of uremic toxin exposure and thereby improve survival. The IDEAL trial directly tested this assumption by randomizing patients to planned early-start or late-start dialysis and found no survival or major clinical benefit to the early-start strategy; most patients randomized to late start were, in practice, started well before their assigned threshold once symptoms developed, and outcomes between the two groups were similar. This finding reoriented practice away from starting dialysis by GFR number alone and toward starting on the basis of symptoms and complications, a shift reflected in essentially all major guideline statements since.

The clinical implication is not that early initiation is uniformly harmful, but that GFR by itself is an insufficient trigger: a patient who is asymptomatic at a GFR of eight is not automatically better served by immediate initiation than one who is symptomatic at a GFR of fourteen, and initiating dialysis in an asymptomatic patient exposes them to the real risks of the therapy itself — access complications, intradialytic hemodynamic stress, and the burden of a three-times-weekly treatment schedule — without a demonstrated corresponding benefit. This reframes the initiation decision as a search for indications, not a countdown against a number.

Absolute and Relative Indications for Urgent Initiation

A small set of findings are treated as absolute indications for urgent initiation because each reflects a uremic complication that is immediately dangerous and reliably reversed by dialysis, and because delaying therapy in their presence carries a clear and preventable risk. The following sequence reflects the order in which these should be actively sought once advanced kidney disease is recognized.

1. Assess for uremic pericarditis — pericardial friction rub, pleuritic chest pain, or tamponade physiology — which constitutes an absolute indication for urgent dialysis regardless of GFR.
2. Assess for uremic encephalopathy — asterixis progressing to confusion, lethargy, or seizure — which is likewise an absolute indication independent of the numeric GFR.
3. Assess for refractory volume overload — pulmonary edema or severe hypertension unresponsive to escalating diuretic therapy — which constitutes an absolute indication when diuretic resistance has been confirmed.
4. Assess for refractory hyperkalemia or metabolic acidosis unresponsive to dietary and medical management, each an absolute indication when conservative measures have been exhausted.
5. In the absence of any absolute indication, weigh relative indications — persistent nausea and anorexia with weight loss, progressive cognitive slowing, and declining functional status — against the patient's own goals and the practical readiness of their chosen access, and initiate on the basis of this composite clinical judgment rather than a fixed GFR threshold.

The distinction between an absolute and a relative indication is not always a matter of a single threshold value; a potassium of 6.2 mEq/L that has been stable at that level for weeks on a fixed medication regimen behaves differently from a potassium of 6.0 mEq/L that has risen from 4.8 mEq/L over three days, even though the second value is numerically lower, because the trajectory in the second case signals an active process — a new ACE inhibitor dose, a dietary change, or worsening acute-on-chronic injury — that may continue to worsen before the next scheduled laboratory check. For this reason, an acutely worsening trend in potassium, bicarbonate, or volume status is weighed as more urgent than a numerically similar but stable value, even when neither yet meets a conventional absolute-indication threshold, and this trend-sensitivity is precisely why the initiation decision is better framed as continuous clinical judgment than as a checklist evaluated once and then set aside.

KEY POINT: GFR is used to anticipate when the initiation conversation will become necessary and to time access referral; it is not, by itself, the trigger that starts dialysis.

Frailty, Comorbidity, and the Initiation Decision in Older Adults

Age alone is a poor guide to the initiation decision, but the frailty that frequently accompanies advanced age in patients with chronic kidney disease changes the calculation in ways that a GFR-and-symptoms framework alone does not capture. A frail older adult carries a materially higher burden from the treatment itself — the vascular access procedure, the intradialytic hemodynamic stress of fluid removal, and the time and transportation demands of a three-times-weekly schedule — than a younger, more physiologically resilient patient with the same laboratory values, and for some frail patients with substantial comorbidity, particularly advanced dementia or severe functional dependence, dialysis initiation does not reliably extend survival once the competing risks of comorbid illness are accounted for, and may not improve, and can sometimes worsen, quality of life relative to conservative kidney management.

Validated frailty and comorbidity indices, alongside a structured discussion of functional status and the patient's own goals, are more informative in this population than GFR trajectory alone, and several nephrology-specific prognostic tools now exist to estimate expected survival on dialysis for older, comorbid patients, allowing that estimate to be weighed openly against the expected trajectory under conservative management. This is not a recommendation against dialysis in older adults broadly — many frail older patients do benefit meaningfully from initiation and tolerate treatment well — but a recommendation that frailty assessment become a routine, explicit part of the initiation discussion for this population rather than an afterthought raised only once a patient has already struggled on treatment.

Practically, this means the modality education and Life-Plan discussion described later in this chapter should, for frail or multimorbid older patients, explicitly include conservative kidney management as a genuine option carrying its own dedicated symptom-management pathway, rather than presenting it as a fallback offered only after dialysis has already been tried and found intolerable. Chapter 3 develops the conservative management pathway, including the advance care planning and symptom control it requires, in full.

Individualizing the Start Decision

Two patients with identical absolute indications may still warrant different timing once their broader context is considered. A patient with a mature, well-functioning arteriovenous fistula who develops early volume overload can be started promptly with a low-risk access already in place, while a patient with equivalent symptoms but no established access and a strong preference for peritoneal dialysis may be better served by an urgent peritoneal catheter placement and a brief bridging period, if their symptoms permit it, rather than a rushed catheter-based hemodialysis start that forecloses their preferred modality. This is precisely the reasoning the ESKD Life-Plan, introduced in the next chapter, is designed to formalize: matching the timing and route of initiation to the individual patient's circumstances rather than defaulting to whichever access is fastest to obtain.

The following case illustrates how symptom-based, individualized timing plays out in practice.

A sixty-eight-year-old woman with diabetic kidney disease and an estimated GFR that has fallen from eighteen to eleven milliliters per minute over four months presents with three weeks of progressive fatigue, poor appetite, and new lower extremity edema unresponsive to an increased diuretic dose. On examination she has bibasilar crackles and mild asterixis but no pericardial rub and is oriented and conversing normally. Her arteriovenous fistula, created eleven weeks earlier in anticipation of this trajectory, is palpably thrilling and has been assessed as usable. Laboratory studies show a potassium of 5.4 mEq/L and a bicarbonate of 18 mEq/L, both stable compared to the prior week rather than acutely worsening, and a chest radiograph confirms mild pulmonary vascular congestion without frank edema. Because she has relative rather than absolute indications — diuretic-resistant volume overload without pulmonary edema, mild asterixis without confusion, and stable rather than acutely dangerous electrolyte derangement — and because her access is ready, the clinical team elects to initiate scheduled hemodialysis using the mature fistula within the next several days rather than treating her as an emergency requiring same-day catheter placement. This decision reflects the chapter's central point: the presence of symptoms warranting initiation does not by itself dictate the urgency or route of that initiation once an access is already prepared.

DIALYSIS RECOGNITION & RESPONSE SYSTEM — Initiation Decision Arcs

The Pattern: A patient with relative indications for initiation and a mature, ready access.

Stem Signature: Diuretic-resistant volume overload without frank pulmonary edema, mild asterixis without confusion, and stable rather than rapidly worsening electrolytes, in a patient whose vascular or peritoneal access has already been created and assessed as usable.

The Decision: Proceed with a scheduled, non-emergent initiation using the prepared access rather than defaulting to urgent catheter placement, preserving the modality and access pathway already established under the patient's Life-Plan.

Trap Logic: The presence of any uremic symptom can prompt reflexive urgent catheter placement; this is unnecessary and carries added infection and central-vein risk when a scheduled start using an already-mature access will achieve the same clinical benefit within days.

Response Anchor: Relative indications with a ready access support a scheduled start; only absolute indications, or relative indications with no usable access, justify an urgent, unplanned one.

The next case illustrates the opposite outcome of the same decision process: a patient whose relative indications, once weighed against her own goals and functional trajectory, support deferring initiation rather than proceeding.

An eighty-four-year-old man with a GFR of nine milliliters per minute, moderate baseline dementia, and a recent decline in ambulatory function following a hip fracture is evaluated for initiation after his family reports several weeks of poor appetite and increasing daytime somnolence. He has no asterixis, no pericardial rub, a potassium of 5.1 mEq/L, and a bicarbonate of 21 mEq/L, all consistent with relative rather than absolute indications, and no vascular access has been created. A frailty assessment documents severe functional dependence and a comorbidity burden associated with a limited expected survival benefit from dialysis in prognostic tools validated for this population. In a structured discussion involving the patient, to the extent his cognition allows, and his family, the team presents both pathways explicitly: initiation with an urgent access procedure and a three-times-weekly treatment burden that his functional status makes difficult to sustain, or a conservative kidney management pathway with active symptom control for uremic anorexia and fatigue. The family, weighing his prior expressed wish to avoid burdensome medical interventions near the end of life against the modest and uncertain survival benefit dialysis would likely offer given his comorbidity profile, elects conservative management. This decision is not a failure to treat; it is the initiation decision reached correctly for this patient, illustrating that the same symptom framework used to justify starting dialysis in the first case can, in a different clinical and personal context, appropriately support not starting it.

CAUTION: Do not treat conservative kidney management as a default fallback offered only after a frail patient has already failed a trial of dialysis. When frailty and limited expected benefit are identified before initiation, present conservative management as a fully developed, actively supported pathway from the outset.

Patient Preparation for Kidney Replacement Therapy

Vein Preservation and Early Access Referral

Because arteriovenous fistula maturation typically requires six to twelve weeks and sometimes longer, and because a substantial minority of fistulas fail to mature adequately on the first attempt, access referral timed to the anticipated need for dialysis — rather than to the actual onset of symptoms — is what allows the scheduled-start scenario described above to be available as an option at all. This requires identifying candidate patients well before kidney failure, typically once GFR falls into the G4 range or trajectory suggests kidney failure within one to two years, and it requires a parallel, easily overlooked intervention: protecting the veins of the non-dominant forearm from venipuncture, intravenous catheter placement, and peripherally inserted central catheters, since each of these can scar or occlude a vein that would otherwise have been suitable for fistula creation.

Vein preservation is best operationalized as a standing order or chart flag rather than left to individual clinician memory, because the patients most likely to need it — those with advanced chronic kidney disease — are frequently hospitalized for unrelated reasons during the very window in which their veins are most valuable to protect. A forearm vein sacrificed for a peripheral intravenous line during an unrelated hospitalization is a preventable cost, not an unavoidable one, and the responsibility for preventing it belongs to every clinician who places a line, not solely to the nephrology team.

Institutions that have successfully reduced avoidable vein sacrifice typically do so with a small number of concrete, low-effort interventions rather than relying on education alone: an electronic chart flag or wristband identifying patients with advanced chronic kidney disease, a default order-set preference for hand or dorsal veins over forearm veins when intravenous access is needed, and a low threshold for ultrasound-guided placement in an alternative site when the non-dominant forearm is the only apparent option. None of these measures depends on the ordering clinician being a nephrologist or even being aware of the patient's kidney disease stage in detail; they depend on the flag being visible at the point of care, which is why the flag itself, not a one-time counseling conversation, is the intervention that actually changes behavior at the bedside.

Modality Education and the Life-Plan Discussion

Patients approaching kidney failure benefit from structured education covering hemodialysis, peritoneal dialysis, and, where appropriate, preemptive transplantation and conservative management well before any one modality becomes the default by circumstance rather than by choice. Absent this education, the path of least resistance — an urgent hemodialysis catheter placed during an unplanned hospitalization — often becomes the modality a patient ends up on, not because it best matches their preferences or clinical situation, but because no other option was actively prepared in time. Deliberate modality education, ideally beginning when GFR falls to approximately twenty milliliters per minute or one year before anticipated kidney failure, is what converts the initiation decision from a default into an actual choice.

This education is most effective when it engages the full range of what a modality decision entails — not just the mechanics of treatment but its effect on employment, travel, home space requirements, and caregiver burden — and when it is revisited rather than delivered once and considered complete, since a patient's circumstances and preferences can shift meaningfully in the months between an initial conversation and the actual start of therapy. The next chapter develops this modality-selection process, formalized as the ESKD Life-Plan, in full.

A structured, multidisciplinary education program — typically involving a nephrologist, a dedicated kidney disease educator or nurse, a dietitian, and social work — consistently outperforms a single physician conversation at improving both patient knowledge and satisfaction with the eventual modality choice, in part because it spreads the necessarily large amount of information across multiple encounters rather than compressing it into one visit already burdened with other clinical concerns. Programs that succeed at increasing preemptive transplantation referral and home-modality uptake tend to share a common feature: they present hemodialysis, peritoneal dialysis, and transplantation as parallel options from the earliest conversation, rather than introducing home modalities only after an in-center hemodialysis default has already been established by circumstance.

Psychosocial and Nutritional Preparation

The nutritional demands of dialysis differ enough from those of pre-dialysis chronic kidney disease management that dietary counseling begun only after initiation leaves patients managing an abrupt transition on top of everything else that initiation itself demands. Pre-dialysis counseling that anticipates the shift — relaxed protein restriction, introduction of potassium and phosphate awareness appropriate to the anticipated modality, and fluid allowance planning specific to hemodialysis versus peritoneal dialysis — allows patients to begin adjusting before the additional burden of a new treatment schedule is added on top.

Psychosocial preparation deserves equal weight and is often given less. A new dialysis dependency changes a patient's relationship to work, caregiving responsibilities, and independence, and unaddressed anxiety or depression around this transition is common and can measurably affect a patient's engagement with early treatment, including attendance at scheduled sessions and adherence to fluid and dietary guidance. Screening for these concerns before initiation, and connecting patients with social work and, where indicated, mental health support in advance rather than only reactively after problems emerge, is a preparation step as concrete as vein preservation or modality education, even though it is less procedural in character.

A brief, validated depression or anxiety screening instrument administered at the same visit as modality education adds little time to the encounter and identifies a meaningful proportion of patients who would otherwise enter dialysis with unaddressed psychological distress, distress that is itself associated with lower treatment adherence and, in several outcome studies, with higher hospitalization rates in the first year of therapy. Practical caregiver logistics deserve the same explicit attention: a patient planning to pursue home hemodialysis or peritoneal dialysis needs a realistic assessment of caregiver availability and home space well before the access procedure is scheduled, since discovering a logistical barrier only after committing to a home modality forces a late, disruptive switch to in-center care at precisely the point when the patient is least prepared to absorb another change.

Figure 1.3

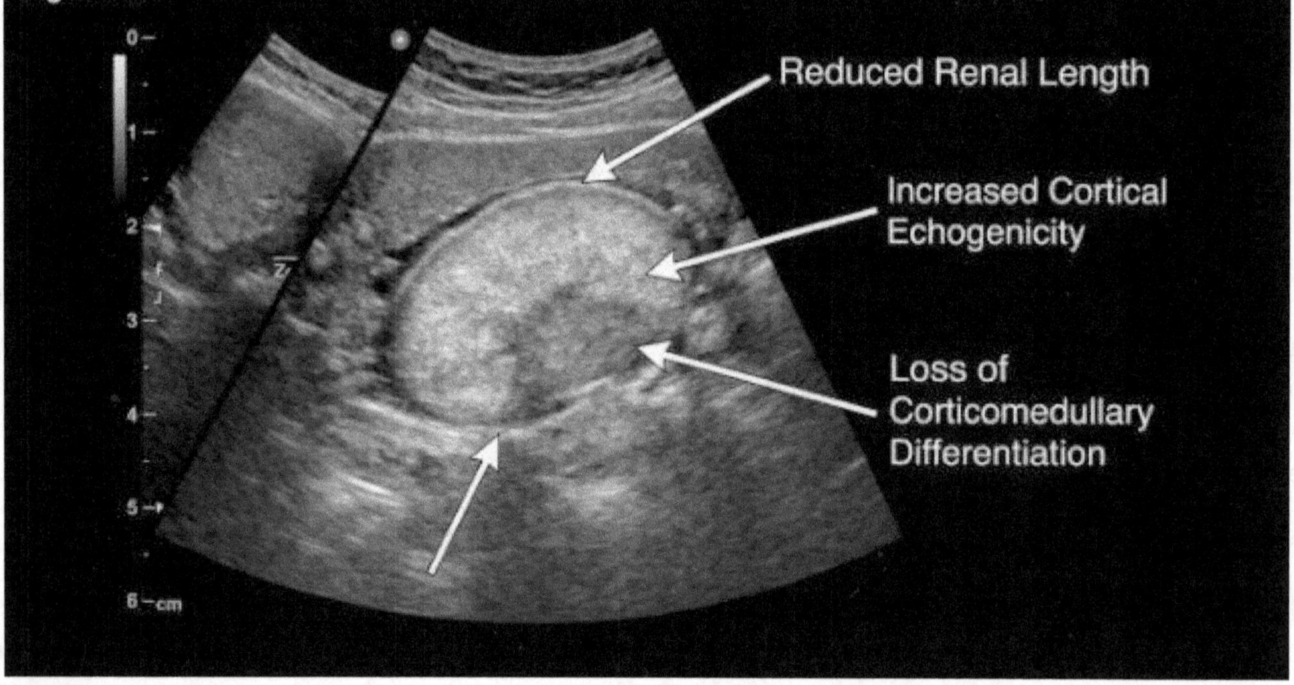

EVIDENCE: The IDEAL trial found no survival or major clinical advantage to planned early-start dialysis compared with planned late-start dialysis guided by symptoms, supporting a symptom- and complication-based approach to timing rather than a fixed GFR threshold.

DIALYSIS RECOGNITION & RESPONSE SYSTEM — Initiation Decision Arcs

The Pattern: A patient approaching kidney failure who has not yet been referred for access or modality education.

Stem Signature: GFR in the G4 range or a trajectory projecting kidney failure within one to two years, with no vascular or peritoneal access referral yet placed and no modality education yet delivered.

The Decision: Refer for access evaluation and begin modality education now, at G4, rather than waiting for G5 or for symptoms to appear — fistula maturation and informed modality choice both require a runway measured in months.

Trap Logic: A reassuringly stable GFR in the G4 range can make referral feel premature, but trajectory, not the current number, determines whether the six-to-twelve-week runway for access maturation will be available when it is actually needed.

Response Anchor: Begin access referral and modality education at G4, not G5 — waiting for symptoms forfeits the runway that makes a scheduled, patient-chosen start possible.

DIALYSIS RECOGNITION & RESPONSE SYSTEM — Initiation Decision Arcs

Rapid Creatinine Rise: Rule out reversible acute-on-chronic injury before accepting a new creatinine as chronic baseline or accelerating the initiation timeline on the basis of it.

Pleuritic Chest Pain in Advanced CKD: Treat as uremic pericarditis until proven otherwise; a pericardial friction rub is an absolute indication for urgent initiation regardless of GFR.

Relative Indications With a Ready Access: Proceed with a scheduled start using the prepared access rather than defaulting to urgent catheter placement.

Approaching Kidney Failure Without Referral: Refer for access and begin modality education at G4, guided by trajectory rather than waiting for the numeric threshold of kidney failure.

Summary and Key Concepts

Chronic kidney disease is staged by both GFR and albuminuria category, and the two interact multiplicatively to determine overall risk of progression.

Rate of decline, not a single GFR value, characterizes a patient's trajectory and should trigger a search for reversible acute-on-chronic contributors when unexpectedly rapid.

Uremic pericarditis, uremic encephalopathy, refractory volume overload, and refractory hyperkalemia or acidosis are absolute indications for urgent initiation regardless of numeric GFR.

The IDEAL trial demonstrated no benefit to early initiation by GFR threshold alone, supporting a symptom- and complication-driven approach to timing.

Vein preservation, access referral, modality education, and nutritional and psychosocial preparation should begin at the G4 stage or with a trajectory projecting kidney failure within one to two years, not at the onset of symptoms.

CHAPTER 2: THE ESKD LIFE-PLAN: MODALITY SELECTION AND PATIENT-CENTERED CARE

Learning Objectives

Describe the ESKD Life-Plan and its P-L-A-N framework for aligning modality choice and access planning to an individual patient's trajectory.

Compare hemodialysis, peritoneal dialysis, and preemptive transplantation across clinical outcomes, lifestyle burden, and patient autonomy.

Apply shared decision-making principles to structure a modality education encounter and to address decisional conflict when it arises.

Sequence vascular or peritoneal access creation so that it matches the modality chosen under the patient's Life-Plan rather than defaulting to whichever access is fastest to obtain.

Recognize when a patient's Life-Plan requires active revision rather than passive continuation of a plan made under different circumstances.

Chapter Overview

Chapter 1 established when replacement therapy becomes necessary. This chapter addresses a question that, in a well-prepared patient, should already be substantially answered by the time that necessity arrives: which therapy, delivered through which access, chosen by whom. The ESKD Life-Plan reframes modality selection from a single decision made at a single visit into a structured, revisited process that treats the patient's own goals as the organizing principle around which clinical options are arranged, rather than treating the patient as the recipient of a modality chosen primarily on logistical convenience.

Principles of the Patient Life-Plan

Origins and Purpose of the ESKD Life-Plan

The Life-Plan concept emerged from a recognition, reflected in the 2019 KDOQI Vascular Access guideline update, that access decisions made in isolation from a patient's broader modality trajectory frequently produced access that was mismatched to what the patient actually needed by the time it matured. A fistula created reflexively in every patient approaching kidney failure, without first asking whether that patient was a transplant candidate likely to receive a kidney within the fistula's maturation window, or whether the patient had already expressed a strong preference for peritoneal dialysis, represented effort and procedural risk spent on an access the patient might never use as intended. The Life-Plan corrects this by inverting the sequence: establish the patient's anticipated modality trajectory first, then derive the access plan from it, rather than creating access first and fitting the modality decision around whatever access happens to exist.

This inversion matters most for patients near the boundary between competing reasonable options — a young, otherwise healthy patient with a living donor already identified, for whom preemptive transplantation may arrive before any dialysis access is needed at all, or an older patient with moderate frailty for whom peritoneal dialysis may preserve residual function and autonomy longer than hemodialysis would. In both cases, defaulting to fistula creation as the reflexive first step risks consuming vascular resources, procedural time, and patient tolerance for procedures on a plan that does not match where the patient is actually headed.

Adoption of the Life-Plan framework has been associated, in observational data following the 2019 guideline update, with a modest but measurable increase in preemptive transplantation rates and a reduction in the proportion of patients who begin hemodialysis with a central venous catheter rather than a mature fistula or graft, both outcomes consistent with the framework succeeding at its intended purpose of aligning access decisions to actual modality trajectories rather than defaulting to the fastest available option under time pressure. These gains are concentrated in centers that have operationalized the framework as a structured, tracked referral pathway rather than treating it as an informal principle invoked inconsistently, underscoring that the Life-Plan delivers its benefit through systematic application, not through good intentions alone.

The P-L-A-N Framework: Patient Life-Plan and Access Needs

The P-L-A-N framework names its two components explicitly: the Patient Life-Plan, an individualized projection of the modalities a patient is likely to need or want over the anticipated course of their kidney disease, and the Access Needs derived from it, meaning the specific vascular or peritoneal access, or sequence of accesses, that supports that projected trajectory. A Life-Plan is not a single modality choice frozen at one point in time; it more often resembles a sequence — for example, peritoneal dialysis in the near term while a living donor evaluation proceeds, transitioning to transplantation if a donor is confirmed suitable, with hemodialysis held in reserve as a contingency if the peritoneal membrane fails or the transplant evaluation does not proceed as anticipated.

Constructing a Life-Plan requires integrating several categories of information that are not usually gathered together in a single encounter: the patient's medical trajectory and transplant candidacy, their personal goals and lifestyle constraints, the practical feasibility of each modality given their home situation and support system, and the realistic timeline over which each option could actually be implemented. Because this integration is broader than a single clinical variable, the Life-Plan is best constructed collaboratively across the nephrology team — physician, access coordinator, transplant referral coordinator, and modality educator — rather than by any one clinician working from their own narrow view of the patient's situation.

In practice, this collaborative construction is most efficient when a single team member, often a dedicated access coordinator or advanced practice provider, is designated to own the Life-Plan document itself —

tracking which components have been completed, which remain outstanding, and when the plan is next due for scheduled review — rather than leaving ownership diffuse across the team, which in practice tends to mean no one individual is accountable for noticing when the plan has become outdated or incomplete, and the trigger events for revision described later in this chapter go unrecognized until a clinical crisis forces the issue rather than a scheduled, proactive review catching the change well in advance.

KEY POINT: The Life-Plan determines the Access Needs, not the reverse. Resist defaulting to fistula creation before the anticipated modality trajectory has actually been established.

Life-Plan as a Living Document Rather Than a One-Time Decision

A Life-Plan constructed at the moment a patient reaches G4 chronic kidney disease reflects that patient's circumstances at that moment, and circumstances change: a living donor evaluation may fail, a peritoneal membrane may develop ultrafiltration failure after several years of otherwise successful use, or a patient's functional status may decline enough that a previously chosen home modality becomes impractical. Treating the Life-Plan as fixed once written invites exactly the mismatch the framework was designed to prevent, only shifted later in the patient's course rather than eliminated. Scheduled Life-Plan review — reasonably timed to major transitions such as a failed transplant evaluation, a peritonitis episode, or a significant change in functional status — keeps the plan aligned with the patient's actual trajectory rather than with an earlier snapshot of it.

DIALYSIS RECOGNITION & RESPONSE SYSTEM — Life-Plan Alignment Arcs

The Pattern: A patient's clinical trajectory has diverged from the modality plan constructed at an earlier visit.

Stem Signature: A transplant evaluation is discontinued, a peritoneal membrane develops declining ultrafiltration capacity, or a functional decline makes a previously chosen home modality newly impractical — in a patient whose Life-Plan has not been revisited since it was originally written.

The Decision: Trigger a scheduled Life-Plan review rather than allowing the original plan to continue by default; reassess modality trajectory and revise the Access Needs plan to match the patient's current, not historical, circumstances.

Trap Logic: Continuing an established modality out of institutional inertia can look identical to a deliberately chosen, still-appropriate plan; the distinguishing feature is whether the plan has been actively reconsidered against the patient's current trajectory or simply continued unexamined.

Response Anchor: A major clinical transition is itself the trigger for Life-Plan review — do not wait for the plan to visibly fail before reconsidering it.

Comparing Hemodialysis, Peritoneal Dialysis, and Transplantation

Clinical Outcomes Across Modalities

Preemptive kidney transplantation, performed before dialysis is ever started, is associated with the best long-term survival and graft outcomes among the three modalities, because it avoids the cumulative vascular and cardiovascular burden that even a brief period of dialysis dependence appears to impose, an effect that grows more pronounced the longer dialysis precedes transplantation. Between hemodialysis and peritoneal dialysis, outcome comparisons are less clearly separated: peritoneal dialysis is associated with better preservation of residual kidney function in the initial years of therapy, plausibly because it avoids the intermittent large-volume fluid shifts and hemodynamic stress that recurring hemodialysis sessions impose on residual nephrons, while overall mortality between the two modalities is similar once analyses account for the differences in comorbidity between the populations who typically select each one.

This similarity in aggregate mortality is easy to misread as clinical equivalence in every individual case, but it obscures meaningful subgroup differences: patients with significant residual kidney function benefit disproportionately from peritoneal dialysis's gentler physiologic profile in the early period, while patients with extensive peritoneal adhesions from prior abdominal surgery, or a home environment unsuited to sterile technique, are poorly matched to peritoneal dialysis regardless of the aggregate mortality data. Modality comparison is therefore most useful as a starting framework to be adjusted for the individual patient's anatomy, comorbidity, and home circumstances, not as a rule applied uniformly.

The mortality curves for hemodialysis and peritoneal dialysis also diverge in shape rather than merely in overall magnitude, a distinction that matters for how the comparison is presented to patients. Several large registry analyses show a survival advantage favoring peritoneal dialysis in the first one to two years of therapy, a period during which residual kidney function and cardiovascular stability are typically better preserved on peritoneal dialysis, with the curves converging or in some analyses reversing modestly in favor of hemodialysis after several years, coinciding with the period when peritoneal membrane function and ultrafiltration capacity in some patients begin to decline. This time-dependent pattern supports peritoneal dialysis as a particularly favorable first modality for patients anticipating a multi-year dialysis course, with a hemodialysis transition planned proactively — as described later in this chapter — rather than deferred until membrane failure forces it.

Health-related quality of life, measured using validated instruments that assess physical functioning, symptom burden, and emotional well-being, shows a less consistent pattern across modalities than mortality does, with most comparative studies finding broadly similar overall quality of life between hemodialysis and peritoneal dialysis once results are averaged across full patient populations, but with individual patients reporting starkly different experiences depending on how well their chosen modality matches their personal circumstances. This averaging effect is itself instructive: it confirms that neither modality is intrinsically superior for quality of life in the abstract, and that the meaningful variation lies almost entirely in the fit between a specific patient's life and a specific modality's demands — the central premise underlying the Life-Plan's emphasis on individualized rather than population-level modality selection.

Lifestyle, Autonomy, and Quality-of-Life Considerations

In-center hemodialysis imposes a fixed, externally set schedule — typically three sessions weekly at a designated time — that structures the patient's week around the treatment rather than fitting the treatment around the patient's existing obligations, which can conflict substantially with employment, caregiving responsibilities for young children or aging parents, and travel. Peritoneal dialysis and home hemodialysis shift treatment timing into the patient's own control, an advantage that matters most to patients who value employment continuity or who have caregiving responsibilities that a fixed in-center schedule would disrupt, but that advantage is inseparable from a corresponding increase in the patient's own responsibility for sterile technique, equipment management, and self-troubleshooting between clinic visits.

Patients vary considerably in how they weigh this trade between externally structured but professionally supervised treatment and self-directed but self-managed treatment, and neither preference reflects better or worse clinical judgment on the patient's part; a patient who prioritizes the reassurance of trained staff managing every treatment session over the schedule flexibility of a home modality is expressing a legitimate value, not a failure to understand the options. The modality educator's task is to make each option's actual day-to-day texture concrete enough that the patient can weigh it against their own priorities, rather than presenting options as an abstract comparison of clinical statistics divorced from what living with each modality actually feels like.

Employment continuation rates differ meaningfully across modalities in observational data, with home-based therapies associated with higher rates of continued employment than in-center hemodialysis, an association plausibly explained by the ability to schedule treatment around a workday rather than around it, though the direction of causation is not fully settled, since patients with more flexible employment or stronger baseline health may also be more likely to select home modalities in the first place. Caregiver burden follows a related but distinct pattern: home hemodialysis in particular typically requires a trained care partner for at least the initial period of treatment, a requirement that immediately excludes patients without an available or willing partner from that specific option regardless of their own preference, and that imposes a real burden on the partner who takes on the role, a burden that deserves direct acknowledgment and support planning rather than being treated as incidental to the patient's own decision.

Preemptive Transplantation Within the Life-Plan

Because preemptive transplantation offers the strongest outcomes among the three modalities, referral for transplant evaluation should occur early enough in the trajectory of chronic kidney disease to allow the evaluation, and any living donor identification process, to complete before dialysis becomes necessary, typically once GFR falls into the G4 range, mirroring the timing recommended for vascular access referral in the previous chapter. Where a suitable living donor is not available, referral for deceased-donor waitlisting still confers benefit, since accumulated waiting time before dialysis initiation is credited toward waitlist priority in many allocation systems, meaning early referral itself shortens the effective waiting period even when transplantation cannot occur preemptively.

A dialysis modality chosen under the Life-Plan should be selected, where transplant candidacy is confirmed, with an eye toward compatibility with an anticipated future transplant rather than in isolation: peritoneal dialysis does not preclude subsequent transplantation and in some analyses is associated with comparable or superior early graft outcomes to hemodialysis, likely reflecting its gentler hemodynamic profile and better preservation of the patient's overall physiologic reserve heading into transplant surgery, though the difference narrows once analyses adjust for the underlying comorbidity differences between patients selecting each modality.

Sensitization — the development of antibodies against a broad range of potential donor tissue types, most commonly from prior transplantation, pregnancy, or blood transfusion — substantially narrows the pool of compatible donors and can extend an otherwise straightforward transplant candidacy into a multi-year waiting process regardless of a patient's medical fitness. Because sensitization status is knowable well in advance through routine antibody testing, incorporating it into the Life-Plan early allows a more realistic transplant timeline to inform the dialysis modality decision: a highly sensitized patient with a long anticipated wait is a better candidate for a modality chosen for its multi-year durability and quality of life than for one chosen primarily as a brief bridge, since the bridge in this case may extend considerably longer than initially anticipated.

Dimension	Hemodialysis (In-Center)	Peritoneal Dialysis	Preemptive Transplantation
Treatment Location and Schedule	Fixed clinic schedule, typically three sessions weekly	Home-based, patient-directed daily schedule	One-time surgical procedure, then outpatient follow-up
Residual Kidney Function	Declines more rapidly with intermittent large-volume shifts	Better early preservation in most patients	Native kidney function replaced by graft function
Access Type	Arteriovenous fistula, graft, or central venous catheter	Peritoneal catheter	None required if preemptive
Primary Patient Responsibility	Attend scheduled sessions; interdialytic diet and fluid limits	Daily exchanges or cycler setup; sterile technique	Immunosuppression adherence and monitoring
Best-Suited Patient Profile	Prefers professionally supervised treatment; limited home support	Values schedule autonomy; adequate home space and support	Suitable candidate with available donor or acceptable wait time

Figure 2.1: Comparative Anatomy of Hemodialysis and Peritoneal Access Routes

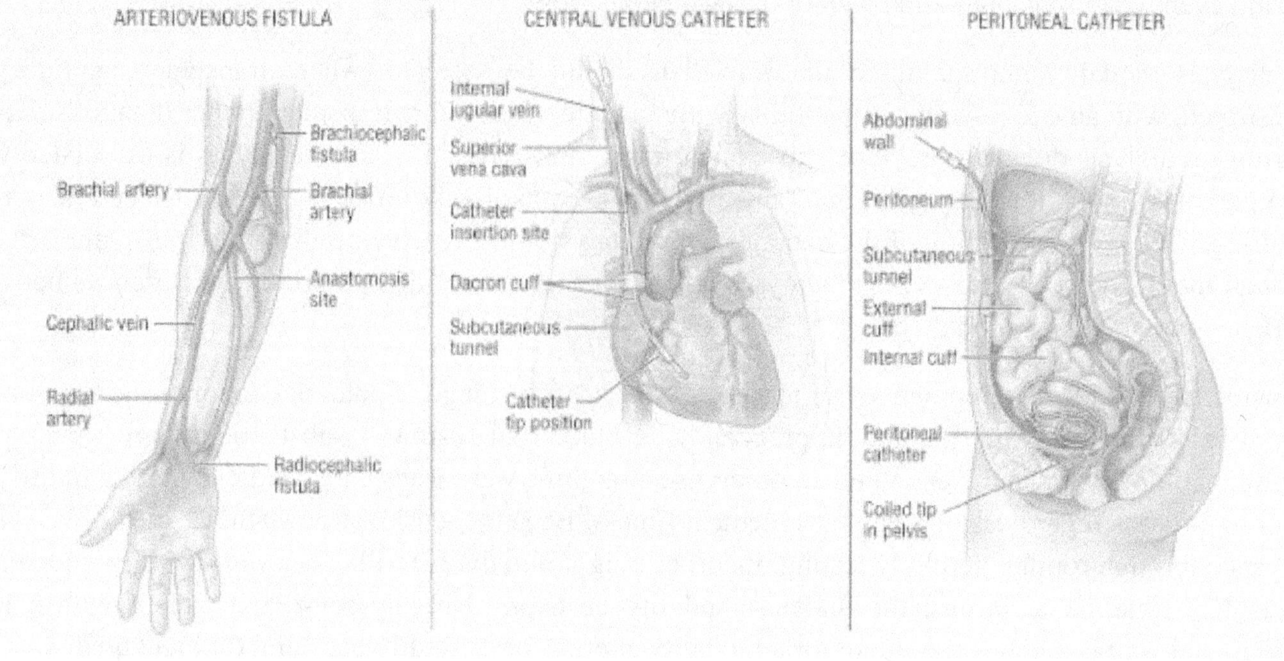

Shared Decision-Making and Modality Education

Principles of Shared Decision-Making in Nephrology

Shared decision-making in the modality context means neither the clinician unilaterally recommending a single option nor the clinician presenting a neutral menu of choices without guidance, but a structured exchange in which the clinician contributes clinical expertise about what is medically feasible and likely to succeed for this particular patient, while the patient contributes expertise about their own values, priorities, and tolerance for the burdens each option imposes. This model differs from a purely informational consent process in that it explicitly invites the patient's values to shape which option is ultimately recommended, rather than treating patient preference as a factor to be accommodated only after a clinically preferred option has already been identified.

Decision aids — structured tools that lay out each modality's typical outcomes, burdens, and lifestyle implications in a consistent, balanced format — improve the quality of this exchange by ensuring that all three options are presented with comparable depth, correcting for the tendency, common when modality education is delivered informally, to describe the option a given clinician is most familiar with or most enthusiastic about in more detail and more favorable terms than the alternatives.

The most effective decision aids used in nephrology combine standardized outcome data with structured value-clarification exercises that prompt the patient to rank their own priorities — schedule flexibility, minimizing hospital visits, preserving independence, minimizing caregiver burden — before the modality discussion proceeds to matching those stated priorities against each option's actual profile. This sequencing, priorities elicited before options are matched to them, reduces the tendency for a patient to reverse-engineer their stated priorities to justify a modality they were already leaning toward for less examined reasons, such as having a family member on a particular modality or a vague impression formed from unrelated media exposure to dialysis.

Structuring the Modality Education Encounter

An effective modality education encounter typically proceeds through a recognizable sequence: establishing the patient's current understanding and any preconceptions before presenting new information, so that existing misconceptions can be directly addressed rather than left to coexist alongside new information; presenting all three modalities with comparable depth using a decision aid or structured framework; explicitly eliciting the patient's own priorities and constraints, including caregiving responsibilities, employment, and home environment; and closing with a concrete plan for the next step, whether that is a follow-up visit, a home assessment, or referral for further evaluation, rather than leaving the conversation open-ended.

Because the volume of information involved routinely exceeds what most patients can absorb and retain from a single encounter, this structure is more effective delivered across two or more visits, with an initial encounter focused on establishing baseline understanding and eliciting priorities, and a subsequent visit focused on the specific modality or modalities that emerged as the patient's leading options after the first conversation. This staged approach also allows written materials or a home visit from a modality educator to occur between encounters, giving the patient time to process information and generate questions rather than being asked to decide during the same visit the information is first presented.

Family members and caregivers, where the patient wishes to include them, are best invited into this process from the initial encounter rather than only after a preliminary decision has been reached, since a modality choice made without input from the person who will share substantially in its daily burden — particularly for home hemodialysis, which typically requires a trained care partner — risks being reconsidered or reversed once that burden becomes concrete rather than hypothetical. Structuring at least one portion of the education encounter for the caregiver's questions specifically, separate from the patient's own, surfaces caregiver-specific concerns — confidence in performing technical tasks, anxiety about managing a medical emergency at home — that the patient may not think to raise on the caregiver's behalf.

Addressing Decisional Conflict and Ambivalence

Some patients arrive at a modality decision readily once presented with balanced information; others experience genuine decisional conflict, torn between options that each carry real advantages and real costs relative to their own priorities, and a smaller number remain ambivalent even after extended education, deferring the decision indefinitely. Recognizing which pattern a given patient is in matters practically: readily decided patients can proceed to access planning promptly, while patients experiencing genuine conflict benefit from explicit acknowledgment that the difficulty reflects the options' actual trade-offs rather than a deficiency in the patient's understanding, and from additional decision-support resources rather than repetition of the same information already presented.

A fifty-four-year-old man with a GFR of seventeen milliliters per minute and no living donor identified attends his second modality education visit still undecided between home hemodialysis and peritoneal dialysis, having found both options' outcome data reassuring and both options' daily demands intimidating. Rather than presenting the same comparative information a third time, the modality educator arranges a home visit with a peritoneal dialysis nurse to assess his kitchen storage space and a parallel conversation with a current home hemodialysis patient willing to describe the treatment's actual daily texture. Following both encounters, he selects peritoneal dialysis, citing the concreteness of seeing his own kitchen accommodate the supplies as the deciding factor — information no verbal description had previously supplied. This illustrates that persistent ambivalence after adequate verbal education often reflects a need for more concrete, experiential information rather than a need for more repetition of the same comparative statistics.

CLINICAL PEARL: When verbal modality education has been thorough but the patient remains undecided, a home assessment or a conversation with a current patient on the modality in question often resolves ambivalence that further repetition of comparative outcome data will not.

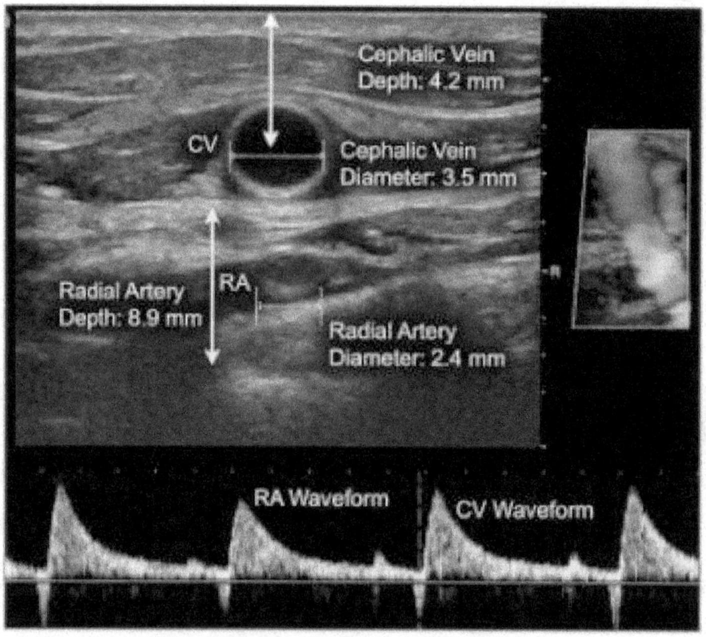

Figure 2.2: Preoperative Vascular Mapping Ultrasound for Access Planning.

DIALYSIS RECOGNITION & RESPONSE SYSTEM — Life-Plan Alignment Arcs

The Pattern: A patient presents persistent, unresolved ambivalence after standard modality education.

Stem Signature: The patient has received balanced comparative information across two or more encounters, finds each option's outcome data reassuring, but remains unable to commit to a modality, often citing the daily demands of each option as similarly intimidating in the abstract.

The Decision: Escalate from verbal comparative education to concrete, experiential resources — a home assessment, a peer-patient conversation, or a hands-on equipment demonstration — rather than repeating the same comparative statistics a further time.

Trap Logic: Persistent ambivalence can be mistaken for a need for more data or a more detailed explanation, when the actual barrier is the abstractness of verbal description rather than a gap in factual understanding.

Response Anchor: Repeated verbal education rarely resolves ambivalence that concrete, experiential exposure to the modality's daily reality can resolve in a single encounter.

Access Needs Planning Aligned to the Life-Plan

Special Considerations for the Late-Referred Patient

Not every patient enters dialysis care with the benefit of a Life-Plan constructed at G4 chronic kidney disease; a meaningful proportion of patients are first identified as having advanced kidney disease only at the point of an unplanned hospitalization for uremic symptoms, with no prior nephrology follow-up, no modality education, and no access of any kind in place. For these patients, the Life-Plan framework still applies, but compressed into days rather than months, and the immediate priority shifts from the deliberate, unhurried process described earlier in this chapter to establishing safe, temporary access — almost always a non-tunneled or tunneled central venous catheter — while the actual Life-Plan conversation begins in parallel rather than being completed first.

This compressed sequence carries real costs that are worth naming explicitly rather than treating the late-referred pathway as simply a faster version of the standard one: a catheter placed under urgent circumstances carries materially higher infection risk than a mature fistula, and it is placed before the modality education that would ideally have shaped the choice of a longer-term access has had time to occur. Recognizing this, the nephrology team's task with a late-referred patient is to treat the urgent catheter explicitly as a temporary bridge from the outset, initiating modality education and, where hemodialysis is the eventual choice, permanent access evaluation within the first days of the hospitalization rather than allowing the catheter to become a de facto long-term solution simply because no alternative was arranged before the need became acute.

Late referral is not evenly distributed across patient populations; it is disproportionately common among patients with limited access to primary care, language or health-literacy barriers to understanding an earlier chronic kidney disease diagnosis, and lower socioeconomic status more broadly, meaning that the compressed, catheter-first pathway described here falls disproportionately on populations already facing other structural disadvantages in their care. Addressing this pattern is only partly a matter of what happens once a late-referred patient reaches the hospital; it is also a matter of earlier primary-care-level chronic kidney disease detection and nephrology referral, a systems-level intervention outside any single hospitalization but one that a nephrology program committed to the Life-Plan framework's goals should track and work to improve at the population level, not only address reactively one late-referred patient at a time.

CAUTION: A catheter placed urgently in a late-referred patient should be documented and tracked explicitly as a temporary bridge, with permanent access evaluation initiated within days — not allowed to persist by default in the absence of an active Life-Plan conversation.

DIALYSIS RECOGNITION & RESPONSE SYSTEM — Life-Plan Alignment Arcs

The Pattern: A patient is identified with advanced kidney disease only at the point of an unplanned hospitalization, with no prior Life-Plan of any kind.

Stem Signature: Uremic symptoms prompting hospital presentation, no established nephrology follow-up, no modality education, and no vascular or peritoneal access in place at the time an absolute or relative indication for initiation is identified.

The Decision: Place a central venous catheter as an explicitly temporary bridge, and begin modality education and permanent access evaluation in parallel within the same hospitalization, rather than completing the full Life-Plan conversation before any access decision is made.

Trap Logic: A late-referred patient's urgent catheter can look, superficially, like a settled access decision simply because it is already in place; the distinguishing action is whether permanent access planning is actively initiated within days or the catheter is allowed to persist unexamined.

Response Anchor: Treat every late-referred catheter as a bridge with an active permanent-access plan attached from day one, not as a default long-term solution.

Matching Access Type to Chosen Modality

Once a modality has been chosen under the Life-Plan, the access plan follows directly: a patient selecting hemodialysis proceeds to vascular access evaluation and creation, sequenced as described in Part III of this book; a patient selecting peritoneal dialysis proceeds to peritoneal catheter placement, sequenced to allow adequate healing time before the catheter is used; and a patient pursuing preemptive transplantation with a confirmed living donor and a favorable timeline may reasonably defer any dialysis access creation altogether if the transplant is expected to occur before dialysis becomes necessary. This sequencing prevents the common mismatch of creating a fistula in a patient who ultimately receives a preemptive transplant before the fistula is ever cannulated, exposing the patient to a procedure and a maturation period that ultimately served no clinical purpose.

A thirty-six-year-old woman with a GFR of sixteen milliliters per minute and a fully evaluated, medically cleared living donor — her sister, with a confirmed compatible crossmatch — is scheduled for preemptive transplantation eight weeks from her current visit. Her nephrology team, applying the Life-Plan framework, elects to defer any dialysis access creation entirely rather than placing a fistula "just in case," reasoning that her trajectory suggests she will likely reach transplantation before dialysis becomes necessary, and that a fistula created now would, in the most likely scenario, mature only to go unused. A contingency plan is documented explicitly rather than left implicit: if she develops an absolute indication for urgent initiation before the transplant date, or if the transplant is unexpectedly delayed beyond a defined threshold, a central venous catheter will be placed as a short-term bridge, accepting its higher infection risk as a reasonable trade-off given the short anticipated duration of use. Her transplant proceeds as scheduled, and she never requires a dialysis access of any kind — an outcome the Life-Plan framework identified as the most probable path from the outset, rather than one arrived at by chance after unnecessary access creation had already occurred.

KEY POINT: Deferring access creation is itself a Life-Plan decision, not an absence of one — it requires an explicit, documented contingency plan for what will be done if the anticipated timeline changes, not simply an assumption that no access will be needed.

Where transplant timing is uncertain — a living donor evaluation still in progress, or a deceased-donor wait of unpredictable duration — the Life-Plan supports proceeding with dialysis access creation as a bridging measure rather than withholding access while awaiting a transplant that may not materialize on the anticipated timeline. In these bridging cases, peritoneal dialysis is often favored specifically because catheter removal at the time of a subsequent transplant is a comparatively minor procedure relative to fistula ligation, making it a lower-cost bridge for a patient whose ultimate destination is transplantation rather than long-term dialysis dependence.

Sequencing Access Creation Within the Life-Plan Timeline

Because arteriovenous fistula maturation and peritoneal catheter healing both require a runway of weeks before the access can be safely used, access creation should be timed against the projected date of dialysis initiation established in Chapter 1's trajectory assessment, not against the date access creation happens to be convenient to schedule. A fistula created too early relative to actual need risks a period of patency without use, during which stenosis can develop before the access is ever cannulated; a fistula created too late forces reliance on a central venous catheter as a bridge, with its attendant infection and central-vein risk, for longer than necessary. The Life-Plan's projected initiation date, revised as the patient's trajectory is reassessed, is what allows access creation to be timed to this narrow window rather than defaulting to either extreme.

In practice, this timing is best coordinated through a shared referral pathway that flags patients for surgical evaluation once their trajectory suggests initiation within four to six months, allowing time for surgical consultation, vessel mapping, the creation procedure itself, and an adequate maturation interval before the access is needed, with routine follow-up to confirm maturation rather than assuming a technically successful creation procedure guarantees a usable access. A meaningful proportion of newly created fistulas fail to mature adequately for cannulation, and this failure is identified far earlier, with more time to pursue a second attempt or an alternative access, when maturation is actively assessed on a defined schedule rather than discovered only when the access is needed and found not to be ready.

Revising Access Plans When the Life-Plan Changes

An access plan derived from an earlier Life-Plan requires explicit reconsideration whenever the underlying Life-Plan changes, rather than being allowed to continue on its original trajectory by default. A patient whose living donor evaluation fails after a peritoneal dialysis bridging catheter was placed in anticipation of near-term transplantation now has an effectively indefinite peritoneal dialysis timeline and may benefit from revisiting whether peritoneal dialysis remains the best long-term modality, rather than continuing on a plan whose original justification — a short bridge to transplantation — no longer applies. Similarly, a patient whose peritoneal membrane develops declining ultrafiltration capacity after several years may need vascular access creation initiated well before the membrane fails outright, so that a hemodialysis access is mature and ready by the time the transition becomes necessary rather than being started reactively once peritoneal dialysis has already failed.

Operationalizing this kind of revision consistently requires a defined trigger list rather than relying on any individual clinician to remember to revisit the Life-Plan at the right moment — a failed transplant evaluation, a peritonitis episode, a documented decline in functional status, or a peritoneal equilibration test showing transporter category migration are all reasonable trigger events that can be built into a clinic's standard workflow, generating an automatic prompt for Life-Plan review rather than depending on the finding being noticed and acted upon informally. Centers that build these triggers into structured order sets or registry flags report more consistent Life-Plan revision than centers relying on individual clinician vigilance alone, for the same reason that vein-preservation flags outperform education-only approaches: a systemic prompt embedded at the point of care is more reliable than memory.

The following case illustrates this revision principle in practice. A forty-one-year-old woman on peritoneal dialysis for three years, originally started as a bridge to a living-donor transplant that did not proceed after the donor was found medically unsuitable, is found on routine peritoneal equilibration testing to have transitioned from an average to a high transporter category, with declining ultrafiltration on her current prescription despite escalating dextrose concentration. Rather than continuing to escalate the peritoneal prescription indefinitely, her nephrology team recognizes this as a signal that her Life-Plan requires active revision: a repeat transplant evaluation is initiated given her improved candidacy since her prior workup, and, because a suitable donor is not immediately available, vascular access evaluation is initiated in parallel so that a fistula has time to mature before her peritoneal ultrafiltration failure becomes clinically limiting. This dual-track revision — pursuing transplant re-evaluation while simultaneously securing a hemodialysis bridge — reflects the Life-Plan's function as a continuously updated plan rather than a decision made once and left unexamined for the remainder of the patient's course.

EVIDENCE: The KDOQI 2019 Vascular Access guideline update introduced the ESKD Life-Plan and its P-L-A-N framework specifically to reduce access creation that is mismatched to a patient's actual modality trajectory, shifting practice away from reflexive fistula-first approaches applied uniformly to all patients approaching kidney failure.

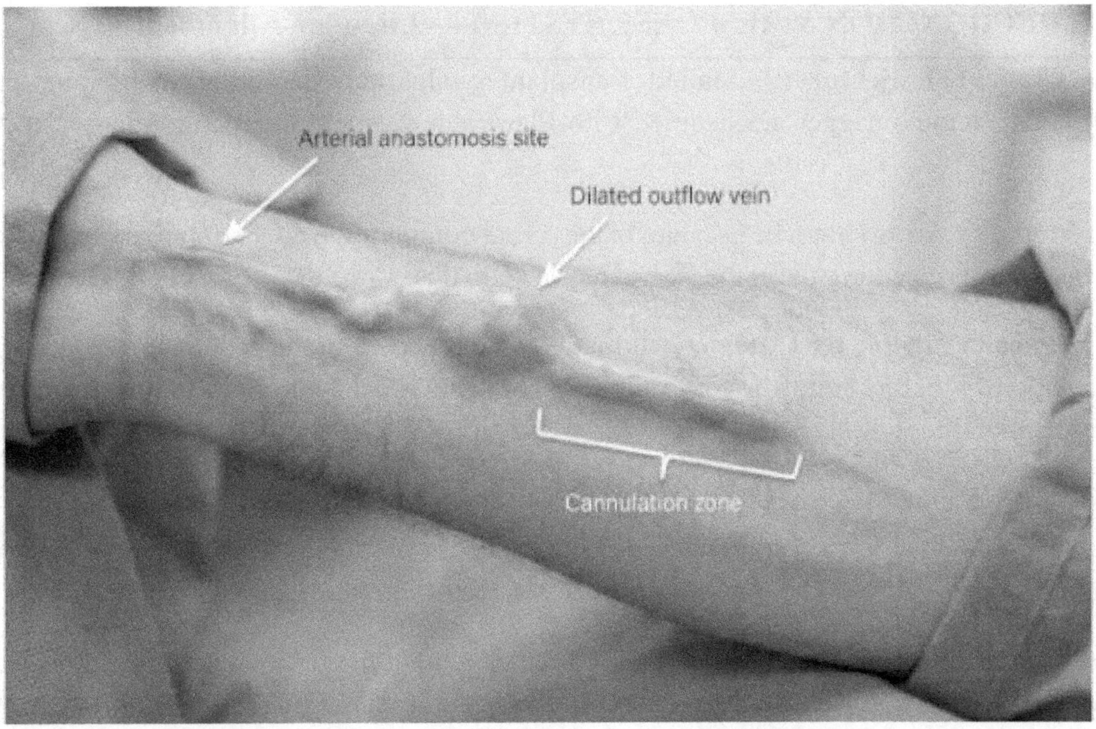

DIALYSIS RECOGNITION & RESPONSE SYSTEM — Life-Plan Alignment Arcs

The Pattern: A peritoneal dialysis patient shows early signs of declining membrane function on routine testing.

Stem Signature: A peritoneal equilibration test shows transition toward a higher transporter category, accompanied by declining ultrafiltration despite escalating dextrose concentration, in a patient with no active hemodialysis access.

The Decision: Initiate hemodialysis access evaluation now, in parallel with any transplant re-evaluation, so that a mature access is available before peritoneal ultrafiltration failure becomes clinically limiting, rather than waiting for outright technique failure to trigger access creation reactively.

Trap Logic: Escalating the peritoneal prescription can appear to solve the problem in the short term, masking the underlying membrane transport change and delaying the access planning that the patient's actual trajectory now requires.

Response Anchor: A rising transporter category with declining ultrafiltration is the trigger to begin the next access in the Life-Plan sequence — not a cue to simply escalate the current prescription further.

Diverging Clinical Trajectory: A failed transplant evaluation, declining membrane function, or functional decline should trigger a scheduled Life-Plan review, not a silent continuation of the existing plan.

Persistent Modality Ambivalence: Escalate from verbal comparative education to concrete, experiential resources rather than repeating the same comparative statistics.

Rising Peritoneal Transporter Category: Initiate the next access in the sequence — typically vascular access evaluation — before ultrafiltration failure becomes clinically limiting, rather than escalating the current prescription indefinitely.

Summary and Key Concepts

The ESKD Life-Plan inverts the traditional sequence of access-first planning, deriving Access Needs from an individualized projection of the patient's modality trajectory rather than the reverse.

Preemptive transplantation offers the strongest outcomes among the three modalities; peritoneal dialysis and hemodialysis show comparable aggregate mortality with meaningful subgroup differences favoring peritoneal dialysis for early preservation of residual kidney function.

Shared decision-making structures the modality conversation as a genuine exchange between clinical expertise and patient values, supported by balanced decision aids rather than informal, unevenly detailed presentations of each option.

Persistent decisional ambivalence after adequate verbal education often responds to concrete, experiential resources — a home assessment or peer-patient conversation — rather than repeated comparative statistics.

Access creation should be sequenced to the Life-Plan's projected modality and initiation timeline, and the Life-Plan itself requires active revision, not passive continuation, whenever a patient's clinical trajectory materially changes.

CHAPTER 3: CONSERVATIVE AND PALLIATIVE KIDNEY MANAGEMENT

Learning Objectives

Define conservative kidney management and distinguish it from both standard dialysis care and generic end-of-life hospice care.

Identify patients for whom conservative kidney management is likely to offer comparable or superior quality of life relative to dialysis, using validated prognostic and frailty assessment.

Apply pharmacologic and non-pharmacologic strategies to control the uremic symptom burden that persists without renal replacement therapy.

Structure an advance care planning conversation and document goals of care in a way that remains usable as a patient's condition evolves.

Recognize when withdrawal from established dialysis may represent an appropriate, considered patient decision rather than a reversible crisis requiring more aggressive intervention.

Chapter Overview

The first two chapters of this book addressed how a patient arrives at kidney replacement therapy and which modality that therapy should take. This chapter addresses the alternative that a meaningful proportion of patients ultimately choose, or should be offered the chance to choose: continuing without dialysis at all, through a structured program of conservative kidney management, or, having started dialysis, later deciding that continuing it no longer serves the patient's own goals. Both paths require the same clinical rigor as initiation itself — they are not the absence of a plan but a different plan, with its own symptom-management demands, its own decision points, and its own risk of being handled poorly when treated as an afterthought to the dialysis-focused chapters that surround it.

Defining Conservative Kidney Management

What Conservative Kidney Management Is and Is Not

Conservative kidney management is an active, structured treatment pathway for patients with kidney failure who choose not to pursue dialysis or transplantation, built around pharmacologic and dietary management of uremic symptoms, careful volume and electrolyte control using medications rather than renal replacement, and ongoing nephrology follow-up rather than discharge from specialty care. It is not the withholding of treatment; a well-run conservative management program requires as much clinical attention as a dialysis program, directed toward a different endpoint — maximizing comfort and function for the time the patient has, rather than maximizing filtration clearance.

It is also distinct from generic hospice or end-of-life care, though the two overlap and often merge as a patient's illness progresses. Hospice care in most systems requires a prognosis of six months or less and centers explicitly on comfort at the end of life; conservative kidney management can begin much earlier in a patient's trajectory, sometimes years before death, and centers on active management of a chronic condition using a different treatment modality than dialysis rather than on end-of-life care specifically. A patient beginning conservative management is not necessarily entering hospice, and conflating the two in patient communication risks patients declining a reasonable long-term treatment choice because they associate it, inaccurately, with imminent death.

The nomenclature itself matters clinically, not merely semantically. Referring to this pathway as "no treatment" or "comfort care only" in the medical record or in conversation with the patient understates what the pathway actually involves and can discourage patients from choosing it even when it is the option best matched to their goals, while also risking undertreatment by clinicians who read the label and conclude that active symptom management is unnecessary. Consistent use of the term conservative kidney management, understood throughout the treating team as an active pathway with its own defined content, protects against both failure modes, and should be reflected consistently in chart documentation, clinic scheduling templates, and verbal handoffs between covering clinicians so that every member of the team, not only the primary nephrologist, understands the pathway the same way.

Candidacy and Patient Selection for Conservative Management

No single criterion identifies every patient for whom conservative management is the better choice, but several converging factors make the option progressively more likely to offer comparable or superior outcomes to dialysis: advanced age combined with significant frailty, a high burden of comorbid illness independent of the kidney disease itself, severe functional dependence, and, most directly, a low estimated survival benefit from dialysis on a validated nephrology-specific prognostic tool. Several such tools, incorporating variables including age, comorbidity count, functional status, and serum albumin, have been developed specifically to estimate expected survival on dialysis in older or frail populations and to support exactly this kind of individualized comparison against the expected trajectory under conservative management.

The largest body of comparative evidence, drawn from multinational prospective cohorts including the EQUAL study following older patients with advanced chronic kidney disease across several European countries, shows that dialysis extends survival on average across the studied population, but that this survival benefit shrinks considerably, and in some subgroups disappears or reverses, among the oldest and most comorbid patients, particularly those with significant functional dependence or dementia at the time the decision is made. This pattern is the empirical foundation for treating candidacy assessment as genuinely individualized rather than applying dialysis as a default to every patient reaching kidney failure regardless of expected benefit.

Candidacy assessment is not, however, a one-time gate that a patient passes or fails; it is better understood as continuously informing an ongoing conversation, revisited as the patient's trajectory clarifies, in the same way the Life-Plan itself is revisited in Chapter 2. A patient initially assessed as a reasonable dialysis candidate may, following a major functional decline from an unrelated illness, shift toward better alignment with conservative management, and the reverse can occur as well — a patient initially favoring conservative management, after adequate symptom control and reassurance, may reconsider dialysis once its actual demands are better understood through the modality education process. Reassessment at defined intervals, not merely at symptom crisis, keeps the candidacy conversation aligned with the patient's actual, evolving circumstances.

An eighty-nine-year-old woman with a GFR of ten milliliters per minute, moderate frailty, and a comorbidity profile including heart failure and prior stroke with residual mild cognitive impairment is referred for a modality decision after a family member requests "everything be done." A structured prognostic assessment estimates limited survival benefit from dialysis given her comorbidity burden, and a capacity evaluation confirms she retains decision-making capacity for this specific choice despite her mild cognitive impairment. In a joint conversation involving the patient, her family, and the conservative care team, she states clearly that she values remaining at home with her family over any intervention that would require frequent travel to a dialysis center, and that she understands this choice will likely shorten her life relative to dialysis. Her family, initially resistant, is offered a separate meeting with the palliative team to discuss the prognostic data and their own concerns, after which they support her decision. She is enrolled in conservative kidney management with proactive symptom planning, remains stable and comfortable at home for eleven months, and dies without ever having required hospitalization for a uremic complication — an outcome her team attributes directly to the early, proactive symptom management the conservative pathway provided rather than a reactive response to crises as they arose.

The Multidisciplinary Conservative Care Team

Conservative kidney management is delivered most effectively by a team structured similarly to the modality education and Life-Plan teams described in the previous chapter: a nephrologist providing ongoing medical management of the kidney disease itself, a palliative care specialist or palliative-trained nephrology provider directing symptom control, a dietitian adapting nutritional guidance to a non-dialysis trajectory, and social work supporting the psychosocial and practical dimensions of the decision. Absent this structure, conservative management risks becoming, in practice, the absence of any coordinated care at all, with the patient's nephrology follow-up tapering off once dialysis is declined and no equivalent structure replacing it.

Embedding a palliative care clinician within the nephrology team, rather than referring patients out to a separate palliative care service only near the end of life, has been associated in several health-system evaluations with earlier and more consistent goals-of-care conversations and with symptom management that begins proactively rather than reactively once symptoms have already become severe. This integration model reflects the same principle underlying the Life-Plan more broadly: outcomes improve when a structured process is built into routine workflow rather than depending on an individual clinician remembering to initiate a referral at the right moment.

Regular interdisciplinary team meetings, distinct from individual clinic visits with the patient, allow the nephrology, palliative care, dietary, and social work team members to align on a shared understanding of each conservatively managed patient's trajectory and current priorities, reducing the risk that one discipline escalates or de-escalates an aspect of care without the rest of the team being aware of the change. This coordination becomes increasingly important as a patient's condition evolves and the balance of the team's involvement shifts, typically with palliative care's role expanding as the patient moves closer to the end of life and nephrology's role narrowing to management of the kidney disease itself, a transition that proceeds more smoothly when the whole team tracks it together rather than each discipline managing its own portion of care in isolation.

KEY POINT: Conservative kidney management is an active treatment pathway with its own defined clinical content, not the absence of treatment, and it is distinct from hospice care, though the two may eventually converge as illness progresses.

Ethical and Legal Foundations of Treatment Refusal

The ethical foundation supporting a patient's choice of conservative management over dialysis is the same foundation supporting any competent adult's right to decline a recommended medical treatment, grounded in the principle of patient autonomy that governs consent law across essentially every jurisdiction in which this book is likely to be used. A patient with intact decision-making capacity who has been adequately informed of the expected consequences of declining dialysis, including the expected symptom trajectory and timeline, is legally and ethically entitled to make that choice, and the clinical team's role is to ensure the decision is genuinely informed and genuinely autonomous, not to substitute its own judgment about which choice is objectively correct.

Decision-making capacity, in this context, is assessed functionally rather than globally: a patient may lack capacity to manage complex financial affairs while retaining full capacity to understand and weigh the specific, relatively concrete choice between dialysis and conservative management, provided they can demonstrate understanding of their situation, appreciation of the consequences of each option, and the ability to reason through the choice and communicate a consistent decision. Formal capacity evaluation, ideally involving a clinician experienced in capacity assessment, is warranted when the patient's cognitive status is uncertain or when the decision represents an unexplained departure from previously expressed values, but capacity should not be questioned reflexively merely because a patient's choice diverges from what the clinical team would recommend, since disagreement with a recommendation is not itself evidence of impaired decision-making.

For patients who lack capacity and have not previously documented their preferences, decisions fall to a legally authorized surrogate decision-maker, who is ethically and, in most jurisdictions, legally obligated to represent the patient's own previously expressed or reasonably inferred wishes rather than the surrogate's own preferences for the patient. This substituted-judgment standard is precisely why the advance care planning conversations described later in this chapter matter so much practically: a surrogate asked to guess what a patient would have wanted, absent any prior documented conversation, is placed in a considerably more difficult position than one who can point to a specific, previously expressed preference, and is also more likely to experience lasting guilt or uncertainty about whether the decision made truly reflected the patient's own wishes.

DIALYSIS RECOGNITION & RESPONSE SYSTEM — Conservative Care Decision Arcs

The Pattern: A patient with advanced kidney disease is being assessed for conservative kidney management candidacy.

Stem Signature: Advanced age with significant frailty, high comorbidity burden, and a low estimated survival benefit from dialysis on a validated prognostic tool, often accompanied by low mood, poor appetite, and apparent resignation that could reflect either the patient's considered assessment of their situation or an undertreated depressive or pain syndrome.

The Decision: Screen explicitly for depression and inadequately controlled symptoms before finalizing a conservative management recommendation, treating any identified depression or pain aggressively, and revisit the candidacy conversation once those are addressed rather than accepting apparent resignation at face value.

Trap Logic: Reversible depression or poorly controlled uremic symptoms can closely mimic a genuinely considered preference for conservative management; the two are distinguished by whether the patient's outlook and stated preference change once mood and symptoms are actively treated.

Response Anchor: Treat depression and uncontrolled symptoms before finalizing a conservative management decision — an apparently settled preference for comfort-focused care should persist once those confounders are addressed, not simply be accepted at the point of maximal distress.

Symptom Burden and Quality of Life Without Dialysis

Common Uremic Symptoms in Conservative Management

Patients managed conservatively experience a symptom profile that overlaps substantially with the uremic manifestations described in Chapter 1 — fatigue, anorexia, pruritus, nausea, and, as filtration declines further, cognitive slowing and eventually uremic encephalopathy — but without dialysis to periodically correct the underlying metabolic derangement, these symptoms tend to progress more steadily rather than being interrupted and partially reversed on a recurring treatment schedule. This distinction shapes symptom management strategy considerably: rather than anticipating a symptom-free interval after each dialysis session, as a hemodialysis patient does, the conservative management team anticipates a gradually rising symptom burden and plans pharmacologic escalation accordingly, on a trajectory rather than a cyclical pattern.

Pain is under-recognized in this population relative to its actual prevalence, in part because clinicians and patients alike may attribute generalized discomfort to "just the kidney disease" without a systematic pain assessment identifying a specific, treatable source — peripheral neuropathy, musculoskeletal pain from renal osteodystrophy, or unrelated comorbid conditions such as osteoarthritis, each of which responds to a different management approach. Routine, structured pain assessment, using the same validated instruments applied in other palliative care contexts, identifies a treatable component of the symptom burden in a substantial proportion of conservatively managed patients who would otherwise have that pain absorbed into an undifferentiated sense of generalized uremic malaise.

Dyspnea, driven by a combination of volume overload, anemia, and metabolic acidosis, is one of the more distressing symptoms in advanced conservative management and one of the more amenable to targeted intervention even without dialysis: careful diuretic titration, correction of anemia within a range appropriate for a non-dialysis patient, and, in refractory cases, low-dose opioid therapy directed specifically at the sensation of breathlessness rather than at pain, can each meaningfully reduce dyspnea's contribution to overall symptom burden. Family and caregivers benefit from explicit education that dyspnea, while distressing to witness, is a treatable symptom in this context rather than an inevitable, unmanageable feature of dying with kidney failure.

Sleep disturbance and restless legs, driven by a combination of uremic toxin accumulation, iron deficiency, and disrupted circadian signaling, compound the fatigue already present from anemia and general uremic burden, and are frequently under-reported by patients who assume poor sleep is simply an unavoidable feature of their illness rather than a specific, addressable symptom. Structured sleep assessment as part of routine conservative management follow-up identifies these treatable contributors, and correction of iron deficiency in particular, even without full anemia correction, can meaningfully improve restless legs symptoms in a substantial proportion of affected patients.

Pharmacologic and Non-Pharmacologic Symptom Control

Symptom management in conservative kidney management draws on a mixture of medications dosed with particular attention to reduced renal clearance, since many standard symptom-control agents accumulate active metabolites in kidney failure and require either dose reduction or selection of an alternative agent with a clearance pathway less dependent on the kidneys, and non-pharmacologic measures that in several trials perform comparably to medication for specific symptoms such as pruritus. A structured, symptom-by-symptom approach, matching intervention to the specific mechanism driving each symptom rather than treating "uremia" as an undifferentiated target, produces more consistent relief than broad, non-specific comfort measures applied uniformly.

Symptom	Non-Pharmacologic Measures	Pharmacologic Options (Renal Dosing Required)
Uremic Pruritus	Emollients, cool ambient temperature, gabapentin-sparing skin care routines	Gabapentin or pregabalin at reduced dose; topical agents; consider phototherapy in refractory cases
Nausea and Anorexia	Small, frequent meals; dietitian-guided flavor and texture modification	Antiemetics selected for minimal renal clearance dependence; appetite stimulants used selectively

Dyspnea	Positioning, fan-directed airflow, anxiety-reduction techniques	Careful diuretic titration; anemia correction within an appropriate target; low-dose opioid for refractory dyspnea
Uremic Pain	Physical therapy for musculoskeletal contributors; heat or cold application	Agents selected and dosed for reduced renal clearance; avoid accumulation-prone agents
Fatigue	Structured activity pacing; sleep hygiene support	Anemia correction; review and reduce sedating medications where feasible

Because polypharmacy is common in this population and each additional medication carries its own burden of side effects and administration complexity, symptom management under conservative care is most effective when guided by an explicit principle of matching treatment intensity to the symptom's actual impact on the patient's quality of life rather than pursuing complete symptom elimination at the cost of sedation or additional pill burden. A patient who reports mild, tolerable pruritus that does not interfere with sleep or daily activity may reasonably prefer a simple emollient regimen over an additional systemic medication, and eliciting this preference explicitly, rather than assuming maximal pharmacologic control is always the patient's goal, is itself part of a patient-centered conservative management approach.

Comparative Quality of Life and Survival Data

Quality-of-life comparisons between conservative management and dialysis in appropriately matched, typically older and more comorbid populations generally show comparable overall quality of life between the two pathways, with conservative management showing a modest advantage in some studies on measures of physical burden and treatment-related time cost, and dialysis showing an advantage on measures more directly tied to symptom control from the metabolic correction dialysis itself provides. As with the modality comparisons in Chapter 2, aggregate similarity conceals substantial individual variation, and the appropriate response to that variation is the same: match the pathway to the individual patient's actual priorities rather than assuming population-level averages resolve any given patient's decision.

Hospitalization burden differs more consistently than overall quality of life: several cohort studies find that conservatively managed patients spend meaningfully less time hospitalized in their final year of life than matched dialysis patients, likely reflecting both the absence of dialysis-related complications requiring hospital management — vascular access infections, intradialytic emergencies, and treatment-related hospitalizations discussed throughout this book — and a greater tendency for conservative management to be paired with structured symptom management that keeps patients comfortable at home rather than requiring inpatient escalation. This reduced hospitalization burden is frequently among the considerations patients weigh most heavily once it is presented concretely, since abstract survival statistics are less immediately meaningful to many patients than the practical question of how much of their remaining time will be spent in a hospital rather than at home.

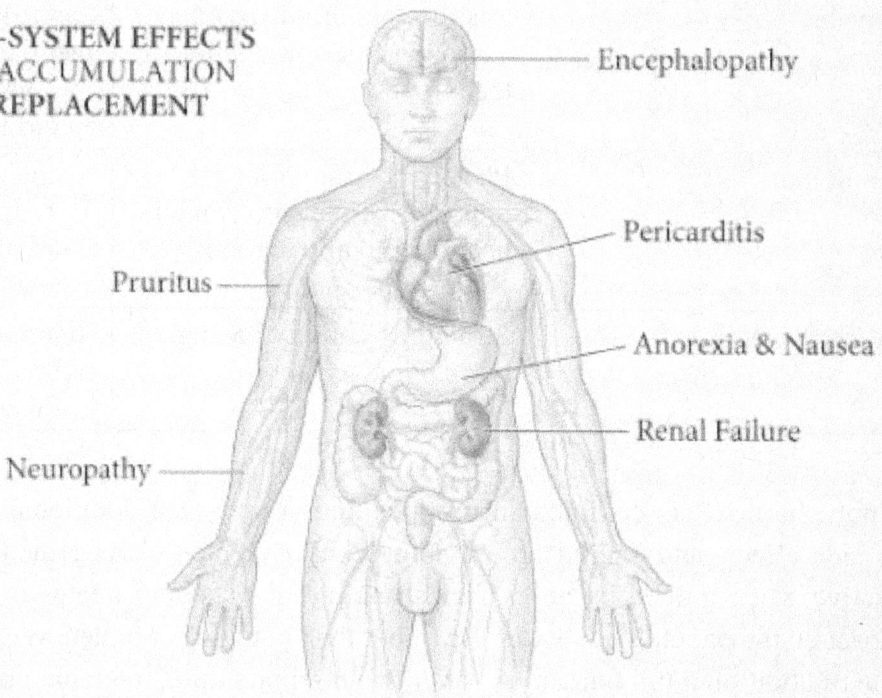

FIGURE 3.1: MULTI-SYSTEM EFFECTS OF UREMIC TOXIN ACCUMULATION WITHOUT RENAL REPLACEMENT

Advance Care Planning and Goals of Care

Initiating the Advance Care Planning Conversation

Advance care planning is frequently delayed until a medical crisis forces the conversation, at which point the patient may be too acutely ill to participate meaningfully and the discussion falls to family members attempting to infer preferences that were never explicitly documented. Initiating this conversation proactively, ideally at the same point in the trajectory that modality education and Life-Plan discussions begin, allows it to occur when the patient can participate fully and allows preferences to be revisited and refined over subsequent visits rather than captured hastily under pressure.

A useful opening framework asks the patient what matters most to them given their kidney disease and overall health — independence, time at home, cognitive clarity, freedom from specific interventions they consider unacceptable — rather than beginning with a checklist of specific interventions to accept or decline in the abstract. Interventions can then be discussed concretely in light of the goals the patient has already articulated, which tends to produce more coherent, internally consistent preferences than working through an intervention checklist first and inferring goals afterward from the pattern of choices made.

Clinicians frequently underestimate how willing most patients are to engage in this conversation once it is framed as an extension of good clinical care rather than as a signal that the clinician has given up on treating them; surveys of patients with advanced kidney disease consistently find that most want to discuss prognosis and goals of care and that most feel this conversation happens later than they would have preferred, not earlier. This finding argues directly against the common clinician concern that raising advance care planning will alarm or distress patients — in most cases, patients are relieved that the conversation is finally occurring rather than distressed that it has begun.

Cultural and religious frameworks shape how patients and families interpret both the conservative management pathway and the broader advance care planning conversation, and effective communication requires eliciting rather than assuming a given patient's framework, since considerable variation exists even within a single cultural or religious tradition. Some traditions and family structures emphasize collective, family-centered decision-making over individual patient autonomy as it is typically framed in Western medical ethics, and a rigid insistence on eliciting the patient's preference in isolation from family input, in a cultural context where decisions are customarily made collectively, can itself be experienced as a failure of culturally competent care rather than as a neutral, universally appropriate default. Asking a patient directly how they would like decisions to be made, and who they would like involved, before proceeding with the standard advance care planning format, accommodates this variation more effectively than applying a single fixed approach to every patient regardless of background.

Documenting Goals of Care and Treatment Preferences

Preferences elicited in conversation are only useful to the care team encountering the patient during a future crisis if they are documented in a form that is both specific enough to guide real decisions and accessible to whichever clinician is on call at the time, which in practice usually means a structured advance directive or portable medical order form specific to the jurisdiction, completed and entered into the medical record rather than recorded only as free-text narrative in a clinic note that a covering clinician may not locate quickly during an emergency. General statements such as "do not want heroic measures" are of limited practical use without translation into the specific, actionable orders — code status, hospital transfer preferences, and dialysis continuation or withdrawal preferences specifically — that a covering team can act on directly.

For patients already on dialysis who are engaging in advance care planning, documentation should address dialysis continuation explicitly and separately from general resuscitation preferences, since a patient may reasonably want continued dialysis but decline cardiopulmonary resuscitation, or vice versa, and the two decisions are frequently conflated in generic advance directive templates that were not designed with a dialysis-dependent population specifically in mind. A dialysis-specific portable order addressing this distinction directly reduces the ambiguity that would otherwise fall to a covering clinician to resolve under time pressure.

Portable medical order forms of this kind, in widespread use across many health systems under various jurisdiction-specific names, differ from a standard advance directive in that they are actionable orders signed by a clinician, intended to be honored immediately by any emergency responder or covering clinician encountering the patient, rather than a statement of the patient's wishes requiring further interpretation before being translated into orders. Because these forms are designed for immediate portability across care settings — home, ambulance, emergency department, and inpatient unit alike — ensuring the patient or family keeps a copy readily accessible, in addition to the copy filed in the medical record, meaningfully increases the likelihood that documented preferences are actually available and honored at the moment they are needed, rather than existing only in a chart that a responding team may not have immediate access to.

Reassessing Goals as Illness Progresses

Goals of care documented at one point in a patient's trajectory should not be treated as permanently fixed, both because patients' preferences can genuinely change as their illness progresses and because a preference articulated when relatively well may not anticipate circumstances that arise later, such as a major functional decline or a new comorbid diagnosis. Scheduled reassessment, timed to the same trigger events that prompt Life-Plan revision in Chapter 2 — a significant hospitalization, a marked functional decline, or a defined interval such as annually — keeps documented goals aligned with the patient's actual, current preferences rather than an earlier snapshot that may no longer reflect them.

This reassessment is particularly important when a patient's cognitive status is expected to decline, since advance care planning completed while the patient retains full decision-making capacity provides the clearest guide for decisions made later, once capacity may be compromised, and delaying this conversation until cognitive decline is already underway forecloses the opportunity to hear the preference directly from the patient rather than inferring it secondhand from family recollection.

A practical trigger schedule, similar in spirit to the Life-Plan revision triggers described in Chapter 2, helps ensure this reassessment actually occurs rather than being deferred indefinitely: a major hospitalization, a new diagnosis substantially affecting prognosis, a documented decline in functional status, or simply the passage of a defined interval such as one year are each reasonable prompts to revisit previously documented goals with the patient directly, confirming that the existing documentation still reflects their current preferences or updating it where it no longer does. Building this trigger schedule into the same registry or chart-flag infrastructure used for Life-Plan revision allows both processes to be tracked together rather than as separate, easily neglected administrative tasks.

CAUTION: A generic advance directive that does not address dialysis continuation or withdrawal specifically leaves this decision ambiguous exactly when it matters most; use a dialysis-specific portable order whenever available rather than relying on general resuscitation preferences alone.

DIALYSIS RECOGNITION & RESPONSE SYSTEM — Conservative Care Decision Arcs

The Pattern: A patient and family express differing preferences during a goals-of-care discussion.

Stem Signature: The patient states a clear preference — for example, to decline further escalation of care — while family members present express distress and advocate for continued aggressive treatment, sometimes speaking over or for the patient during the encounter.

The Decision: Prioritize the documented, directly expressed preference of a patient who retains decision-making capacity, while offering the family a separate, structured meeting to process their distress and understand the reasoning behind the patient's choice, rather than allowing the family's more vocal objection to override a competent patient's stated preference in the moment.

Trap Logic: A distressed family's objection can be mistaken for evidence that the patient's stated preference is not genuinely considered; the two are distinguished by directly confirming the preference with the patient themselves, in a setting separate from the family's distress, rather than deferring to whichever party is speaking most forcefully.

Response Anchor: A capacitated patient's directly expressed preference governs the plan; family distress is addressed through dedicated support, not by overriding the patient's own stated goals.

Transitioning Between Active Therapy and Conservative Care

Recognizing When Dialysis Withdrawal May Be Appropriate

Withdrawal from established dialysis, distinct from never having started it, is a recognized and, in some settings, common pathway to death for dialysis-dependent patients, accounting for a meaningful proportion of deaths in this population in registry data. A request to withdraw from dialysis deserves the same careful evaluation as an initial conservative management candidacy assessment, distinguishing a considered, stable preference reflecting the patient's own assessment of their situation from a reversible crisis — an untreated depressive episode, inadequately controlled pain, an acute delirium, or a transient loss of hope during a difficult but survivable complication — that, once addressed, may resolve the request.

Several features help distinguish a considered withdrawal request from a crisis-driven one: a considered request tends to be stable across more than one conversation rather than voiced only during a single acute distressing episode, is consistent with previously expressed values and goals rather than representing an abrupt reversal, and persists after acute reversible contributors — uncontrolled pain, untreated depression, or delirium — have been actively addressed. None of these features alone is definitive, but their convergence supports treating the request as a genuine, considered decision deserving of respect rather than an emergency to be overridden.

Clinicians sometimes experience discomfort honoring a withdrawal request precisely because dialysis is, unlike many terminal illnesses, a treatment that can technically be continued indefinitely, which can make withdrawal feel more like an active choice to hasten death than the natural progression of an untreatable disease does. This discomfort is understandable but should not itself become a reason to withhold the same respect for patient autonomy that governs every other treatment decision in this book — a competent patient's informed decision to stop a treatment they are legally and ethically entitled to decline carries the same weight whether that treatment is dialysis, chemotherapy, or mechanical ventilation.

The Withdrawal Process and Expected Trajectory

Once a withdrawal decision has been confirmed as considered and stable, the clinical team's focus shifts to anticipating and proactively managing the symptoms that will emerge as residual kidney function alone can no longer maintain metabolic balance, typically over a period ranging from several days to roughly two weeks depending on the patient's residual native kidney function at the time dialysis is stopped. Patients with little to no residual function generally decline more rapidly than those retaining meaningful residual clearance, and this expected timeline should be discussed explicitly with the patient and family in advance so that the trajectory, when it occurs, is anticipated rather than alarming.

Symptom management following withdrawal draws on the same pharmacologic and non-pharmacologic strategies described earlier in this chapter, escalated proactively rather than reactively as uremic symptoms, volume overload, and eventually uremic encephalopathy progress, with hospice enrollment, where the anticipated trajectory falls within the eligibility window, providing an established structure for this escalating symptom management in the home or a comparable setting. Coordinating hospice enrollment before, rather than after, dialysis is actually stopped avoids a gap in symptom-management coverage during the earliest and sometimes most uncomfortable days following withdrawal.

The physiological sequence following withdrawal generally mirrors, in accelerated and unopposed form, the natural progression toward kidney failure described in Chapter 1: potassium and acid-base derangement accumulate over days, volume overload progresses as urine output, if any remains, cannot keep pace with ongoing fluid intake, and uremic toxin accumulation eventually produces progressive somnolence that, in most patients, deepens gradually into a comfortable, unresponsive state before death rather than producing the acute distress that family members sometimes fear in advance. Anticipatory guidance describing this expected gradual transition to families in advance measurably reduces their distress once the trajectory actually unfolds, since the pattern, though unfamiliar to most families, is a predictable and generally comfortable one rather than an acute crisis requiring emergency intervention.

Supporting Patients and Families Through Transition

A withdrawal decision, however considered and appropriate, is rarely experienced by family members as a neutral clinical event, and explicit emotional and informational support for the family — clear explanation of what to expect, an accessible point of contact for questions as the trajectory unfolds, and acknowledgment of the grief the decision understandably provokes even when family members support it — measurably improves the family's experience of this period and their subsequent bereavement course in studies of end-of-life care more broadly. Nephrology teams that have cared for a patient over years of dialysis treatment often experience their own sense of loss at this transition, and acknowledging this within the team, rather than treating withdrawal purely as an administrative endpoint, supports the staff who will continue caring for other patients facing similar decisions.

A seventy-two-year-old man on hemodialysis for six years, with progressive heart failure and increasing difficulty tolerating his treatment sessions due to intradialytic hypotension despite prescription adjustments described in later chapters, raises the question of stopping dialysis during a routine clinic visit, stating that he is tired of feeling unwell around every treatment and no longer believes the burden is worth the time it buys him. Over two subsequent visits, his nephrology team confirms the request is stable across conversations, screens for and finds no evidence of untreated depression, and explores his understanding of the expected trajectory following withdrawal, which he articulates accurately and without apparent ambivalence. His family, initially distressed, receives a dedicated meeting with the palliative care team to process their reaction separately from the decision itself, and ultimately supports his choice once his reasoning is explained directly to them. Dialysis is discontinued with hospice enrolled in advance, and he dies comfortably at home nine days later with symptom control escalated proactively throughout, an outcome his team documents as reflecting a well-supported, considered decision rather than a crisis inadequately addressed. This case is revisited by the team afterward in a brief debrief, standard practice for withdrawal decisions in this program, both to confirm that the process was followed as intended and to give the involved staff a structured opportunity to process their own reactions to a patient they had cared for across six years of treatment, reflecting the same acknowledgment of staff experience described earlier in this chapter.

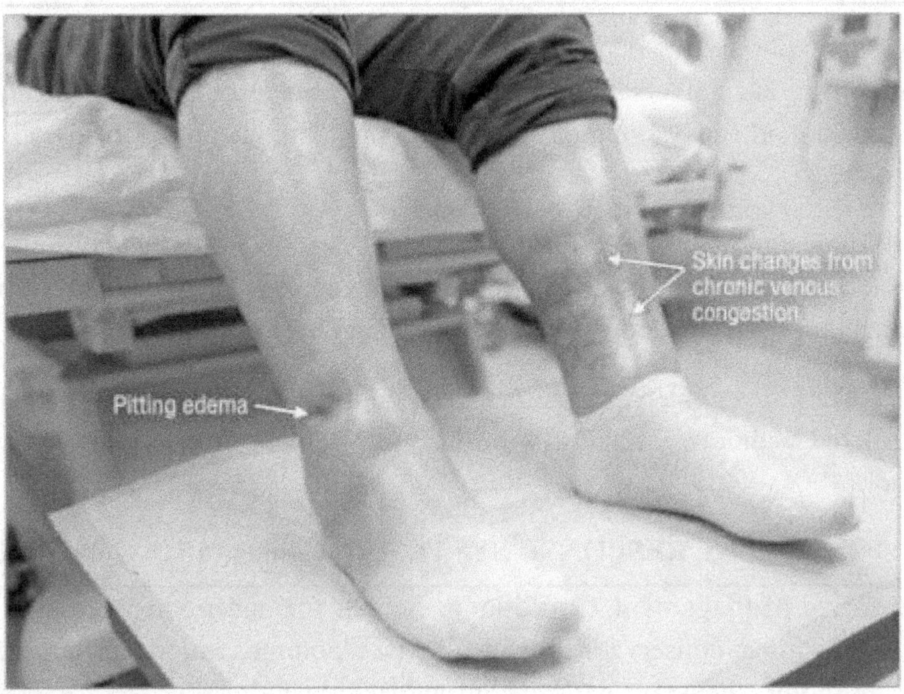

Figure 3.3: Pulmonary Congestion on Chest Radiograph in a Conservatively Managed Patient

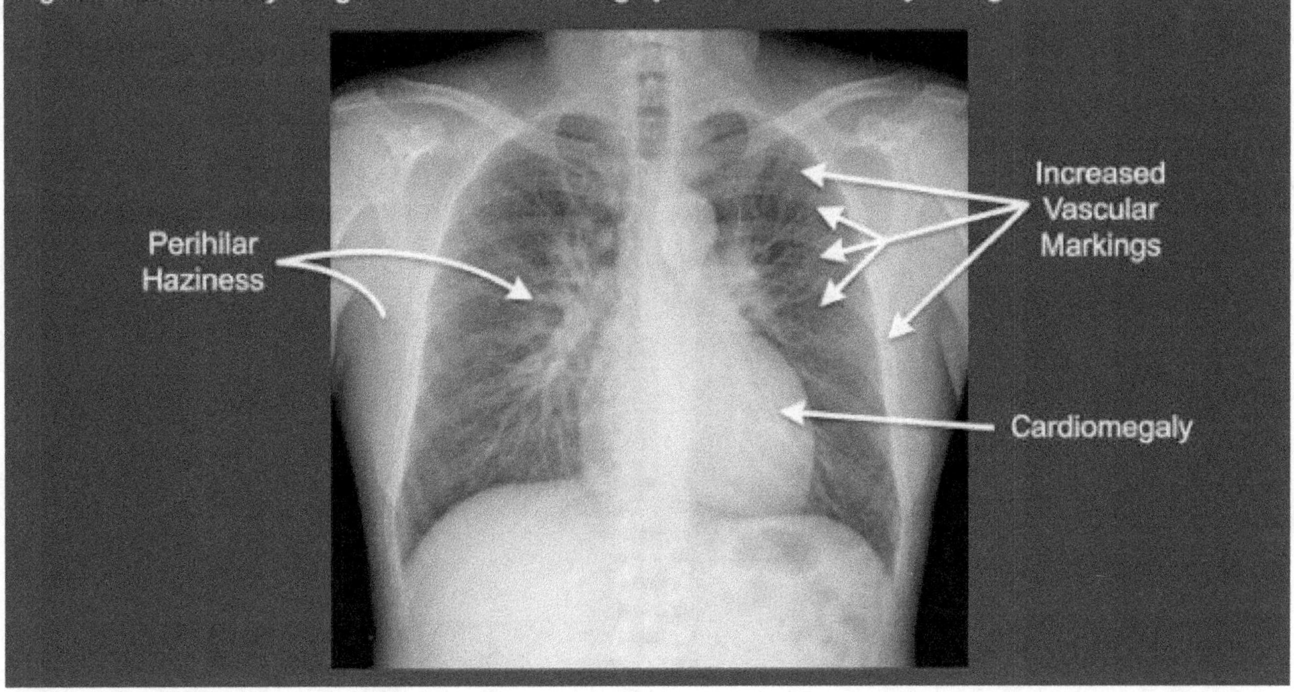

DIALYSIS RECOGNITION & RESPONSE SYSTEM — Conservative Care Decision Arcs

The Pattern: An established dialysis patient voices a request to stop treatment.

Stem Signature: A stated wish to discontinue dialysis, which may arise during a difficult but medically survivable complication, an acute mood disturbance, or as a stable, repeatedly expressed preference consistent with the patient's previously stated values.

The Decision: Screen explicitly for depression, uncontrolled pain, and delirium; confirm the request's stability across more than one conversation; and, once confirmed as considered and stable, honor it with the same clinical rigor and proactive symptom-management planning applied to any other major treatment decision in this book.

Trap Logic: A withdrawal request voiced during an acute, reversible crisis can closely resemble a stable, considered preference in the moment it is first expressed; the distinguishing step is confirming persistence after the acute contributor has been addressed, not accepting the first expression of the request as final.

Response Anchor: Treat reversible contributors first, confirm stability across repeated conversations, then honor a considered withdrawal request with the same respect given to any other informed patient decision in this book.

DIALYSIS RECOGNITION & RESPONSE SYSTEM — Conservative Care Decision Arcs

Assessing Conservative Management Candidacy: Screen for and treat depression and uncontrolled symptoms before finalizing a conservative management recommendation; an apparent preference for comfort-focused care should persist once those confounders are addressed.

Family-Patient Preference Conflict: A capacitated patient's directly expressed preference governs the plan; support family distress separately rather than allowing it to override the patient's stated goals.

A Request to Withdraw From Dialysis: Treat reversible contributors first, confirm stability across repeated conversations, then honor a considered withdrawal request with full clinical rigor and proactive symptom planning.

Summary and Key Concepts

Conservative kidney management is an active, structured treatment pathway distinct from both standard dialysis care and generic hospice care, requiring its own coordinated multidisciplinary team.

Candidacy is best assessed using validated prognostic tools alongside frailty and comorbidity data, and should be reassessed as a patient's trajectory evolves rather than decided once and fixed permanently.

Uremic symptoms without dialysis tend to progress steadily rather than cycle with treatment, and structured, symptom-specific pharmacologic and non-pharmacologic management can control this burden effectively when guided by mechanism rather than treated as undifferentiated malaise.

Advance care planning is most effective when initiated proactively, framed around the patient's own goals before specific interventions are discussed, and documented in a dialysis-specific, actionable format rather than general narrative language.

Dialysis withdrawal is a recognized, respected pathway when a request is confirmed as stable and considered after reversible contributors such as depression, uncontrolled pain, and delirium have been actively addressed and treated.

CHAPTER 4: PHYSIOLOGY OF SOLUTE AND FLUID REMOVAL IN HEMODIALYSIS

Learning Objectives

Distinguish diffusion, convection, and ultrafiltration as the three physical mechanisms by which hemodialysis removes solutes and fluid.

Explain why small-solute clearance, middle-molecule clearance, and protein-bound toxin clearance each follow different kinetics and require different technical strategies.

Describe the sodium gradient between blood and dialysate and its role in both solute clearance and intradialytic hemodynamic stability.

Relate ultrafiltration rate to vascular refilling capacity and interdialytic weight gain in the context of fluid management.

Explain the physiologic basis of bicarbonate-based dialysate and the risks associated with rapid acid-base correction.

Chapter Overview

Every clinical decision made at the hemodialysis machine — which dialyzer to select, what dialysate composition to prescribe, how aggressively to remove fluid — rests on a small number of physical principles governing how solutes and water cross a semipermeable membrane. This chapter develops those principles in enough depth that the prescription-writing content of Chapter 6 and the adequacy calculations of Chapter 7 will read as applications of known physiology rather than as memorized rules. Diffusion, convection, and ultrafiltration are not interchangeable terms for the same process; each removes a different category of substance by a different physical mechanism, and understanding why is what allows a clinician to reason through an unfamiliar clinical scenario rather than simply pattern-matching to a remembered protocol.

Diffusion, Convection, and Ultrafiltration

Diffusive Solute Transport Across the Dialyzer Membrane

Diffusion is the movement of solute molecules from a region of higher concentration to one of lower concentration, driven entirely by the concentration gradient across the dialyzer membrane and requiring no bulk movement of fluid to occur. In hemodialysis, blood carrying a high concentration of urea, creatinine, and other accumulated solutes flows on one side of the membrane while dialysate, formulated to be essentially free of these waste solutes, flows on the other, usually in a countercurrent direction that maximizes the concentration gradient along the entire length of the membrane rather than allowing it to collapse toward equilibrium at the outflow end as would occur with parallel flow.

The rate of diffusive clearance for a given solute depends on the concentration gradient, the membrane's surface area and permeability to that specific solute, and, critically, the solute's molecular size: small molecules such as urea, with a molecular weight around sixty daltons, diffuse readily through the pores of essentially any clinically used dialyzer membrane, while progressively larger molecules diffuse more slowly because their size increasingly restricts their passage through the membrane's pore structure. This size-dependent restriction is the physiological reason small solutes are cleared far more efficiently by diffusion than the middle molecules discussed later in this chapter, and it is not a limitation that can be overcome simply by running a diffusion-based treatment longer, since the rate-limiting step is the solute's ability to enter and cross the pore, not merely the duration of exposure.

Blood flow rate and dialysate flow rate both influence diffusive clearance by determining how quickly fresh, solute-free dialysate and solute-rich blood are delivered to the membrane surface, replenishing the concentration gradient that diffusion depends on; below a certain flow rate, clearance is limited by how quickly blood or dialysate can be delivered to the membrane rather than by the membrane's intrinsic permeability, while above that threshold, further increases in flow yield progressively smaller clearance gains because the membrane's own diffusive capacity, not delivery rate, becomes the limiting factor. This diminishing-returns relationship is why simply increasing blood flow rate indefinitely is not an effective strategy for improving clearance once the membrane itself has become the rate-limiting step.

A further, more subtle influence on diffusive transport arises from the Gibbs-Donnan effect: because plasma proteins carry a net negative charge and cannot cross the dialyzer membrane, they exert a modest electrochemical influence on the distribution of small, diffusible charged solutes across the membrane, slightly altering the effective concentration gradient for ions such as chloride and bicarbonate relative to what a simple concentration-difference calculation alone would predict. This effect is generally small enough to be accounted for in the dialysate formulation process by manufacturers rather than requiring adjustment by the prescribing clinician, but it is part of why dialysate electrolyte concentrations are not simply set equal to a physiologically normal serum value and instead reflect empirically validated formulations that account for these membrane-transport nuances.

Convective Transport and Solute Drag

Convection removes solute by an entirely different mechanism: as fluid is driven across the membrane by a pressure gradient, solutes small enough to pass through the membrane's pores are carried along with that fluid movement, a phenomenon termed solvent drag. Unlike diffusion, convective clearance is far less dependent on molecular size within the range of molecules the membrane's pores can accommodate at all, because the solute is not migrating independently down its own concentration gradient but is instead swept along with the bulk fluid movement, meaning that convection can clear a broader range of molecular sizes, including some middle molecules that diffusion clears only poorly, provided the membrane's pore structure permits their passage.

The magnitude of convective clearance is governed primarily by the volume of fluid moved across the membrane, meaning that achieving clinically meaningful convective clearance of middle molecules requires substantially larger fluid exchange volumes than are needed for standard fluid removal alone, which is why techniques that emphasize convection, such as hemodiafiltration, deliberately move and then replace large volumes of fluid rather than relying on the smaller net ultrafiltration volume needed simply to manage a patient's fluid balance. This distinction between the fluid volume needed for convective solute clearance and the fluid volume needed for weight management is a common source of confusion, since both involve moving fluid across the same membrane but for functionally different clinical purposes.

The degree to which a given solute is carried along with convective fluid flow is described by its sieving coefficient, a value between zero and one representing the fraction of the solute's plasma concentration that appears in the ultrafiltrate; a sieving coefficient near one indicates the solute passes through the membrane essentially unimpeded by convective flow, while a sieving coefficient near zero indicates the membrane effectively excludes it regardless of how much fluid volume is moved. Albumin, whose retention in the blood is essential to maintaining oncotic pressure and avoiding its loss into the ultrafiltrate, has a sieving coefficient designed to be very low in properly functioning dialysis membranes, illustrating that convective membrane design must simultaneously permit passage of the middle molecules convection is meant to clear while excluding proteins the patient needs to retain, a design tension that limits how large a pore size can be used regardless of how much convective clearance of larger middle molecules might otherwise be achieved.

Ultrafiltration: Separating Fluid Removal From Solute Clearance

Ultrafiltration refers specifically to the net removal of fluid from the patient's blood across the dialyzer membrane, driven by a pressure gradient, usually created by applying negative pressure on the dialysate side relative to the blood side, termed transmembrane pressure. It is important to separate this concept, fluid removal for the purpose of correcting a patient's volume overload, from the convective solute clearance discussed above: a standard hemodialysis prescription typically removes several liters of fluid net over a treatment, an amount sufficient for meaningful fluid management but modest relative to the much larger fluid exchange volumes used specifically to drive convective middle-molecule clearance in hemodiafiltration.

The rate at which fluid can safely be removed is constrained not by the membrane's capacity, which can accommodate far higher ultrafiltration rates than are typically prescribed, but by the patient's own physiology — specifically, the rate at which fluid can refill the vascular space from the interstitial and intracellular compartments to replace the volume being removed from the blood. This vascular refilling rate, discussed further later in this chapter, is the physiological ceiling on safe ultrafiltration rate, and exceeding it is the central mechanism underlying the intradialytic hypotension discussed in detail in Chapter 13.

Vascular refilling depends on the interstitial compartment's hydraulic conductance and on the oncotic and hydrostatic pressure gradients between the interstitial and vascular spaces, both of which shift as ultrafiltration proceeds: as plasma volume contracts relative to the interstitial reservoir, the pressure gradients favoring refilling change, and in some patients this relationship becomes less favorable later in a treatment, producing a pattern in which hypotension risk is disproportionately concentrated in the final portion of a session as the interstitial reservoir available to refill the vascular space becomes progressively depleted. This time-dependent pattern is part of the physiological rationale for the sodium profiling strategy discussed later in this chapter, which aims to support refilling specifically during the treatment phases when the interstitial reservoir is becoming less able to support it on its own.

KEY POINT: Diffusion clears small solutes efficiently but middle molecules poorly; convection can clear a broader size range but requires much larger fluid exchange volumes than ultrafiltration for weight management alone requires.

A forty-nine-year-old man on conventional hemodialysis for four years, with a consistently adequate Kt/V above the standard target, reports worsening fatigue, diffuse joint discomfort, and pruritus that have not responded to the symptom-management measures described in Chapter 3. Investigation reveals a markedly elevated beta-2 microglobulin level, and imaging of his shoulders shows early changes consistent with dialysis-related amyloidosis, a recognized complication of chronic middle-molecule accumulation. Because his vascular access can support the higher blood flow rate required, his nephrology team transitions him from conventional high-flux hemodialysis to online hemodiafiltration, adding a substantial convective exchange volume to his existing diffusive clearance. Over the following several months, his beta-2 microglobulin level falls meaningfully, and his joint symptoms and pruritus both improve, illustrating the clinical relevance of the distinction developed in this chapter: his Kt/V, a small-solute metric, had never signaled a problem, because the problem was never in the domain diffusion-dominant clearance addresses well.

Combining Diffusion and Convection in Modern Hemodialysis

Standard hemodialysis relies predominantly on diffusion, with the modest ultrafiltration needed for fluid management contributing only a small amount of convective clearance as a secondary effect. Hemodiafiltration deliberately combines both mechanisms: a high-flux membrane permits substantial diffusive clearance of small and some middle molecules, while a large-volume convective exchange, with sterile replacement fluid infused to offset the large fluid volume removed, adds meaningful clearance of middle molecules that diffusion alone would clear poorly. This combined approach reflects a deliberate engineering trade-off, since achieving substantial convective clearance safely requires infrastructure — ultrapure dialysate and a validated replacement fluid production system — that a standard hemodialysis setup does not require, which is why hemodiafiltration is not universally available across every dialysis facility despite its theoretical clearance advantages for middle molecules.

Figure 4.1: Countercurrent Diffusive and Convective Transport Across the Dialyzer Membrane

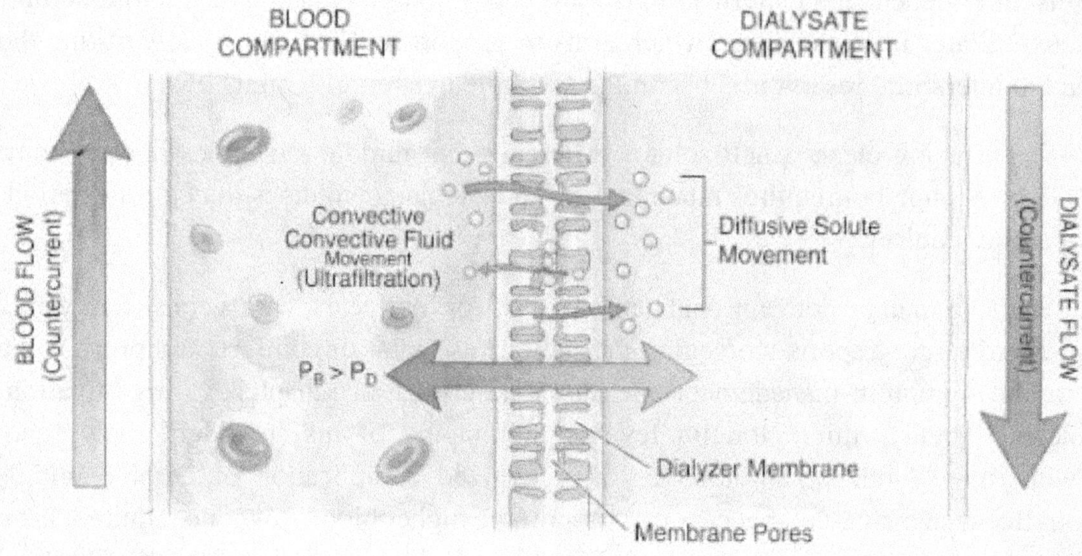

Solute Clearance and Middle Molecule Removal

Small-Solute Clearance and Its Determinants

Urea, with its small molecular size and free distribution across total body water, is the reference solute for small-solute clearance and the basis of the Kt/V adequacy calculation developed fully in Chapter 7. Its clearance during a standard hemodialysis treatment is governed predominantly by blood flow rate, dialysate flow rate, and the dialyzer's mass transfer area coefficient, a property reflecting the combined effect of membrane surface area and permeability, and is relatively insensitive to the fine details of membrane material once a given membrane's mass transfer coefficient for urea is known. Creatinine, somewhat larger than urea but still readily diffusible, follows a broadly similar clearance pattern, which is why urea reduction ratio and creatinine-based clearance estimates track each other reasonably well across most standard treatments.

Because small-solute clearance responds strongly to blood flow rate up to the point where membrane-limited clearance takes over, achieving adequate blood flow through a well-functioning vascular access, discussed in Part III of this book, is a prerequisite for achieving prescribed small-solute clearance regardless of how carefully the remainder of the prescription is calculated; a prescription that assumes a blood flow rate the patient's access cannot actually sustain will underdeliver clearance relative to what the calculation predicts, a mismatch that is often first identified only when a measured adequacy value falls short of the prescribed target, discussed further in Chapter 7.

Urea concentration measured immediately at the end of treatment underestimates the patient's true post-treatment equilibrium urea level because urea clearance during treatment occurs predominantly from the blood compartment, while urea continues to move out of less well-perfused tissue compartments into the blood for some time after treatment ends, producing a rebound rise in blood urea over the thirty to sixty minutes following treatment completion. This post-dialysis urea rebound is the physiological reason equilibrated Kt/V calculations, which account for this compartment redistribution, differ modestly from single-pool Kt/V calculations based on an immediate post-treatment sample, and why the distinction between the two calculation methods, developed further in Chapter 7, matters for accurately characterizing a given patient's true delivered dialysis dose rather than an artificially favorable value produced by measuring urea before redistribution has completed.

Middle Molecules and the Limits of Diffusive Clearance

Middle molecules, generally defined as solutes with a molecular weight between roughly five hundred and sixty thousand daltons, include compounds such as beta-2 microglobulin that accumulate in kidney failure and are implicated in several of the chronic complications discussed later in this book, including certain forms of amyloidosis and contributions to the broader uremic symptom burden described in Chapter 3. Their intermediate size places them at a physiological disadvantage under diffusion-dominant clearance: they are too large to cross standard membranes as readily as small solutes, yet still small enough that a high-flux membrane's larger pores permit some diffusive passage, producing clearance that is real but substantially lower than that achieved for small solutes under the same treatment conditions.

Because middle-molecule clearance responds more strongly to treatment duration and to convective clearance strategies than to blood flow rate alone, strategies aimed specifically at improving middle-molecule removal — longer or more frequent treatments, discussed in the context of home and intensive hemodialysis in Chapter 20, and hemodiafiltration's convective exchange described above — target different levers than the strategies used to optimize small-solute clearance. A prescription optimized purely for small-solute Kt/V may therefore leave middle-molecule clearance comparatively under-addressed, which is part of the rationale, still an area of active clinical investigation, for considering treatment frequency and convective strategies as complementary rather than redundant to standard adequacy targets, an approach discussed in greater practical detail when home and intensive hemodialysis regimens are covered in Chapter 20.

Beta-2 microglobulin itself has become a useful surrogate marker for middle-molecule clearance more broadly in both clinical practice and research, analogous to the role urea plays as the reference solute for small-solute clearance, precisely because it is readily measured, well characterized, and representative of the broader class of middle molecules implicated in long-term dialysis complications. A rising or persistently elevated beta-2 microglobulin level in a patient already meeting standard small-solute adequacy targets is therefore a reasonable prompt to consider whether treatment modifications aimed specifically at middle-molecule clearance, rather than further small-solute Kt/V optimization, would better address the patient's overall toxin burden.

Protein-Bound Uremic Toxins and Their Clearance Challenge

A further category of accumulated solute, protein-bound uremic toxins such as indoxyl sulfate and p-cresyl sulfate, presents a clearance challenge distinct from either small-solute or middle-molecule removal: these toxins circulate substantially bound to plasma proteins, particularly albumin, and only the small free, unbound fraction is available to cross the dialyzer membrane by either diffusion or convection, regardless of the membrane's pore size or the treatment's convective volume. Because protein binding, not molecular size, is the rate-limiting factor for this category of toxin, standard strategies that improve small-solute or middle-molecule clearance produce comparatively little improvement in protein-bound toxin removal, and specialized strategies — including adsorptive membranes or techniques that transiently displace toxin from its protein-binding site — remain largely investigational rather than standard clinical practice at the time of this writing.

This clearance gap is clinically relevant because protein-bound uremic toxins are increasingly implicated in the cardiovascular disease burden that dominates long-term dialysis mortality, discussed in Chapter 24, meaning that a patient's dialysis adequacy, however well small-solute clearance targets are met, does not fully correct this particular category of accumulated toxin. Recognizing this distinction helps set realistic expectations: an adequately dialyzed patient by conventional Kt/V criteria has not necessarily cleared protein-bound toxins to a comparable degree, and the residual cardiovascular risk this leaves unaddressed is an active area of ongoing clinical research rather than a solved problem current dialysis technology fully resolves.

Extending treatment duration, rather than increasing blood or dialysate flow rate, offers a modest additional benefit for protein-bound toxin removal in some studies, plausibly because a longer treatment allows more cycles of toxin dissociation from its protein-binding site and subsequent diffusion of the transiently free fraction, even though the overall clearance achieved remains well below what is possible for small solutes over the same treatment duration. This partial, duration-dependent benefit is one of several considerations, alongside the middle-molecule clearance advantages discussed earlier, that support longer or more frequent hemodialysis regimens, covered in Chapter 20, as a complementary strategy to standard adequacy targets rather than as a redundant intensification of the same clearance already being achieved.

Solute Category	Representative Examples	Approximate Molecular Weight	Primary Clearance Mechanism
Small Solutes	Urea, creatinine, potassium	60–113 Da	Diffusion, highly efficient
Middle Molecules	Beta-2 microglobulin, parathyroid hormone	500–60,000 Da	Convection more effective than diffusion; improved by high-flux membranes and

			longer or more frequent treatment
Protein-Bound Toxins	Indoxyl sulfate, p-cresyl sulfate	Variable, small unbound fraction	Limited by protein binding rather than size; poorly cleared by standard diffusion or convection

DIALYSIS RECOGNITION & RESPONSE SYSTEM — Solute Physiology Arcs

The Pattern: A patient achieves an adequate small-solute Kt/V but continues to report significant uremic symptom burden.

Stem Signature: Urea reduction ratio and Kt/V both meet or exceed standard adequacy targets, yet the patient reports persistent fatigue, pruritus, or other uremic symptoms that would typically be expected to improve with adequate clearance.

The Decision: Consider that small-solute adequacy does not guarantee comparable clearance of middle molecules or protein-bound toxins, and evaluate whether treatment frequency, duration, or convective strategy adjustment, rather than further escalation of the standard Kt/V target, is the more appropriate response to this symptom pattern.

Trap Logic: A persistently symptomatic patient with an adequate Kt/V can be mistaken for a treatment-adherence or access-function problem, prompting unnecessary re-investigation of the access or session attendance, when the actual explanation may be the inherent limitation of diffusion-dominant clearance for larger or protein-bound solutes.

Response Anchor: An adequate small-solute Kt/V does not rule out an undertreated middle-molecule or protein-bound toxin burden as a contributor to persistent uremic symptoms.

Sodium and Fluid Balance During Treatment

Sodium Kinetics and the Dialysate Sodium Gradient

Sodium, unlike urea, is present in the blood at a concentration that is deliberately kept close to the dialysate sodium concentration in most standard prescriptions, because sodium is the primary determinant of plasma osmolality and therefore of the osmotic gradient that governs fluid shifts between the intracellular and extracellular compartments. A large sodium gradient between blood and dialysate would drive rapid diffusive sodium movement that, in turn, would produce abrupt osmotic fluid shifts poorly tolerated by most patients, which is why standard dialysate sodium concentrations are set close to a typical patient's own serum sodium rather than at a fixed physiologic normal value that might differ substantially from an individual patient's baseline.

Because dialysate sodium is nonetheless usually set slightly higher than a typical patient's predialysis serum sodium, a small net diffusive sodium gain typically occurs over the course of a treatment, an effect that, left unaddressed, would work against rather than support the fluid removal ultrafiltration is meant to achieve, since sodium gain draws water with it and expands rather than contracts extracellular volume. Dialysate sodium prescription is therefore not simply a matter of matching the patient's serum value but a deliberate balance between minimizing hemodynamic instability from an overly aggressive sodium gradient and avoiding a sodium load that undermines the treatment's fluid removal goal.

This balance is sometimes described in terms of the dialysate-to-serum sodium gradient, or sodium set point, and clinicians adjusting a patient's dialysate sodium prescription typically do so incrementally rather than through large single adjustments, monitoring the effect on intradialytic tolerance and interdialytic weight gain over several treatments before concluding whether a given change has achieved its intended effect. A patient whose dialysate sodium is lowered specifically to reduce interdialytic thirst and fluid gain, for example, may initially tolerate treatment less well hemodynamically if the change is made too abruptly relative to their accustomed sodium gradient, illustrating that sodium prescription changes, like most of the physiologic adjustments described in this chapter, are generally best made gradually and reassessed empirically rather than through a single large correction.

Sodium Profiling and Its Clinical Rationale

Sodium profiling, in which the dialysate sodium concentration is deliberately varied over the course of a treatment — typically starting higher and declining toward the end of the session — aims to support vascular refilling early in treatment, when the largest fluid volume is typically removed, while reducing the sodium load delivered later in the session when less aggressive support is needed. The physiological rationale rests on using a modestly higher early sodium gradient to help maintain plasma osmolality and thereby support fluid movement from the interstitial space into the vascular compartment, offsetting some of the hemodynamic stress of rapid ultrafiltration during the period when it occurs most intensively.

Profiles vary in their specific shape — some step down sodium concentration in discrete increments over the course of treatment, while others decline more continuously — and the choice of shape is generally guided by the specific dialysis machine's programming capability and by empirical observation of which pattern a given patient tolerates best, rather than by strong evidence favoring one specific profile shape over another for the population as a whole. Because the physiological goal is matching sodium support to the period of greatest ultrafiltration-related hemodynamic stress, profiles are most useful when their timing is actually aligned with a given patient's own ultrafiltration pattern, which is not necessarily uniform across the treatment if, for example, a large portion of the prescribed fluid removal is deliberately front-loaded or back-loaded within the session.

Sodium profiling's clinical benefit is most apparent in patients prone to intradialytic hypotension, discussed at length in Chapter 13, but it carries a genuine trade-off: the same higher early sodium exposure that supports blood pressure can also increase thirst and interdialytic fluid intake if used indiscriminately or extended too far into the treatment, potentially worsening the very fluid overload the treatment is meant to correct over the following interdialytic interval. This trade-off is why sodium profiling is generally reserved for patients demonstrating a clear hemodynamic benefit from it rather than applied as a universal default across all patients.

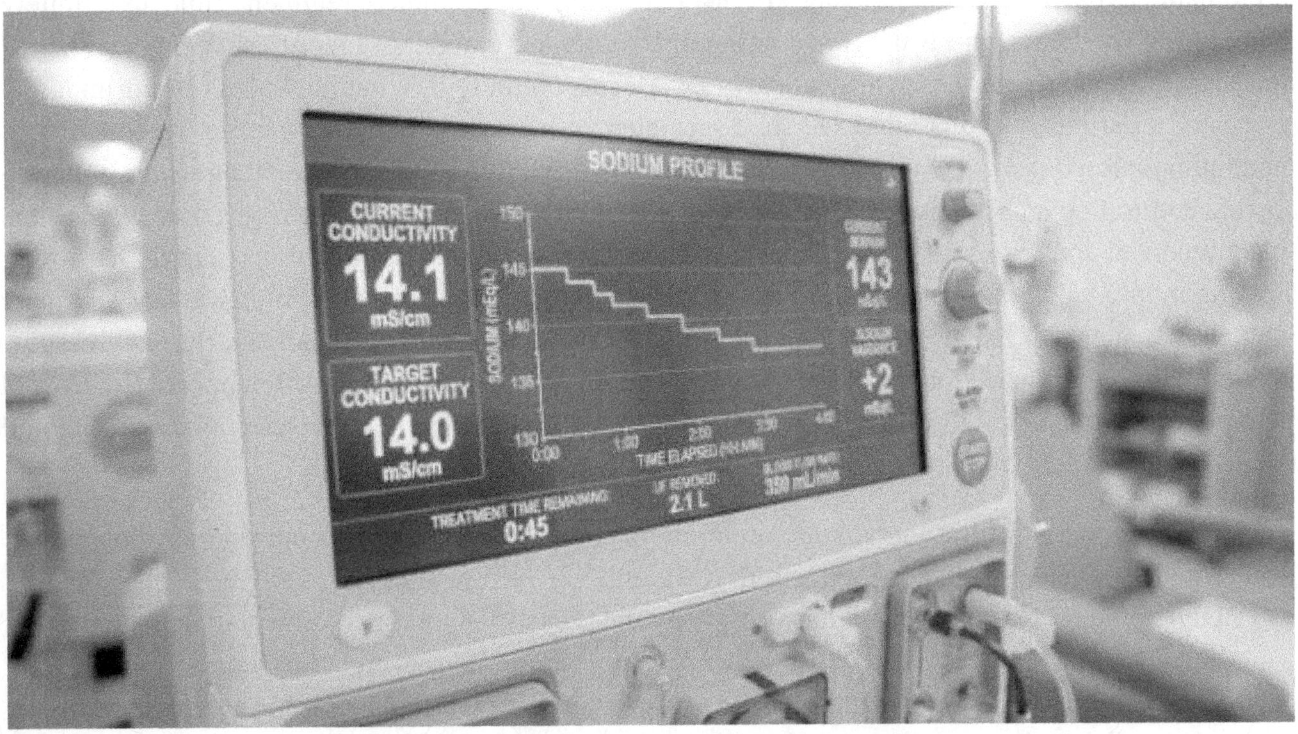

Ultrafiltration Rate, Vascular Refilling, and Interdialytic Weight Gain

The vascular refilling rate — the speed at which fluid moves from the interstitial and intracellular compartments back into the vascular space to replace plasma volume being removed by ultrafiltration — varies considerably between patients and even within the same patient depending on their current degree of volume overload, with more fluid-overloaded patients generally able to refill more readily than euvolemic patients because they have a larger interstitial fluid reservoir to draw from. This variability is why a fixed ultrafiltration rate that one patient tolerates comfortably may produce significant hypotension in another, and why ultrafiltration rate, discussed further in the prescription-writing content of Chapter 6, is properly individualized rather than applied as a uniform value across all patients regardless of their current volume status.

Interdialytic weight gain, the fluid accumulated between treatments from dietary sodium and fluid intake, directly determines how much ultrafiltration a given treatment must accomplish to return the patient to their target weight, meaning that a patient with large interdialytic weight gains requires either a higher ultrafiltration rate within a fixed treatment time, with its attendant hemodynamic risk, or a longer treatment time to remove the same volume at a gentler, better-tolerated rate. This relationship is a central reason dietary sodium and fluid counseling, addressed further in Chapter 25, is not a peripheral nutritional concern but a direct determinant of how safely a patient's fluid removal can be accomplished at each treatment.

A sixty-one-year-old woman on a standard three-times-weekly hemodialysis schedule consistently gains four to five kilograms between her longer weekend interdialytic interval and her Monday treatment, requiring an ultrafiltration rate that repeatedly approaches the upper limit of what she tolerates without symptomatic hypotension. Rather than simply extending her Monday treatment time indefinitely to accommodate the larger removal volume at a gentler rate, her care team identifies, through a structured dietary review, that her weekend fluid intake is driven substantially by a habitual pattern of drinking large volumes of a particular sports beverage she associates with staying hydrated, a belief reasonable in the general population but poorly suited to someone with no urine output to eliminate the resulting fluid load. Targeted counseling addressing this specific behavior, rather than generic fluid-restriction advice she had already received and found difficult to apply, reduces her weekend weight gain by roughly half over the following month, allowing her Monday ultrafiltration rate to fall comfortably within her known tolerance without any change to her treatment time or prescription. This outcome illustrates that addressing the behavioral driver of interdialytic weight gain directly, once identified, is often more effective than repeating the same general dietary advice or simply adjusting the treatment prescription to accommodate an unaddressed underlying pattern.

1. Estimate the ultrafiltration volume required by comparing the patient's current pre-dialysis weight to their established target, or dry, weight.
2. Divide the required ultrafiltration volume by the prescribed treatment time to calculate the ultrafiltration rate, expressed per hour or per kilogram of body weight per hour.
3. Compare the calculated rate against the patient's individual tolerance, informed by their history of intradialytic symptoms and their typical vascular refilling capacity, rather than against a single fixed threshold applied uniformly to all patients.
4. Where the required ultrafiltration volume would exceed a rate the patient is known to tolerate, consider extending treatment time or, where the underlying driver is large interdialytic weight gain, addressing dietary sodium and fluid intake directly rather than accepting a poorly tolerated ultrafiltration rate as unavoidable.

CLINICAL PEARL: When a patient repeatedly requires an ultrafiltration rate near or above their known tolerance threshold, the more durable fix is often reducing interdialytic weight gain through dietary counseling, not simply increasing treatment time indefinitely.

Acid-Base Correction on Hemodialysis

Buffer Systems Used in Modern Dialysate

Patients with kidney failure develop a progressive metabolic acidosis because the kidneys' normal role in regenerating bicarbonate and excreting the daily acid load from dietary and metabolic sources is lost, and correcting this acidosis is one of hemodialysis's essential functions alongside solute clearance and fluid removal. Modern dialysate uses bicarbonate as its primary buffer, delivered as a concentrate mixed with the acid concentrate and water at the point of treatment, having almost entirely replaced the acetate-based dialysate used in earlier decades of dialysis practice, because acetate itself required hepatic metabolism to bicarbonate and produced hemodynamic instability and nausea in a meaningful proportion of patients, effects that bicarbonate-based dialysate largely avoids.

Because bicarbonate can precipitate with calcium and magnesium if combined directly in a single concentrated solution, bicarbonate-based dialysate is prepared from two separate concentrates, an acid concentrate containing calcium, magnesium, and a small amount of acetate to prevent bacterial growth, and a bicarbonate concentrate, mixed with treated water by the dialysis machine at the time of treatment rather than stored premixed, a practical detail with direct implications for water treatment system requirements discussed in Chapter 5.

The bicarbonate concentrate itself is susceptible to bacterial growth if stored improperly, since it provides a nutrient source that acetate's mild antimicrobial property, retained in small quantity within the acid concentrate specifically to address this vulnerability, helps control; dialysis facilities therefore follow defined protocols for concentrate storage duration, container handling, and periodic microbiological surveillance of the mixed dialysate itself, since endotoxin or bacterial contamination introduced through this pathway can produce a systemic inflammatory response in patients despite the dialyzer membrane's intact physical barrier against direct bacterial passage, a topic developed further alongside broader water treatment standards in the next chapter.

Bicarbonate Kinetics and the Risks of Rapid Correction

Bicarbonate diffuses from dialysate into blood down its concentration gradient in essentially the same manner as any other small solute, correcting the patient's metabolic acidosis over the course of treatment, but this correction occurs considerably faster than the compensatory respiratory changes and intracellular buffering the body would use to adjust to a comparable pH change occurring gradually, creating a mismatch between the rapidity of the serum pH correction and the slower equilibration of intracellular and cerebrospinal fluid pH. This mismatch is the physiological basis for a transient paradoxical acidosis within the central nervous system during rapid bicarbonate correction, since carbon dioxide, generated as bicarbonate buffers accumulated acid, crosses the blood-brain barrier more readily than bicarbonate itself, transiently lowering cerebrospinal fluid pH even as serum pH is rising.

This phenomenon is most clinically relevant in patients with severe, longstanding acidosis undergoing their first several hemodialysis treatments, in whom overly rapid bicarbonate correction has been associated with a dialysis disequilibrium-like presentation of headache, nausea, and in severe cases altered mental status or seizure, a risk that overlaps with but is mechanistically distinct from the more general dialysis disequilibrium syndrome driven primarily by rapid urea clearance and osmotic water shift into the brain. Recognizing that both processes can contribute to a similar clinical picture in a new dialysis patient is part of why initial hemodialysis treatments are conventionally shortened and conducted at reduced blood flow rate, gradually escalating over the first several sessions rather than delivering a full-intensity prescription from the outset.

The carbon dioxide generated during bicarbonate buffering also has a direct respiratory dimension worth noting: as serum bicarbonate rises during treatment, the buffering reaction that consumes hydrogen ion and regenerates carbon dioxide can transiently increase the carbon dioxide load the patient must eliminate through ventilation, an effect generally well tolerated by patients with normal respiratory reserve but one that deserves attention in patients with significant underlying pulmonary disease, whose ability to compensate for this transient carbon dioxide generation through increased minute ventilation may be more limited. This is one of several reasons a patient's respiratory status and overall physiologic reserve, not only their kidney disease itself, informs how aggressively acid-base correction should proceed during any individual treatment.

Individualizing the Dialysate Buffer Prescription

The dialysate bicarbonate concentration is prescribed, within a standard range, based on the patient's typical predialysis bicarbonate level and the degree of correction that has been observed to be well tolerated, with the goal of achieving a postdialysis bicarbonate within a normal to near-normal range without producing a metabolic alkalosis by the time of the next treatment, an outcome that can occur if the prescribed dialysate bicarbonate is set too high relative to a given patient's typical predialysis level and residual metabolic acid production between treatments.

Because interdialytic acid accumulation continues at a relatively steady rate between treatments, largely reflecting a patient's ongoing dietary protein intake and residual endogenous acid production, a patient whose predialysis bicarbonate consistently runs low despite an apparently adequate dialysate bicarbonate prescription may be more efficiently helped by evaluating their protein intake and residual kidney function than by escalating dialysate bicarbonate concentration indefinitely, since dialysate bicarbonate can only correct acidosis at the time of treatment and cannot address a between-treatment acid accumulation rate that exceeds what a standard prescription is designed to offset.

This same reasoning extends to the less common but clinically important scenario of a patient whose predialysis bicarbonate runs persistently high rather than low, which may reflect a dialysate bicarbonate prescription set too generously relative to the patient's actual interdialytic acid production, or, in some cases, a superimposed respiratory or metabolic alkalosis process unrelated to the dialysate prescription itself, such as chronic diuretic use or a primary respiratory disorder; distinguishing between these possibilities before adjusting the dialysate prescription downward prevents inappropriately undertreating an acidosis that the dialysate correction was never actually causing in the first place.

CAUTION: Escalating dialysate bicarbonate concentration in a chronically low-bicarbonate patient without first evaluating dietary acid load and interdialytic accumulation risks producing postdialysis alkalosis without addressing the underlying cause of the low predialysis value.

Figure 4.3: Extracorporeal Hemodialysis Circuit Schematic

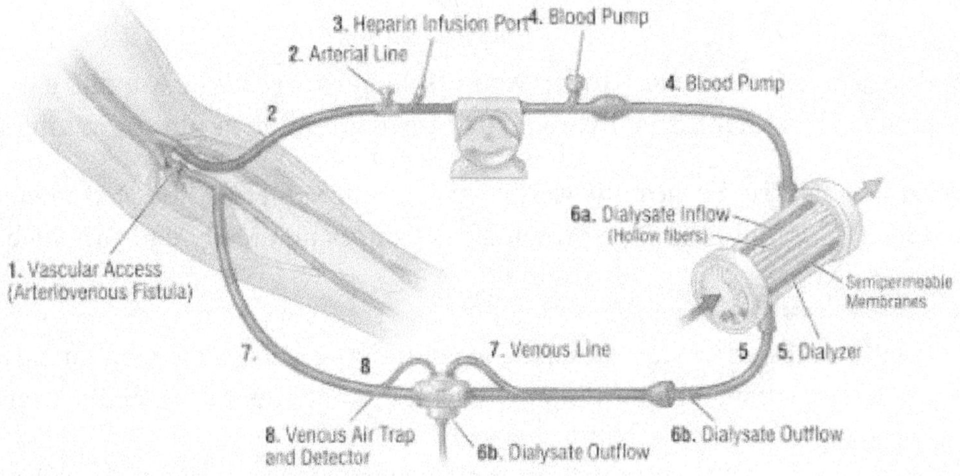

Figure 4.3: Extracorporeal Hemodialysis Circuit Schematic

DIALYSIS RECOGNITION & RESPONSE SYSTEM — Solute Physiology Arcs

The Pattern: A patient beginning their first several hemodialysis treatments with severe, longstanding pre-treatment acidosis and uremia develops headache and nausea during or shortly after treatment.

Stem Signature: New-onset headache, nausea, or mild confusion developing during or within hours of an early hemodialysis session in a patient with a markedly elevated pre-treatment blood urea nitrogen and low bicarbonate, typically on one of the first several treatments rather than an established patient on a stable prescription.

The Decision: Recognize this as a disequilibrium-type presentation potentially reflecting both rapid urea-driven osmotic shift and rapid bicarbonate correction, and confirm that initial treatments are being conducted at reduced intensity — shortened duration and reduced blood flow — with gradual escalation over subsequent sessions rather than delivering a full-intensity prescription to a new, severely uremic patient.

Trap Logic: This presentation can resemble an unrelated acute neurologic event or an intradialytic hypotensive episode; the distinguishing context is the timing relative to a new, high-intensity first treatment in a severely uremic patient rather than an established patient on a stable, previously well-tolerated prescription.

Response Anchor: Severely uremic, acidotic patients begin hemodialysis at reduced intensity with gradual escalation — this is a preventive prescription choice, not merely a response to symptoms once they occur.

Adequate Kt/V With Persistent Symptoms: An adequate small-solute Kt/V does not rule out an undertreated middle-molecule or protein-bound toxin burden as the explanation for persistent uremic symptoms.

Ultrafiltration Rate Near Tolerance Limit: Address large interdialytic weight gain through dietary counseling as a durable fix, rather than only escalating treatment time or ultrafiltration rate.

New Patient With Severe Pre-Treatment Acidosis: Begin treatment at reduced intensity with gradual escalation to prevent a disequilibrium-type presentation from rapid urea and bicarbonate correction.

Summary and Key Concepts

Diffusion clears small solutes efficiently down a concentration gradient; convection clears a broader size range by carrying solute along with bulk fluid movement, but requires substantially larger fluid exchange volumes to do so meaningfully.

Middle molecules and protein-bound uremic toxins are cleared far less efficiently than small solutes under standard diffusion-dominant hemodialysis, and an adequate small-solute Kt/V does not guarantee comparable clearance of either category.

Dialysate sodium is set close to, though usually slightly above, a typical patient's serum sodium to avoid destabilizing osmotic shifts, and sodium profiling trades improved intradialytic hemodynamic stability against a risk of increased interdialytic thirst and fluid gain.

Safe ultrafiltration rate is limited by the patient's individual vascular refilling capacity rather than by the dialyzer membrane's capacity, and large interdialytic weight gain is often better addressed through dietary counseling than through escalating ultrafiltration rate alone.

Bicarbonate-based dialysate corrects metabolic acidosis effectively but can produce a transient central nervous system paradoxical acidosis when correction is too rapid, which is why new, severely uremic patients begin dialysis at reduced treatment intensity with gradual escalation.

CHAPTER 5: DIALYZERS, MEMBRANES, AND WATER TREATMENT SYSTEMS

Learning Objectives

Classify dialyzer membranes by material, flux, and surface area, and relate each characteristic to the clearance mechanisms described in Chapter 4.

Select a dialyzer appropriate to a given patient's prescription and weigh the considerations relevant to reprocessed versus single-use dialyzers.

Describe the components of a hemodialysis water treatment system and the water and dialysate quality standards they are designed to meet.

Recognize the clinical presentations produced by water treatment failure and distinguish them from other causes of intradialytic symptoms.

Interpret the major categories of dialysis machine safety alarms and respond appropriately at the bedside.

Chapter Overview

Chapter 4 established the physical mechanisms of diffusion, convection, and ultrafiltration in the abstract. This chapter turns to the physical equipment that implements those mechanisms: the dialyzer membrane itself, the water treatment system that produces the enormous volume of purified water a dialysis session requires, and the machine safety systems that monitor the treatment throughout. None of these are inert infrastructure; each carries its own failure modes, each is a common source of intradialytic symptoms when something goes wrong, and each is a decision point a clinician managing a dialysis unit needs to understand rather than treat as a fixed background condition outside clinical control. Several of the cases in this chapter share a common structural lesson worth stating at the outset: a failure affecting shared infrastructure — a water system, a reprocessing unit, a formulary decision — tends to present as a cluster of similarly affected patients rather than as an isolated single-patient event, and recognizing that clustering promptly is often the single most useful diagnostic step available to the clinician or charge nurse first encountering it.

Membrane Composition and Flux Classification

Membrane Materials and Biocompatibility

Early dialyzer membranes were manufactured from cellulose, a material derived from cotton linters that, in its unmodified form, activates the complement cascade on contact with blood through hydroxyl groups exposed on the membrane surface, producing a measurable degree of intradialytic leukopenia and a low-grade inflammatory response with each treatment. Modified cellulosic membranes, in which these reactive hydroxyl groups are chemically substituted, reduce this complement activation considerably, and synthetic membranes, manufactured from polymers such as polysulfone, polyethersulfone, and polyacrylonitrile, are generally considered more biocompatible still, activating complement and triggering intradialytic inflammatory markers less than even modified cellulosic membranes.

This biocompatibility distinction, prominent in an earlier era of dialysis membrane research, has narrowed in clinical significance as synthetic membranes have become the dominant material in contemporary practice across most health systems, but it remains relevant when interpreting older literature and when a patient on a legacy cellulosic membrane presents with symptoms suggestive of complement-mediated intradialytic reaction, discussed later in this chapter. Synthetic membranes also tend to have more favorable protein adsorption characteristics, meaning uremic toxins and inflammatory mediators bind to the membrane surface itself in addition to being cleared by diffusion and convection, an adsorptive clearance mechanism distinct from the three mechanisms detailed in Chapter 4 and one that contributes modestly to overall solute removal, particularly for larger inflammatory mediators that clear poorly by diffusion or convection alone.

A further category of specialized membranes incorporates surface modifications intended to reduce the extracorporeal circuit's inherent thrombogenicity, most commonly a heparin-grafted or heparin-coated surface that locally reduces clot formation along the membrane and blood-contact surfaces without requiring the same degree of systemic anticoagulation that an unmodified membrane would need. These membranes are most relevant to the anticoagulation-minimization and anticoagulation-free approaches developed in Chapter 8, where patients with an elevated bleeding risk require a circuit that remains patent through the treatment despite reduced or absent systemic heparin, and membrane surface chemistry becomes one of several tools — alongside citrate-based and saline-flush techniques discussed in that chapter — for maintaining circuit patency under those constraints.

Low-Flux Versus High-Flux Membrane Classification

Membranes are classified as low-flux or high-flux based on their hydraulic permeability and, correspondingly, their pore size and the largest molecules they permit to pass. Low-flux membranes, with smaller, more uniform pores, clear small solutes such as urea effectively through diffusion but restrict middle molecule passage considerably, making them poorly suited to a prescription intended to address the middle molecule burden discussed in Chapter 4. High-flux membranes, with larger pores and correspondingly higher water permeability, permit middle molecule passage sufficient to support the convective and diffusive middle-molecule clearance that modern practice generally favors, and are the membrane category required as a foundation for hemodiafiltration, which layers substantial additional convective clearance on top of a high-flux membrane's baseline permeability.

Because high-flux membranes' greater water permeability also increases the risk of backfiltration — the inadvertent movement of dialysate, and any contaminants it may carry, into the blood compartment under certain pressure conditions — their safe use depends on dialysate meeting a higher microbiological purity standard than would be strictly necessary for a low-flux membrane, a dependency that connects membrane selection directly to the water treatment standards discussed later in this chapter rather than treating the two as unrelated topics.

The transition from low-flux to high-flux membranes as the standard of care in most contemporary practice was driven substantially by accumulating evidence that middle molecule clearance, largely unavailable through low-flux membranes regardless of how flow rates and treatment time are optimized, contributes meaningfully to long-term outcomes including cardiovascular morbidity and the dialysis-related amyloidosis historically associated with prolonged beta-2 microglobulin accumulation in patients treated for many years on low-flux membranes. Low-flux membranes retain a narrower role in contemporary practice, most commonly in settings where water quality cannot reliably meet the higher standard high-flux membranes require, underscoring again that membrane flux selection and water treatment infrastructure are linked decisions rather than independent ones.

Membrane Surface Area and Its Clinical Implications

Membrane surface area, typically ranging across commercially available dialyzers from under one square meter to more than two square meters, is a further determinant of diffusive clearance capacity independent of flux classification, since a larger surface area provides more total membrane area across which diffusion can occur for a given blood and dialysate flow rate. Selecting a larger surface area dialyzer is one lever, alongside blood flow rate, dialysate flow rate, and treatment time, for increasing achieved Kt/V in a patient whose vascular access or treatment time constraints limit how far the other levers can be adjusted, though surface area increases beyond a certain point yield diminishing incremental clearance for the same diminishing-returns reasons described for flow rate in Chapter 4.

Larger surface area dialyzers also carry a larger extracorporeal blood volume, a consideration relevant to smaller-bodied patients and pediatric patients, discussed further in Chapter 26, in whom a disproportionately large extracorporeal circuit volume relative to total blood volume can itself contribute to intradialytic hemodynamic instability independent of the ultrafiltration rate. Dialyzer selection is therefore not simply a matter of maximizing clearance capacity in the abstract, but of matching surface area, along with flux and membrane material, to the specific patient's body size, vascular access characteristics, and clinical tolerance.

Priming volume, the volume of saline or blood required to fill the extracorporeal circuit and dialyzer before treatment begins, scales with membrane surface area and is a related but distinct consideration from total extracorporeal blood volume during treatment, since priming determines how much fluid must be given to the patient during circuit setup, or how much of the patient's own blood volume is transiently committed to the circuit during initiation, both of which carry more clinical weight in smaller patients and in patients whose baseline hemodynamic reserve is already limited. Manufacturers publish priming volume alongside surface area and flux classification for every commercially available dialyzer, and this figure should be reviewed explicitly, not merely assumed to be proportionally negligible, when selecting a dialyzer for a smaller or hemodynamically fragile patient.

Figure 5.1: Dialyzer External Housing and Blood/Dialysate Port Configuration

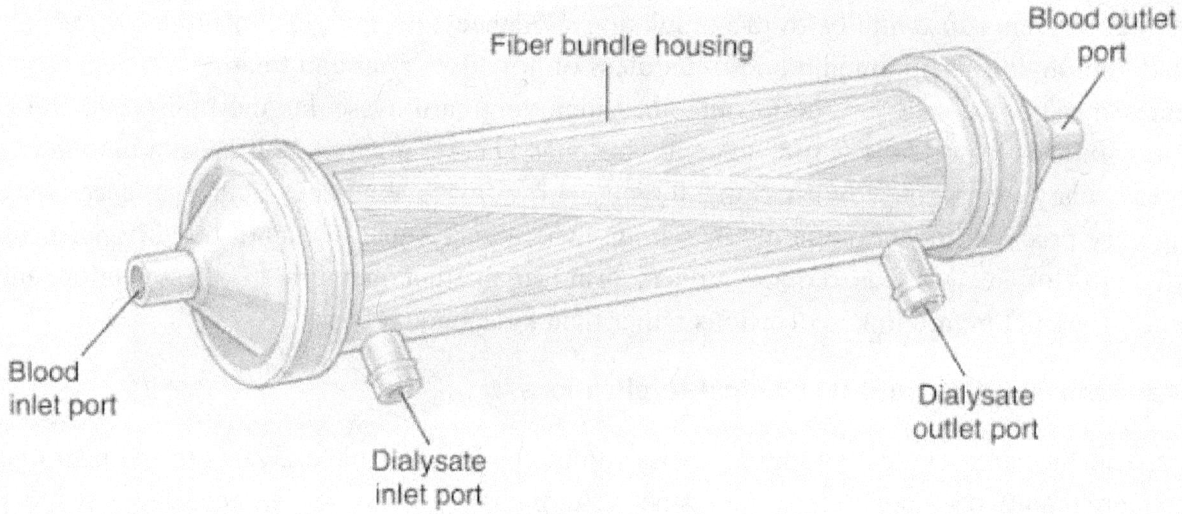

Dialyzer Selection and Reuse Considerations

Matching Dialyzer Characteristics to the Prescription

Dialyzer selection begins from the prescription goals established in Chapter 6 rather than from a default choice applied uniformly across a unit's entire patient population: a patient prescribed hemodiafiltration requires a high-flux membrane with adequate hydraulic permeability to support the convective volume targeted, a patient with a smaller body habitus benefits from a smaller extracorporeal volume dialyzer to limit hemodynamic stress, and a patient with demonstrated sensitivity to a particular membrane material, discussed further below, requires an alternative material regardless of that material's clearance characteristics otherwise being appropriate.

Because these considerations can pull in different directions for a given patient — for example, a larger surface area dialyzer that would improve clearance but also increases extracorporeal volume beyond what a smaller patient tolerates well — dialyzer selection is best treated as an individualized decision revisited whenever a patient's prescription, body size, or tolerance changes materially, rather than a static assignment made once at the start of a patient's dialysis course and left unexamined thereafter.

Individual dialysis units typically maintain a limited formulary of dialyzer models across the flux, surface area, and material categories they stock, rather than an unbounded selection, both for cost and inventory management reasons and because clinical staff become more proficient at recognizing the specific handling characteristics and expected clearance performance of a smaller set of familiar devices than they would with a very large and constantly changing inventory of unfamiliar equipment. This standardization is a reasonable operational compromise provided the formulary spans a range sufficient to cover the clinically meaningful categories described in this chapter — at minimum, a high-flux option suitable for hemodiafiltration and at least two surface area options to accommodate the range of body sizes a unit is likely to treat — rather than being narrowed so far that an individual patient's genuine clinical need cannot be matched within the available formulary.

Single-Use Versus Reprocessed Dialyzers

Dialyzer reuse, in which a single dialyzer is cleaned, disinfected, and used for multiple treatments in the same patient rather than discarded after a single use, was historically motivated primarily by cost considerations and remains practiced in some settings, though its prevalence has declined considerably as single-use dialyzer costs have fallen. Where practiced, reuse follows a defined protocol specifying the maximum number of reuses, the disinfection and sterility testing process between uses, and the performance testing — typically measuring the dialyzer's residual fiber bundle volume or its total cell volume, both of which decline gradually with repeated use and cleaning — used to confirm the dialyzer remains functionally adequate before each subsequent use.

A dialyzer whose measured performance has declined below a defined threshold, most commonly because residual disinfectant, protein deposition on the membrane, or fiber clotting from prior treatments has reduced its effective clearance capacity, must be retired from the reuse protocol rather than continued in service simply because it has not yet reached its maximum permitted reuse count, since the number of prior uses is a proxy for expected performance decline rather than a substitute for directly measuring it. Facilities that practice dialyzer reuse are expected to maintain rigorous, auditable protocols for this testing, since inadequate reprocessing has been directly implicated in outbreaks of bloodstream infection and pyrogenic reaction in settings where protocol adherence lapsed.

A dialysis facility practicing dialyzer reuse experiences a cluster of febrile reactions across several patients over the same week, each occurring within the first hour of treatment and resolving without an identified alternative source of infection on subsequent evaluation. Reviewing the reprocessing records for the implicated dialyzers reveals that a recently installed automated reprocessing unit had been recording disinfectant concentration readings that, on closer audit, fell modestly below the validated effective concentration for a portion of the affected treatment cycles, a discrepancy that had not been caught because the automated system's pass confirmation was being accepted without periodic independent verification of the underlying concentration readings. The facility immediately suspends reuse for all dialyzers processed on the affected unit, reverts to single-use dialyzers while the reprocessing equipment is inspected and recalibrated, and reports the incident through its quality assurance system. This case illustrates a broader principle for any reprocessing or automated safety system in a dialysis unit: an automated pass or fail indicator is only as reliable as the periodic independent verification confirming that the underlying measurement it relies on remains accurate, and audit schedules for this kind of verification deserve the same rigor as the reprocessing protocol itself.

Regulatory oversight of dialyzer reprocessing, where it is practiced, typically requires a designated staff member with specific reprocessing training to oversee the program, written protocols covering cleaning, disinfection, performance testing, and labeling of each reprocessed dialyzer with the specific patient and treatment count it is approved for, and a documented process for immediately removing a dialyzer from service if performance testing at any point fails to meet the defined threshold. Facilities considering whether to adopt or continue a reuse program weigh the cost savings against this additional infrastructure and oversight burden, and the calculation has shifted over recent years as single-use dialyzer costs have declined and the regulatory and staffing burden of maintaining a rigorous reprocessing program has, if anything, increased, contributing to the declining prevalence of reuse in contemporary practice noted earlier in this section, a trend expected to continue as single-use manufacturing costs decline further relative to the fixed staffing and quality-oversight costs a reprocessing program requires regardless of patient volume.

CAUTION: An automated dialyzer reprocessing system's pass indicator should be periodically verified against an independent measurement of disinfectant concentration; a systematic calibration drift can produce a cluster of pyrogenic reactions before the underlying equipment fault is otherwise noticed.

Dialyzer Reactions and Their Prevention

Dialyzer reactions, though uncommon with contemporary synthetic membranes, are traditionally classified into two types with distinct mechanisms and presentations. Type A reactions, an anaphylactoid response typically occurring within the first several minutes of a new treatment, present with dyspnea, urticaria, and, in severe cases, frank anaphylaxis with hypotension, and are most strongly associated with ethylene oxide sterilization residue on the membrane or, less commonly, with an underlying patient sensitivity such as concurrent ACE inhibitor use combined with a negatively charged membrane surface known to activate the kinin system. Type B reactions, milder and more delayed in onset, typically presenting as chest and back discomfort within the first half hour of treatment without the urticaria or severe hypotension of a Type A reaction, are thought to relate to complement activation on membrane contact and are more strongly associated with less biocompatible membrane materials.

Prevention of Type A reactions centers on adequate rinsing of a new dialyzer before use to remove sterilant residue, avoidance of ACE inhibitors in combination with negatively charged membranes in patients with a prior reaction history, and, where a specific sterilization method is implicated, selection of an alternatively sterilized dialyzer for future treatments. Because the timing and clustering of dialyzer reaction symptoms differ meaningfully from the timing of the intradialytic hypotension discussed in Part IV of this book, recognizing this timing pattern is the key discriminating feature that allows a clinician to distinguish a dialyzer reaction from other causes of early intradialytic symptoms rather than treating every early-treatment symptom complex as hypotension by default.

CLINICAL PEARL: A severe reaction within the first few minutes of a new dialyzer's first use, with urticaria and dyspnea, should prompt immediate discontinuation of that treatment and evaluation for a Type A dialyzer reaction rather than empiric treatment for presumed anaphylaxis of unclear source alone.

The Pattern: A patient develops respiratory and cutaneous symptoms within minutes of starting a hemodialysis treatment using a newly opened dialyzer.

Stem Signature: Dyspnea, urticaria, and, in severe cases, hypotension developing within the first five to ten minutes of a treatment using a dialyzer the patient has not previously used, particularly if the patient is concurrently taking an ACE inhibitor.

The Decision: Stop the treatment immediately, do not return the blood in the extracorporeal circuit to the patient if the reaction is severe, treat as an anaphylactoid reaction, and document the specific dialyzer membrane and sterilization method for future avoidance.

Trap Logic: Early intradialytic hypotension from rapid initial fluid shifts can superficially resemble a Type A reaction, but the presence of urticaria and the specific temporal association with a new, previously unused dialyzer point specifically to a dialyzer reaction rather than a hemodynamic cause.

Response Anchor: Severe symptoms within minutes of a new dialyzer's first use, especially with urticaria, are a dialyzer reaction until proven otherwise — stop the treatment and avoid that membrane and sterilization method going forward.

Water Treatment and Dialysate Quality Standards

Water Treatment System Components and Purpose

A single hemodialysis treatment exposes a patient's blood, across the dialyzer membrane, to a volume of dialysate on the order of one hundred twenty liters or more, several orders of magnitude greater than the volume of fluid a patient would ever receive by direct intravenous infusion in the same period, making water purity for dialysate preparation a matter of considerably greater consequence than ordinary tap water safety standards address. A standard water treatment system for hemodialysis typically includes sediment and carbon filtration to remove particulates and chlorine or chloramine, a water softener to remove calcium and magnesium that would otherwise precipitate and damage downstream components, reverse osmosis to remove the great majority of dissolved ions, organic contaminants, and microorganisms, and, in many systems, a final deionization or ultrafiltration polishing step before the purified water is delivered to the dialysis machines themselves.

Each component in this sequence addresses a distinct category of contaminant that, if it reached the dialysate unaddressed, would produce a specific and often severe clinical consequence: inadequate chloramine removal produces oxidative hemolysis, discussed below; inadequate reverse osmosis performance permits aluminum, fluoride, and other trace elements to reach concentrations that, delivered across one hundred twenty liters of dialysate exposure per treatment, become clinically significant even though the same concentration in ordinary drinking water would pose no risk; and inadequate microbiological control permits bacterial endotoxin to accumulate to concentrations capable of producing the pyrogenic reactions discussed in Chapter 14.

Purified water leaving the reverse osmosis and polishing stages is distributed to individual dialysis machines through a loop designed to maintain continuous flow and minimize stagnant segments where bacterial biofilm could otherwise establish and progressively contaminate the system from within; many contemporary systems incorporate an additional ultrafilter immediately upstream of dialysate preparation specifically to remove bacterial endotoxin fragments that could otherwise pass through the rest of the treatment train, providing a final safeguard directly at the point dialysate is produced rather than relying solely on upstream purification. Because biofilm can establish and shed contaminants intermittently rather than producing a constant, easily detected baseline of contamination, routine microbiological monitoring at defined intervals, rather than only when a clinical event prompts investigation, is what allows a developing biofilm problem to be caught before it produces the kind of clinical cluster described in the case below.

Water and Dialysate Quality Standards

Recognized standards bodies, including the Association for the Advancement of Medical Instrumentation and corresponding international standards organizations, publish maximum permissible concentrations for a defined panel of chemical contaminants in water used for hemodialysis, along with microbiological limits for bacterial colony count and endotoxin concentration, distinguishing standard dialysate quality from the more stringent ultrapure dialysate standard required for on-line hemodiafiltration, in which large volumes of dialysate-derived substitution fluid are infused directly into the patient's bloodstream rather than merely bathing the far side of an intact membrane.

Routine water and dialysate testing against these standards, conducted on a defined schedule specified by the applicable regulatory and accreditation framework, is not an optional quality-improvement exercise but a core patient safety requirement, since the consequences of contaminated dialysate are not confined to a single patient the way a medication error typically is, but can affect every patient treated on a contaminated water system on a given day, a pattern illustrated in the case presented later in this section.

Testing responsibility is typically distributed across several parties operating under a documented quality plan: on-site technical staff performing routine chemical and microbiological sampling on a defined schedule, an independent laboratory confirming results periodically to verify the on-site testing's accuracy, and the equipment manufacturer's specifications defining the expected performance of each treatment stage against which observed results are compared. When results from any of these sources fall outside the accepted range, action must follow according to a predefined corrective protocol — typically increased sampling frequency, equipment inspection, and, where the deviation is significant, suspension of treatments on the affected system until the issue is resolved and retesting confirms restored water quality — rather than being noted and left for the next scheduled review cycle.

Consequences of Water Treatment Failure

Chloramine, added to municipal water supplies as a disinfectant and not fully removed by simple carbon filtration if the carbon filter is exhausted or improperly maintained, oxidizes hemoglobin within red blood cells on contact during dialysis, producing an acute hemolytic anemia that presents with fatigue, chest or back pain, and a falling hematocrit disproportionate to any blood loss, typically affecting multiple patients on the same water system simultaneously if the underlying carbon filtration has failed, which is the key feature distinguishing a water treatment failure from an isolated single-patient hemolytic process.

Aluminum contamination, historically associated with encephalopathy and a specific form of adynamic bone disease when reverse osmosis performance was inadequate, is now rare in systems with properly functioning and monitored reverse osmosis, but remains a relevant historical example of how a trace contaminant, delivered across the enormous cumulative dialysate exposure discussed above, can produce toxicity at concentrations that would be inconsequential in any other clinical context. Bacterial endotoxin, even when filtered by an intact dialyzer membrane that itself prevents whole bacteria from crossing into blood, can still provoke a pyrogenic reaction through smaller endotoxin fragments capable of crossing an otherwise intact membrane, particularly with high-flux membranes and the backfiltration risk discussed earlier in this chapter, underscoring why microbiological water quality standards apply even when the membrane itself appears to provide an adequate barrier.

Fluoride contamination, similarly rare in systems with functioning reverse osmosis but historically documented in settings where source water fluoridation levels exceeded what the treatment system was validated to remove, can produce acute symptoms including nausea, cardiac arrhythmia, and hyperkalemia through mechanisms distinct from the hemolysis and encephalopathy associated with chloramine and aluminum respectively, illustrating that different trace contaminants failing to be removed at different stages of the treatment train produce recognizably distinct clinical syndromes rather than a single generic pattern of water treatment failure. This syndrome-specificity is clinically useful: a cluster of patients presenting with a recognizable pattern — hemolysis and anemia, neurologic and bone findings, or cardiac and electrolyte disturbance — can help direct which specific stage of the water treatment system deserves the most urgent inspection, even before a full water quality panel returns.

Because these consequences are severe and disproportionate to the trace concentrations involved, regulatory frameworks in most jurisdictions require documented water treatment maintenance and testing logs to be retained and available for inspection, and require reporting of any water-quality-related adverse event through the facility's patient safety system, a requirement that exists precisely because the case presented in this chapter is not a hypothetical scenario but a recurring, documented failure mode across dialysis facilities historically, one that a rigorous, consistently followed maintenance and testing schedule is specifically designed to prevent.

A dialysis unit's charge nurse notices that three patients scheduled on the same water loop and treated within the same morning shift each report new fatigue, chest tightness, and back pain approximately one hour into treatment, with a repeat hematocrit in the first affected patient showing an acute decline inconsistent with any identified blood loss. Recognizing the temporal clustering across multiple patients on the same water system as the key distinguishing feature from an isolated single-patient hemolytic process, the charge nurse immediately stops all treatments on that water loop, notifies the technical staff to inspect the carbon filtration system, and arranges alternative water access for any patients still requiring treatment that day. Inspection confirms the carbon filter had reached exhaustion beyond its scheduled replacement interval, allowing chloramine to pass into the treated water; the filter is replaced, water quality is retested and confirmed adequate before treatments resume, and the affected patients are monitored and supported with transfusion as clinically indicated, with the incident subsequently reported through the facility's quality and safety system to review the filter replacement scheduling that allowed the exhaustion to occur.

CAUTION: New or worsening symptoms occurring in multiple patients on the same water system within the same shift should prompt immediate suspicion of a water treatment failure and cessation of treatments on that system, rather than management of each patient's symptoms as an isolated, unrelated event.

Figure 5.2: Hemodialysis Water Treatment System Flow Schematic

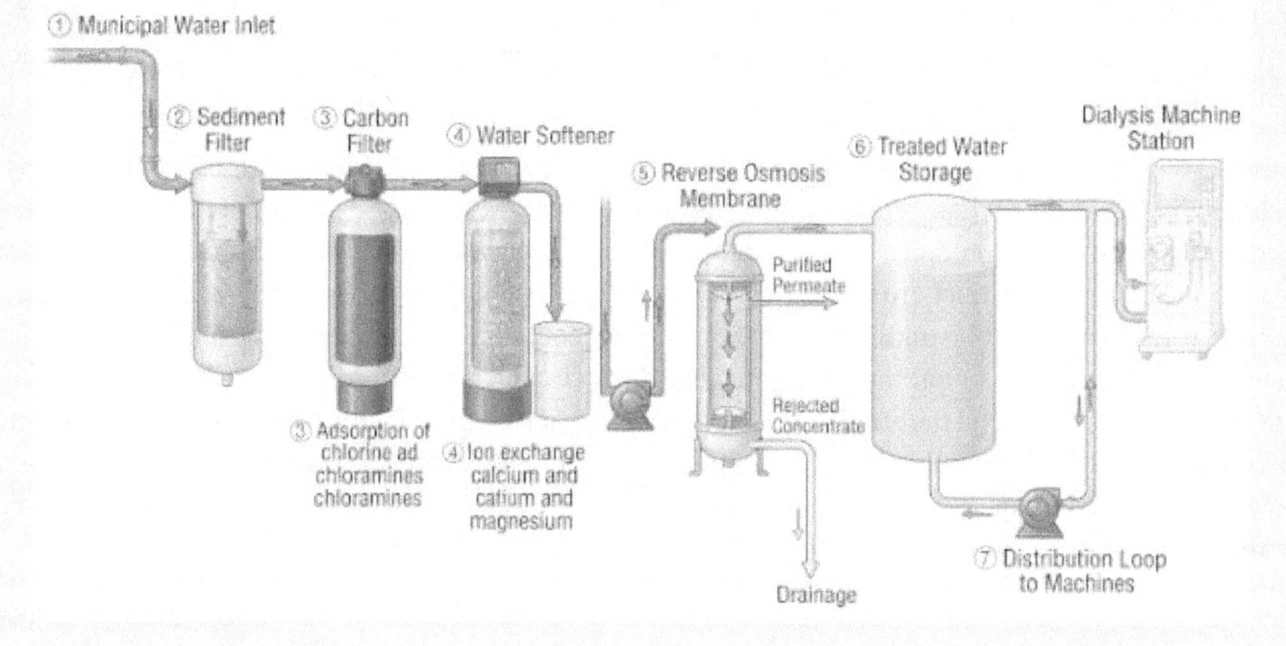

Machine Safety Monitors and Alarms

Air Detection and Venous Line Safety

The air detector positioned on the venous return line is among the most safety-critical monitors on a hemodialysis machine, since air entering the patient's bloodstream in sufficient volume produces the air embolism emergency discussed in Chapter 15, and the detector's function is to identify air in the returning blood line and immediately clamp the venous line while stopping the blood pump, preventing air from reaching the patient before a clinician can even respond manually. Because this detector's proper function depends on correct line positioning and an intact detection sensor, machines perform this check automatically at treatment initiation, and any alarm indicating detector malfunction must be resolved before proceeding rather than bypassed, given the severity of the complication the detector exists specifically to prevent.

Venous line pressure monitoring serves a complementary safety function, since a properly functioning venous needle or catheter maintains a venous pressure within an expected range for the prescribed blood flow rate, and a pressure reading outside that range signals a problem requiring evaluation before the treatment safely continues: a pressure that is too low can indicate needle dislodgement or disconnection, a scenario in which blood loss from the circuit could otherwise proceed unrecognized, while a pressure that is too high can indicate a clot forming in the venous line or a positional problem with the needle or catheter tip against the vessel wall.

Most contemporary air detectors use an ultrasonic sensor that identifies the change in acoustic transmission produced by air bubbles within the blood line, a method sensitive enough to detect even small volumes of microbubbles that would themselves be clinically insignificant but that serve as an early warning that a larger air entrainment event, arising from a loose connection or an emptied line, may be developing. Because this sensitivity means the detector will trigger periodically on clinically trivial microbubble transients during routine treatment, staff response protocol distinguishes a genuine air-in-line event, confirmed by direct visual inspection of the venous line for a visible air column, from a sensor-triggered pause without any visible air present, in which case the line is checked for connection integrity before treatment resumes, rather than treating every air detector alarm identically regardless of what direct inspection actually reveals.

Blood Leak Detection and Conductivity Monitoring

The blood leak detector, positioned in the dialysate outflow line downstream of the dialyzer, identifies blood crossing into the dialysate compartment through a ruptured or damaged membrane fiber, a failure that, left undetected, would result in ongoing blood loss into the dialysate drain, and the detector's alarm triggers automatic cessation of the blood pump and clamping of the blood lines to prevent this loss from continuing. A dialyzer that triggers a blood leak alarm is not reused for that treatment even after the alarm appears to clear, since a membrane that has already ruptured under treatment conditions cannot be relied upon not to rupture further.

Conductivity monitoring continuously verifies that the dialysate produced by the machine's proportioning system matches the prescribed electrolyte concentration, since conductivity correlates closely with total dissolved ion concentration and provides a real-time, continuous check that the machine is mixing concentrate and purified water in the correct ratio; a conductivity reading outside the expected range for the prescribed dialysate composition triggers an alarm and diverts dialysate away from the dialyzer rather than delivering an incorrectly mixed dialysate to the patient, protecting against the electrolyte derangement that an uncorrected proportioning error could otherwise produce.

Blood leak detectors are typically optical, measuring light transmission or scatter through the dialysate outflow stream and detecting the change produced by even small quantities of blood, which is considerably more opaque than clear dialysate. Because a genuine blood leak, once it begins, tends to progress rather than spontaneously resolve as the membrane defect that caused it does not heal during the treatment, the detector's response — immediate blood pump cessation and line clamping — is deliberately conservative, treating any confirmed detection as a stop-and-discard event for that dialyzer rather than attempting to continue treatment at a reduced blood flow rate in the hope that the leak remains small, since there is no reliable way to predict whether a small leak will remain small for the remainder of the treatment.

Responding to Machine Alarms at the Bedside

Because dialysis machine alarms are frequent during routine treatment and the great majority reflect minor, easily corrected issues such as patient movement affecting venous pressure or a kinked line rather than a genuine safety event, effective bedside response depends on rapidly distinguishing alarms that require only a simple mechanical correction from the smaller subset that indicate a genuine safety concern requiring the treatment to be paused or stopped outright. Staff training that emphasizes this triage — checking line position and patient movement first for pressure alarms, verifying air detector and blood leak alarms are addressed according to their specific protocol rather than silenced without evaluation — keeps alarm response efficient without becoming complacent about the alarms that matter most.

Alarm fatigue, the phenomenon by which staff exposed to frequent, mostly benign alarms become desensitized and respond more slowly or less carefully to all alarms including the rare genuinely dangerous ones, is a recognized patient safety concern in hemodialysis units treating many patients simultaneously, and is best addressed through appropriately configured alarm thresholds that minimize nuisance alarms without disabling genuinely protective ones, rather than through staff vigilance alone, which predictably degrades under a high volume of low-value alarms regardless of individual staff conscientiousness.

Units that have measurably reduced alarm fatigue typically do so through a combination of periodic review of alarm log data to identify and adjust threshold settings responsible for the highest volume of nuisance alarms, staff education specifically distinguishing which alarm categories are safety-critical and non-negotiable from which are more often benign and correctable, and physical unit design that supports rapid visual and auditory identification of which specific machine, among several running simultaneously in a shared treatment area, is generating a given alarm. This last consideration matters more than it might initially appear: in a busy unit with many machines running concurrently, the time a staff member spends identifying which machine is alarming before they can even begin to assess the alarm itself is time during which a genuinely urgent event, however rare, continues unaddressed.

New staff orientation in a well-run hemodialysis unit typically includes structured, hands-on training specifically on alarm response, distinct from general dialysis technique training, precisely because the triage judgment described throughout this section — distinguishing a benign, easily corrected alarm from one signaling a genuine safety event — is a skill that develops with deliberate practice and exposure rather than one that can be fully conveyed through a written protocol alone. Simulation-based training, in which trainees practice responding to a range of alarm scenarios including the rare but critical ones they may otherwise not encounter for months or years in routine practice, has been adopted in a growing number of units specifically to accelerate this skill development and to ensure that a new staff member's first encounter with a genuine air-in-line or blood leak event is not also their first time reasoning through the appropriate response under real time pressure.

KEY POINT: Air detector and blood leak alarms are never bypassed or silenced without direct evaluation of their cause; venous and arterial pressure alarms are more often benign but still require a specific check of line position and patency before being cleared.

DIALYSIS RECOGNITION & RESPONSE SYSTEM — Equipment and Water Quality Arcs

The Pattern: Multiple patients treated on the same water system develop new, similar symptoms within the same treatment shift.

Stem Signature: Fatigue, chest or back discomfort, or an unexplained falling hematocrit arising in more than one patient scheduled on the same water loop within the same shift, without an identified source of blood loss in any individual patient.

The Decision: Stop treatments on the implicated water system immediately, notify technical staff to inspect water treatment components — chloramine removal and reverse osmosis performance in particular — and arrange alternative water access before resuming any further treatments on that system.

Trap Logic: An isolated case can resemble a single patient's unrelated hemolytic or cardiopulmonary process; the clustering across multiple patients on the same water system within the same shift is the specific feature that should trigger suspicion of a shared water treatment failure rather than several unrelated individual events.

Response Anchor: Similar new symptoms in multiple patients on the same water system within one shift is a water treatment failure until inspection proves otherwise — stop treatments on that system immediately rather than managing each patient in isolation.

DIALYSIS RECOGNITION & RESPONSE SYSTEM — Equipment and Water Quality Arcs

The Pattern: A venous pressure alarm triggers during an otherwise unremarkable treatment.

Stem Signature: A venous pressure reading outside the expected range for the prescribed blood flow rate, without any accompanying air detection alarm or blood leak alarm, occurring either as an isolated event or with a gradually rising trend over the preceding portion of the treatment.

The Decision: Check needle or catheter position and line patency directly rather than simply resetting the alarm; a low pressure warrants checking for dislodgement or disconnection, while a rising or high pressure warrants checking for clot formation in the line or a positional problem with the access itself.

Trap Logic: A venous pressure alarm can be reflexively treated as a nuisance alarm requiring only a reset, given how frequently pressure alarms occur from simple patient movement; a gradually rising trend across a treatment, rather than a single isolated spike, is the feature that should prompt a more thorough patency check rather than a quick reset and continuation.

Response Anchor: A rising venous pressure trend, as opposed to a single isolated spike, warrants a direct patency check of the access and line — not simply an alarm reset.

Reaction to a New Dialyzer: Severe symptoms with urticaria within minutes of a new dialyzer's first use are a Type A reaction until proven otherwise — stop the treatment and avoid that membrane and sterilization method going forward.

Clustered Symptoms Across Patients on One Water System: Similar new symptoms in multiple patients on the same water system within one shift signal a water treatment failure — stop treatments on that system and inspect immediately.

A Rising Venous Pressure Trend: A gradually rising venous pressure across a treatment, as distinct from a single isolated spike, warrants a direct patency check of the access and line rather than a simple alarm reset.

Summary and Key Concepts

Synthetic membranes are generally more biocompatible than cellulosic membranes, and flux classification, driven by pore size, determines middle molecule passage independent of the diffusive small-solute clearance discussed in Chapter 4.

Dialyzer selection should match membrane material, flux, and surface area to an individual patient's prescription, body size, and tolerance rather than defaulting to a single unit-wide standard, and reprocessed dialyzers require rigorous, auditable performance testing before each reuse.

Type A dialyzer reactions are anaphylactoid and occur within minutes of a new dialyzer's first use; Type B reactions are milder, complement-mediated, and occur somewhat later in treatment.

Water treatment removes distinct categories of contaminants at each stage, and failure at any stage — chloramine, trace elements, or microbiological contamination — produces a characteristic clinical syndrome, often affecting multiple patients on the same water system simultaneously.

Air detector and blood leak alarms represent safety-critical monitors that are never bypassed without direct evaluation, while pressure alarms are more often benign but still warrant a specific check before being cleared.

CHAPTER 6: THE HEMODIALYSIS PRESCRIPTION: WRITING AND ADJUSTING ORDERS

Learning Objectives

List the core components of a complete hemodialysis prescription and explain the clinical rationale behind each.

Individualize dialysate potassium, calcium, bicarbonate, and temperature to a specific patient's clinical status rather than applying a single unit-wide standard.

Reason through the relationship between treatment time, frequency, and ultrafiltration rate when a fixed thrice-weekly schedule proves inadequate for a given patient.

Recognize the clinical signals that warrant a prescription adjustment and sequence multiple simultaneous changes safely.

Document and communicate prescription changes in a way that keeps the entire treating team, across shifts and covering clinicians, working from the same current order.

Chapter Overview

The physiologic mechanisms established in Chapter 4 and the equipment described in Chapter 5 come together in this chapter as a single, concrete artifact: the written hemodialysis prescription, the order set that translates clearance physiology and available technology into a specific, individualized instruction set for a specific patient's specific treatment. A prescription is not a one-time document completed at dialysis initiation and left unchanged; it is a living instruction that requires deliberate construction at the outset and active, reasoned revision as a patient's clinical status evolves, and this chapter addresses both the initial construction and the ongoing revision in turn. Several of the cases and recognition patterns developed throughout this chapter share a common thread worth naming explicitly at the outset: prescription problems frequently masquerade as something else — an adequacy shortfall that looks like it needs more blood flow rather than a recirculation check, a hypotension pattern that looks like it needs sodium profiling rather than a dry weight update, a hyperkalemia pattern that looks like a dietary counseling problem rather than a dialysate concentration review — and the discipline this chapter aims to build is the habit of checking the prescription itself, systematically, before assuming the explanation lies elsewhere.

Components of a Complete Hemodialysis Order

The Core Elements of a Hemodialysis Prescription

A complete hemodialysis prescription specifies, at minimum, the dialyzer to be used, drawing on the membrane and surface area considerations from Chapter 5; the blood and dialysate flow rates; the treatment duration and weekly frequency; the dialysate composition across potassium, calcium, bicarbonate, sodium, and, where relevant, glucose and temperature; the anticoagulation approach, detailed further in Chapter 8; and the ultrafiltration goal for the treatment, derived from the patient's current weight relative to their established dry weight. Omitting any one of these elements from a written order leaves a decision to be made informally at the bedside by whichever staff member happens to be setting up the treatment, introducing variability that a complete, specific prescription is designed to prevent.

Because several of these elements interact with one another in ways already developed in Chapters 4 and 5 — blood flow rate and dialyzer surface area jointly determining achievable clearance, dialysate composition and membrane flux jointly determining safe operating parameters — a prescription is best reviewed as an integrated whole rather than as a checklist of independent line items each considered in isolation. A change to one element, such as switching to a larger surface area dialyzer to improve clearance, may have downstream implications for another, such as increased extracorporeal volume affecting hemodynamic tolerance, that a piecemeal, line-by-line review would risk overlooking, and this integrated view is best supported by a prescription note format that groups related elements together rather than listing every parameter as an undifferentiated flat list in the order a template happens to present them.

The prescription's clinical target, most commonly a defined Kt/V or urea reduction ratio threshold discussed in full in Chapter 7, should also be stated explicitly alongside the specific parameters chosen to achieve it, since documenting the target alongside the means of achieving it allows a covering clinician encountering an unfamiliar patient's chart to understand not only what the current prescription is but why it was set that way, supporting more informed adjustment if the patient's status changes before the original prescribing clinician is available to weigh in.

A useful discipline when writing a new hemodialysis prescription is to state, in the same note as the prescription itself, the specific clinical reasoning connecting each chosen parameter to this particular patient's circumstances, rather than recording only the final numbers with no accompanying rationale. A blood flow rate of a given value chosen because it is the maximum a specific vascular access can safely sustain carries different implications for future adjustment than the same blood flow rate chosen simply because it matches the unit's typical default, and only the first framing tells a future clinician whether increasing that blood flow rate later is a reasonable option to consider or one already ruled out by an access limitation that may not otherwise be immediately apparent from the numeric order alone.

This same principle extends to how a prescription is reviewed over time: a periodic prescription audit, ideally conducted at defined intervals rather than only when a problem prompts it, checking each element against the patient's current clinical status rather than assuming continuity from the original order, catches the kind of drift between a patient's actual circumstances and their written prescription that accumulates gradually and is easy to miss in the absence of a structured review, echoing the same scheduled-reassessment principle introduced for the Life-Plan in Chapter 2, for goals of care in Chapter 3, and for dry weight in Chapter 4.

Vascular Access and Anticoagulation Orders Within the Prescription

The prescription should specify the vascular access to be used and any access-specific instructions — cannulation technique for a fistula or graft, or lock solution and dwell instructions for a catheter, both developed further in Part III of this book — rather than leaving access management to default unit practice, since access-specific complications and preferences, once identified for a given patient, need to travel with the prescription rather than being separately tracked and potentially missed by staff unfamiliar with that patient's specific access history.

Anticoagulation orders, whether a standard heparin protocol, a reduced or citrate-based regimen for a patient with elevated bleeding risk, or an anticoagulant-free approach using periodic saline flushes, are detailed in full in Chapter 8, but their presence as an explicit, individualized component of the prescription bears mentioning here and now: a default heparin order applied without confirming it is appropriate for a given patient's current bleeding risk is among the more common and consequential prescription oversights, particularly in a patient recently started on a new anticoagulant or antiplatelet medication, or recovering from a recent procedure, whose bleeding risk may have changed since the standing anticoagulation order was last reviewed.

Because vascular access type and anticoagulation strategy interact — a central venous catheter, for example, generally requiring a lock solution between treatments that a fistula or graft does not, and a patient with recurrent access clotting potentially benefiting from a more aggressive intradialytic anticoagulation approach than a patient with excellent access flow and no clotting history — reviewing these two prescription elements together, rather than as separately maintained order sets that happen to apply to the same patient, reduces the risk of an internally inconsistent prescription, such as an anticoagulation regimen appropriate for a well-functioning fistula being left unchanged after a patient transitions to a catheter with different clotting risk characteristics.

Standing Orders Versus Individualized Prescriptions

Many dialysis units operate with a standing order template covering the majority of routine prescription elements, into which patient-specific values are entered, an approach that improves efficiency and reduces the risk of omitting a required element entirely, provided the template is treated as a starting structure to be individualized rather than a default to be accepted unmodified for every patient. A standing template's greatest risk is not that it specifies wrong values, but that its convenience discourages the active, patient-specific reconsideration that a genuinely individualized prescription requires, particularly for the dialysate composition elements discussed in the next section, where a default value appropriate for a typical patient may be actively inappropriate for a patient with an atypical potassium, calcium, or bicarbonate trajectory.

Distinguishing which prescription elements are reasonably standardized across most patients — dialysate glucose concentration and typical blood flow ranges, for instance, vary less patient to patient than potassium or ultrafiltration parameters do — from which elements require deliberate individualization for each specific patient allows a unit to use standing templates efficiently without allowing that efficiency to substitute for the individualized clinical judgment the higher-stakes elements require, and this distinction is itself worth documenting explicitly in a unit's own standing order policy.

A dialysis unit transitioning to a new electronic order-entry system adopts a standard template prescription, including a fixed default dialysate potassium concentration intended for a typical patient, applied automatically to every new patient entered into the system unless a clinician actively overrides it. Several weeks after the transition, a review of predialysis potassium values across the unit's patient panel identifies a small cluster of patients running unexpectedly low predialysis potassium, several of whom report new symptoms of fatigue and, in one case, a documented arrhythmia during a recent treatment. Investigation reveals that these patients had a lower dialysate potassium individually appropriate under the unit's prior paper-based ordering system, a prior individualization that was not carried forward when the new system's default template was applied during the transition, silently reverting these patients to the standard default value rather than preserving their previously established individualized order. The unit's medical director implements a mandatory reconciliation review, cross-checking every patient's new electronic prescription against their prior individualized orders before the transition is considered complete, and identifies and corrects several additional silent reversions beyond the ones initially discovered through the potassium review. This case illustrates a hazard specific to standing templates and system transitions: an individualized prescription element, once established for good clinical reason, can be silently lost during a template update or system change unless a deliberate reconciliation step is built into that transition specifically to catch it.

CAUTION: Any transition to a new order-entry system or standing template carries a risk of silently reverting previously individualized prescription elements to a new default; a deliberate reconciliation review comparing prior individualized orders against the new system is required before considering such a transition complete.

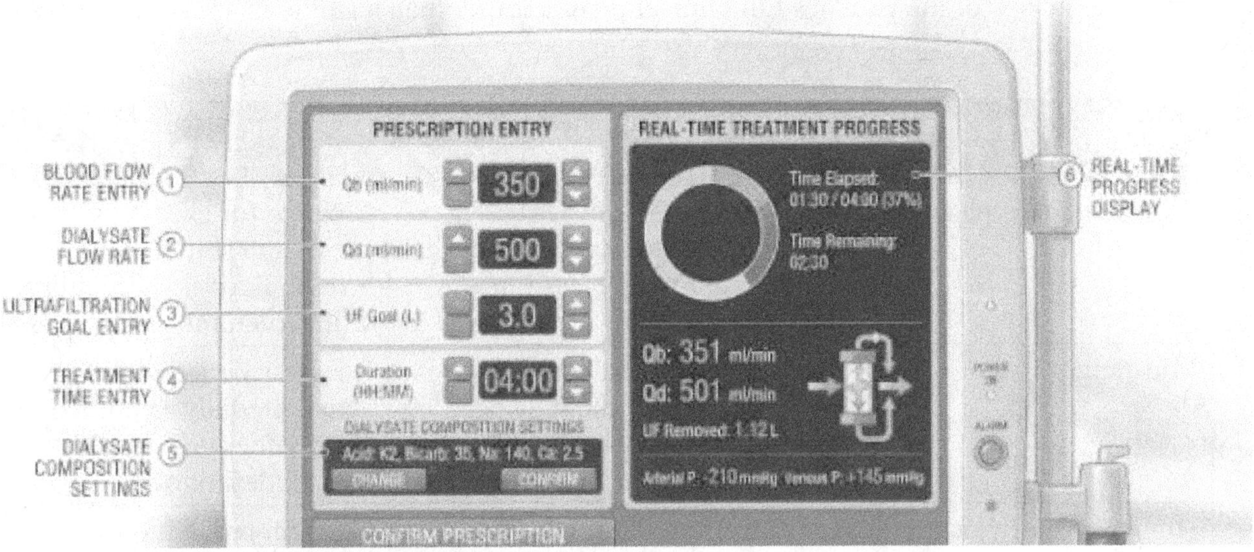

Dialysate Composition and Individualization

Potassium Individualization in the Dialysate

Dialysate potassium concentration is set below the patient's own plasma potassium to drive diffusive potassium removal, but the specific concentration chosen requires deliberate individualization rather than a single default applied to every patient: a patient with a chronically elevated predialysis potassium from dietary intake or medication effects, such as an ACE inhibitor or angiotensin receptor blocker, may require a lower dialysate potassium to achieve adequate removal within a standard treatment, while a patient prone to hypokalemia between treatments, or one with a history of intradialytic arrhythmia, may require a higher dialysate potassium to avoid removing potassium too rapidly or too completely.

Rapid potassium removal carries its own arrhythmia risk independent of the direction of the shift, because the rate of extracellular-to-intracellular potassium redistribution during treatment, not only the absolute predialysis-to-postdialysis potassium change, influences cardiac membrane stability, and this is part of why a very low dialysate potassium is not simply the safest default choice for every hyperkalemic patient regardless of how rapidly it removes potassium; the goal is a potassium trajectory that corrects hyperkalemia over the course of treatment without producing a rate of intracellular shift steep enough to itself destabilize cardiac conduction, particularly in patients with structural heart disease or a history of arrhythmia.

Concurrent digoxin therapy deserves particular attention when individualizing dialysate potassium, since digoxin toxicity risk rises as serum potassium falls, meaning a dialysate potassium concentration that would otherwise be reasonable for a given predialysis potassium level may need to be set modestly higher in a patient on digoxin specifically to avoid precipitating toxicity as potassium declines over the course of treatment. This interaction is easy to overlook when dialysate potassium is selected using predialysis potassium alone as the deciding factor, without cross-referencing the patient's concurrent medication list for an interaction of this kind, reinforcing the broader point that dialysate composition decisions benefit from a holistic review of the patient's full clinical picture rather than a single laboratory value considered in isolation.

Dialysate Potassium Concentration	Typical Clinical Scenario	Key Consideration
Lower end of typical range	Chronically elevated predialysis potassium; large interdialytic potassium accumulation	Monitor for excessively rapid potassium shift and arrhythmia risk, particularly with structural heart disease
Mid-range	Typical predialysis potassium without a specific indication for adjustment	Reassess periodically against actual predialysis potassium trend rather than leaving fixed indefinitely
Higher end of typical range	Recurrent interdialytic hypokalemia; history of intradialytic arrhythmia; concurrent digoxin therapy	Confirm predialysis potassium does not run persistently elevated before selecting a higher concentration

Calcium and Bicarbonate Individualization

Dialysate calcium concentration influences both intradialytic hemodynamic stability, since ionized calcium supports vascular tone and myocardial contractility, and longer-term mineral and bone disorder management detailed in Chapter 23, creating a tension that requires individualized resolution rather than a single default: a higher dialysate calcium supports intradialytic blood pressure but risks contributing to positive calcium balance and vascular calcification over time in a patient already receiving calcium-based phosphate binders or active vitamin D therapy, while a lower dialysate calcium reduces that long-term calcium load but may worsen intradialytic hypotension in a hemodynamically fragile patient.

Bicarbonate individualization, introduced in Chapter 4's discussion of acid-base correction, follows a similar logic of balancing competing considerations: a patient with severe predialysis acidosis benefits from adequate bicarbonate correction to avoid the undercorrection that would leave symptomatic acidosis persisting between treatments, while a patient prone to post-dialysis alkalosis, discussed in Chapter 4, requires a more conservative bicarbonate prescription to avoid overshooting into the alkalosis-related symptoms — including the muscle cramps discussed in Chapter 14 — that excessive correction can produce.

Because calcium and bicarbonate individualization each depend on the same predialysis laboratory trend data used to individualize potassium, reviewing all three parameters together at the same scheduled interval, rather than adjusting one in isolation while leaving the others unreviewed, produces a more internally consistent dialysate prescription overall. A patient whose calcium is adjusted upward for hemodynamic reasons without corresponding attention to their concurrent phosphate binder and vitamin D therapy, discussed in Chapter 23, risks an aggregate calcium exposure across all three sources that no single element considered on its own would have revealed, underscoring why dialysate composition review benefits from a holistic rather than parameter-by-parameter approach.

Dialysate Temperature and Its Hemodynamic Effects

Dialysate temperature, often left at a standard default setting without active consideration, has a measurable effect on intradialytic hemodynamic stability: cooler dialysate, typically set modestly below core body temperature rather than at standard room or body temperature, promotes peripheral vasoconstriction that helps maintain blood pressure during ultrafiltration, and several controlled comparisons have found reduced intradialytic hypotension frequency with cooler dialysate temperature compared to standard settings, particularly in patients with recurrent hemodynamic instability despite otherwise optimized ultrafiltration and sodium prescriptions.

The trade-off with cooler dialysate is reduced patient comfort, since many patients experience the cooler temperature as unpleasant chilliness during treatment, and this comfort cost means cooler dialysate temperature is best reserved for patients with a demonstrated hemodynamic indication rather than applied as a universal default, weighing the physiologic benefit against the patient-reported comfort burden on an individualized basis in the same manner as the other dialysate composition decisions addressed in this section.

Glucose Concentration and Special Dialysate Considerations

Dialysate glucose concentration, typically maintained at a level close to normal fasting plasma glucose rather than at zero, prevents the intradialytic hypoglycemia that would otherwise result from glucose diffusing out of the blood down a concentration gradient into glucose-free dialysate, a particular concern in patients with diabetes on insulin or secretagogue therapy whose glucose regulation is already less robust than a non-diabetic patient's. A dialysate glucose concentration set too low for a given patient's typical intradialytic glucose trend can produce recurrent intradialytic hypoglycemia that is easily misattributed to insulin dosing alone rather than to the dialysate glucose concentration itself, particularly when the hypoglycemia recurs at a consistent point in treatment across multiple sessions.

Beyond glucose, several less commonly adjusted dialysate parameters deserve mention as part of a complete, individualized prescription: dialysate magnesium, generally left at a standard concentration but occasionally adjusted in a patient with a specific magnesium disturbance; and phosphate, which is not typically added to dialysate but can be in the specific circumstance of a patient with severe hypophosphatemia on intensive or frequent hemodialysis regimens, discussed further in Chapter 20, where the cumulative phosphate removal from more frequent treatment can outpace a patient's oral phosphate intake and produce clinically significant hypophosphatemia requiring active correction through the dialysate itself rather than oral supplementation alone.

Each of these less commonly adjusted parameters shares a common practical lesson with the more frequently individualized elements discussed earlier in this section: the default setting appropriate for the great majority of patients should not be assumed to remain appropriate for every patient without exception, and a clinician managing a patient whose clinical trajectory diverges from the typical case — an intensive home hemodialysis regimen, an unusual electrolyte disturbance, a rare drug interaction — should actively reconsider even the dialysate parameters that are rarely adjusted in routine practice, rather than assuming that because a parameter is rarely individualized it is therefore never worth individualizing.

KEY POINT: Dialysate potassium, calcium, bicarbonate, and temperature each involve a genuine clinical trade-off rather than a single universally correct setting; each should be individualized to the specific patient's risk profile and reassessed as that profile changes.

DIALYSIS RECOGNITION & RESPONSE SYSTEM — Prescription Adjustment Arcs

The Pattern: A patient on a standard dialysate potassium prescription is found to have a persistently elevated predialysis potassium despite reported dietary adherence.

Stem Signature: Predialysis potassium consistently above target on serial monthly labs, in a patient reporting adherence to dietary potassium restriction, with no recent medication change and no evidence of missed treatments.

The Decision: Reassess dialysate potassium prescription and the interdialytic interval and treatment time rather than assuming dietary nonadherence by default; consider a lower dialysate potassium concentration, evaluate whether treatment time or frequency is adequate for this patient's potassium generation rate, and reserve dietary counseling escalation for after the prescription itself has been optimized.

Trap Logic: Persistently elevated predialysis potassium is frequently attributed reflexively to dietary nonadherence; an inadequately individualized dialysate potassium prescription or an insufficient treatment time relative to the patient's potassium generation rate can produce an identical laboratory pattern and is more directly correctable.

Response Anchor: Review the dialysate potassium prescription and treatment adequacy before attributing persistent hyperkalemia to dietary nonadherence.

Treatment Time, Frequency, and Ultrafiltration Rate

The Relationship Between Treatment Time and Adequacy

Treatment time interacts with blood flow rate, dialysate flow rate, and dialyzer surface area to determine total achieved small-solute clearance, but it also independently determines the ultrafiltration rate required to remove a given interdialytic fluid gain, since ultrafiltration rate is simply the total volume to be removed divided by the treatment duration. This dual role means treatment time cannot be optimized for clearance alone without also considering its effect on ultrafiltration rate, and a treatment shortened to improve efficiency or patient convenience, without a corresponding reduction in interdialytic weight gain, forces a higher ultrafiltration rate that risks the hemodynamic instability discussed in Chapter 4 and developed further in Part IV of this book.

Extending treatment time, whether through a longer conventional in-center session or through the extended and nocturnal home regimens detailed in Chapter 20, addresses both sides of this relationship simultaneously: it increases the time available for diffusive clearance and reduces the ultrafiltration rate required to remove the same total fluid volume, which is part of why extended-time regimens are associated with improved hemodynamic tolerance and blood pressure control independent of any change in the total weekly clearance delivered.

This dual benefit of extended treatment time is easy to underappreciate when clearance and fluid removal are considered as separate prescription problems rather than as two outcomes of the same single variable; a clinician focused solely on achieving a target Kt/V might conclude that a shorter, more efficient treatment using a larger dialyzer and higher blood flow rate is preferable to a longer treatment achieving the same Kt/V, without recognizing that the shorter treatment, by compressing the same fluid removal into less time, has traded improved clearance efficiency for a higher ultrafiltration rate and its associated hemodynamic cost. Evaluating a proposed treatment time change against both its effect on clearance and its effect on ultrafiltration rate, rather than either dimension in isolation, avoids this incomplete evaluation.

Standard Thrice-Weekly Scheduling and Its Limitations

The conventional thrice-weekly schedule, typically arranged with a two-day gap on one side of the week and a three-day gap on the other, produces an inherently uneven interdialytic interval that concentrates fluid and solute accumulation disproportionately before the longer gap, a pattern reflected in the well-documented increase in cardiovascular events observed in the period following the longer interdialytic interval across large registry studies. This unevenness is a structural feature of the standard schedule itself rather than a failure of any individual patient's adherence, and it is part of the rationale, developed further in Chapter 20, for considering more frequent schedules in patients who experience recurrent complications clustering around the long interdialytic gap specifically, rather than assuming that any given patient's pattern of weekend complications simply reflects worse dietary or fluid adherence over the weekend itself.

Recognizing this pattern in an individual patient — recurrent volume overload, hypertension, or arrhythmia concentrated specifically around the Monday or Tuesday treatment following the long weekend gap, rather than distributed evenly across the week — is itself a diagnostic signal pointing toward the interdialytic interval structure as a contributing factor, distinct from and complementary to the dry weight and dialysate individualization considerations discussed elsewhere in this chapter, and one that an increased treatment frequency, rather than further adjustment of dry weight or dialysate composition alone, may be better positioned to address.

Before concluding that increased frequency is warranted, it is worth confirming that the pattern is genuinely tied to the interdialytic interval structure rather than to an unrelated coincidence of timing, such as a medication taken on a schedule that happens to align with the long-gap treatment, or a dietary pattern specific to weekend eating that a patient may not spontaneously volunteer unless asked directly.

Reviewing several consecutive weeks of the pattern, rather than concluding from a single occurrence, and asking the patient directly about weekend dietary and medication patterns, helps distinguish a genuine interdialytic-interval effect from a coincidental confound that a change in treatment frequency would not actually resolve.

Access Recirculation and Its Effect on Effective Clearance

Vascular access recirculation, in which a portion of blood already returned to the patient through the venous needle is drawn back into the circuit through the arterial needle before it has circulated through the rest of the body, reduces the effective concentration gradient available for diffusive clearance and can produce a substantial gap between the blood flow rate set on the machine and the clearance actually achieved, a gap that is not visible from the machine's flow rate display alone and requires either a dedicated recirculation measurement or a high index of suspicion based on the clinical pattern described below.

Recirculation most commonly arises from needle placement too close together on a fistula or graft, from a significant access stenosis upstream of the arterial needle limiting the flow available to be drawn without pulling from the already-returned venous stream, or from reversed needle placement in which the arterial needle is inadvertently positioned downstream of the venous needle rather than upstream of it. A patient whose measured Kt/V or urea reduction ratio, discussed in full in Chapter 7, falls persistently short of target despite an apparently adequate prescribed blood flow rate and treatment time should prompt consideration of recirculation as a specific, correctable explanation, distinct from simply escalating blood flow rate or treatment time further in response to an adequacy shortfall whose actual cause has not yet been identified.

Calculating and Constraining the Ultrafiltration Rate

Ultrafiltration rate, expressed per unit of body weight, is calculated directly from the total fluid to be removed — current weight minus dry weight — divided by treatment time, and several clinical guidelines and registry analyses have identified a maximum ultrafiltration rate threshold above which intradialytic hypotension, cardiovascular events, and mortality risk rise disproportionately, providing a practical ceiling that should inform prescription decisions rather than treating fluid removal as unconstrained by time so long as the total volume is eventually achieved.

When the fluid volume needed to reach dry weight would require an ultrafiltration rate above this threshold within the scheduled treatment time, the appropriate response is to extend treatment time, add an additional treatment during the week, or, most fundamentally, to address the excessive interdialytic weight gain directly through dietary and fluid counseling, rather than accepting an elevated ultrafiltration rate as an unavoidable consequence of the fixed schedule. Treating an elevated ultrafiltration rate as simply the number required to reach dry weight within the time available, without considering these alternatives, is a common and correctable prescription oversight.

The Pattern: A patient's measured dialysis adequacy falls persistently short of target despite an apparently adequate prescribed blood flow rate and treatment time.

Stem Signature: A Kt/V or urea reduction ratio below target on repeated measurement, in a patient whose prescribed blood flow rate, dialysate flow rate, and treatment time appear more than sufficient to achieve the target on paper, without an obvious alternative explanation such as missed treatments.

The Decision: Evaluate specifically for vascular access recirculation — checking needle placement and spacing, and assessing for access stenosis — rather than responding to the adequacy shortfall by further increasing blood flow rate or treatment time, which will not correct a clearance gap caused by recirculation and may worsen it if the underlying cause is a stenosis limiting available flow.

Trap Logic: An adequacy shortfall despite an apparently sufficient prescription is easily met with an instinctive response of increasing blood flow rate or treatment time further; when recirculation is the actual cause, this response does not address the problem and can escalate access strain without improving measured clearance.

Response Anchor: An unexplained adequacy shortfall despite a seemingly sufficient prescription warrants a specific recirculation evaluation before escalating flow rate or treatment time further.

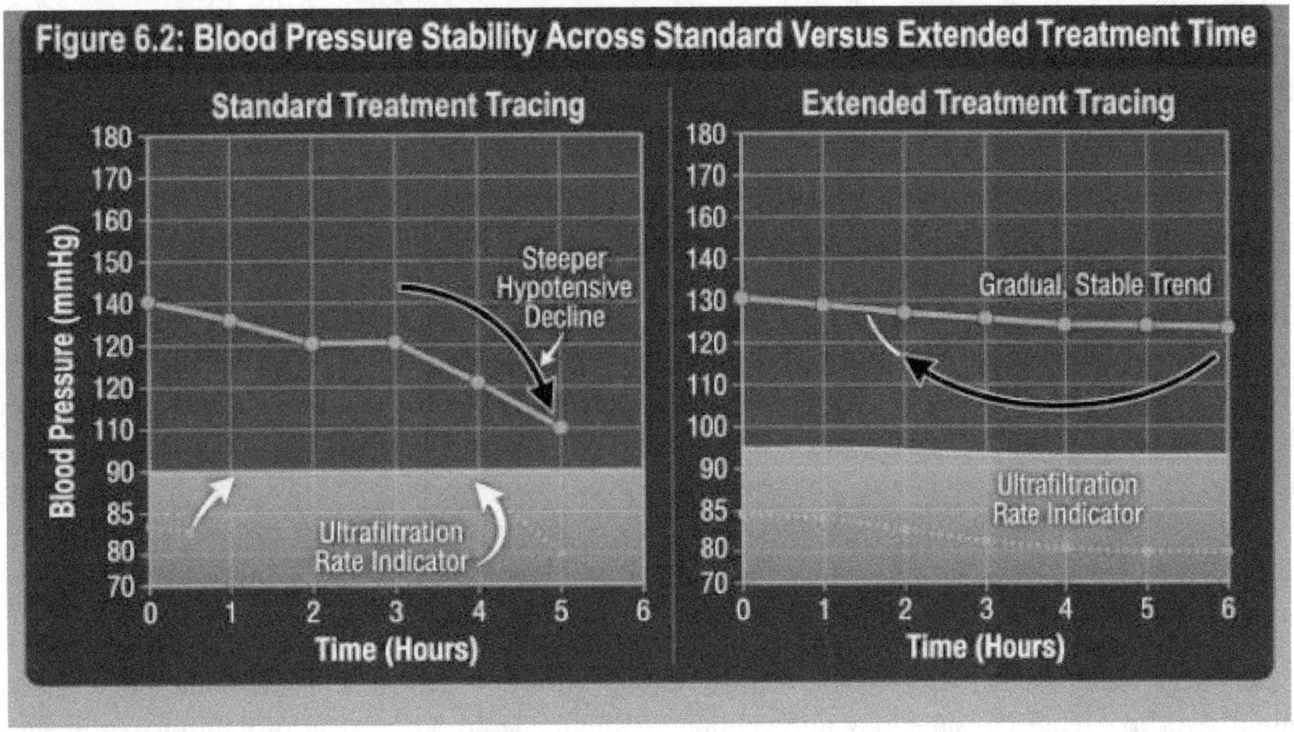

Figure 6.2: Blood Pressure Stability Across Standard Versus Extended Treatment Time

Adjusting the Prescription for Changing Clinical Status

Recognizing When the Prescription Needs Adjustment

A prescription that was appropriate at initiation does not remain appropriate indefinitely, and several recurring signals should prompt active reconsideration rather than continuation of the existing prescription by default: recurrent intradialytic hypotension or hypertension, laboratory values persistently outside target range despite reported adherence, a change in vascular access affecting achievable blood flow, a significant change in body weight or nutritional status affecting dry weight and dialyzer sizing, or a new comorbid diagnosis, such as heart failure, that changes the patient's fluid tolerance.

Because these signals often develop gradually rather than presenting as an acute crisis, they are more reliably caught through scheduled, periodic prescription review — reasonably timed monthly alongside routine laboratory monitoring — than through reactive adjustment only once a signal has become severe enough to prompt an unplanned visit or hospitalization, echoing the same proactive-review principle developed for the Life-Plan in Chapter 2 and for goals of care in Chapter 3.

A structured monthly review checklist, covering each of the prescription elements discussed throughout this chapter alongside the most recent laboratory panel and any intercurrent clinical events since the prior review, gives this process a consistent, repeatable structure rather than depending on whichever clinician happens to be reviewing the chart that month to remember which elements warrant particular attention for a given patient. Units that have adopted a standardized review checklist of this kind report catching prescription-status mismatches earlier and more consistently than units relying on individual clinician judgment alone to decide what to review at each visit, a pattern consistent with the broader theme, repeated throughout this book, that structured, systematized processes outperform good intentions applied inconsistently.

Sequential Versus Simultaneous Parameter Changes

When multiple prescription elements plausibly require adjustment at once — for example, a patient with both recurrent intradialytic hypotension and a rising predialysis potassium — changing several parameters simultaneously makes it difficult to determine afterward which specific change produced which specific effect, complicating any further adjustment that later proves necessary. Sequential adjustment, changing one element, allowing sufficient time to observe its effect over several treatments, and then adjusting the next element only if needed, preserves this diagnostic clarity at the cost of a slower overall adjustment process, a trade-off that is usually worthwhile except in genuinely urgent situations where the clinical situation cannot safely wait for a sequential trial.

In genuinely urgent situations — a patient presenting with both severe hyperkalemia and significant volume overload requiring same-day intervention — simultaneous adjustment of multiple parameters is appropriate and necessary, but even in this urgent context, documenting which parameters were changed and the specific reasoning for each supports a subsequent, calmer review once the acute situation has resolved, allowing the team to determine afterward whether every simultaneous change remains necessary as an ongoing prescription element or whether some were appropriate only for the acute situation and should be reverted once it has resolved.

A reasonable practical guideline for distinguishing an urgent from a non-urgent adjustment situation is whether the clinical consequence of waiting several treatments to observe the effect of a single sequential change would itself pose meaningful risk to the patient: a modestly elevated predialysis potassium trending upward over several months can typically tolerate a sequential approach, while a severely elevated potassium with electrocardiographic changes cannot, and the urgency of the underlying clinical problem, rather than a fixed rule about how many parameters may be changed at once, is what should govern the choice between sequential and simultaneous adjustment in a given case.

Documenting and Communicating Prescription Changes

A prescription change made by one clinician is only reliably implemented if it is documented clearly enough, and communicated actively enough, that every subsequent staff member setting up that patient's treatment — potentially days or weeks later, potentially a covering clinician unfamiliar with the reasoning behind the original change — applies the updated order correctly rather than reverting inadvertently to a prior version still present in an outdated standing template or a staff member's memory of the patient's usual settings. Explicit documentation of both the new parameter and the clinical reasoning behind it, rather than the parameter alone, supports this continuity by allowing a covering clinician to judge whether the reasoning still applies if the patient's situation has changed further since the note was written.

A forty-eight-year-old woman on a stable thrice-weekly hemodialysis prescription develops recurrent intradialytic hypotension over several consecutive treatments following a recent hospitalization for a myocardial infarction, during which her dry weight was not reassessed despite a documented weight change during the admission. Her nephrologist reviews the pattern at the next scheduled monthly review rather than waiting for a further acute event, identifies that her post-hospitalization dry weight has not been updated to reflect a decline in her actual dry body weight following a period of reduced oral intake during the admission, and sequentially adjusts her dry weight downward over two subsequent treatments while monitoring tolerance at each step, rather than making a single large downward adjustment in one step. The intradialytic hypotension resolves following this stepwise adjustment, and the reasoning — dry weight reassessment following a hospitalization affecting weight and volume status — is documented explicitly in her chart, along with a flag prompting reassessment at the next scheduled review rather than assuming the new dry weight will remain accurate indefinitely.

This case is also used, in this unit's practice, as a recurring teaching example for new staff specifically because the failure it illustrates — a hospitalization-related weight change not carried forward into the outpatient dialysis prescription — is common enough across transitions of care generally that recognizing the pattern reliably is a skill worth deliberately building rather than leaving to chance recognition. The unit has since adopted a standing practice of explicitly reviewing dry weight at the first outpatient treatment following any hospitalization, regardless of the reason for admission, rather than relying on the hospitalization discharge summary to flag a weight change that may not have been the primary focus of the inpatient team's attention, and this standing practice is now documented in the unit's own onboarding materials as a specific, named checklist item rather than left as an informal expectation passed along verbally between staff.

CAUTION: A hospitalization involving significant weight change is a trigger for dry weight reassessment at the next dialysis treatment, not an incidental detail to be addressed only if intradialytic hypotension subsequently develops.

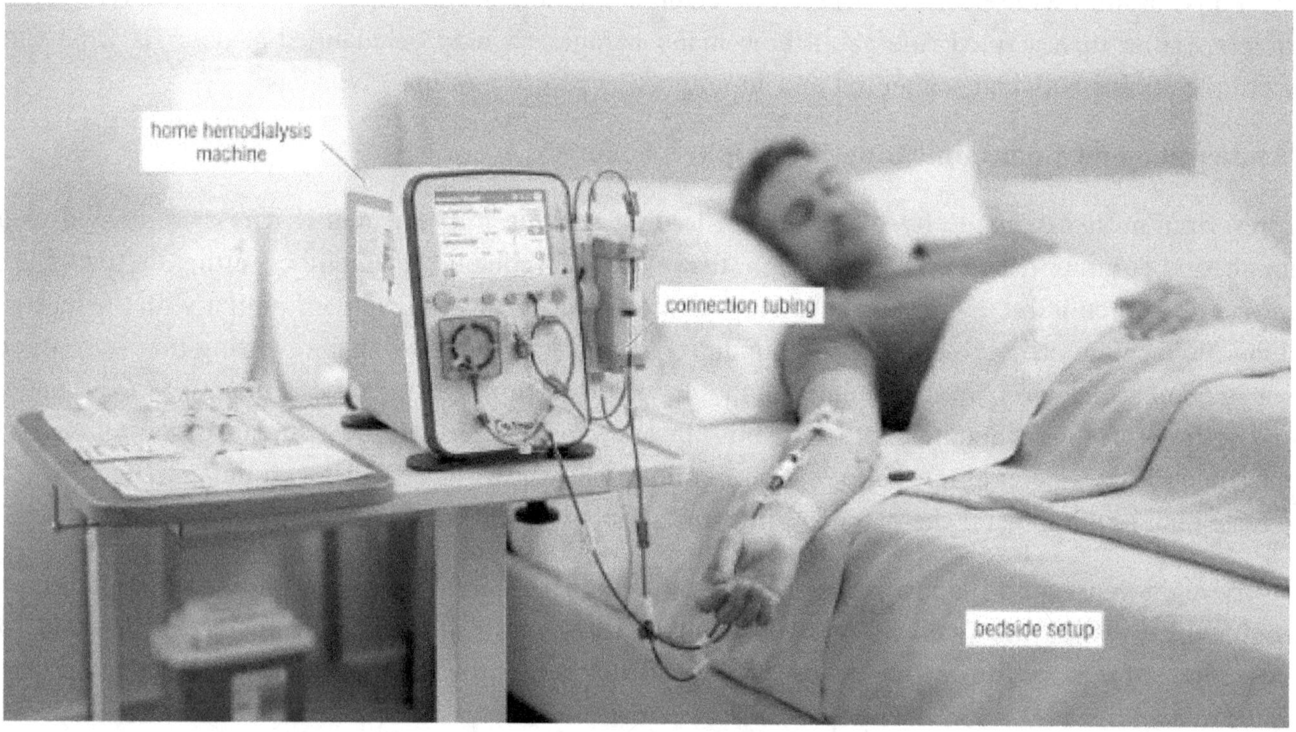

DIALYSIS RECOGNITION & RESPONSE SYSTEM — Prescription Adjustment Arcs

The Pattern: A patient develops new or worsening intradialytic hypotension following a recent hospitalization.

Stem Signature: Recurrent intradialytic hypotension over several treatments beginning shortly after a hospital admission, particularly one involving a documented weight change, in a patient whose dry weight was not reassessed at the time of discharge.

The Decision: Reassess dry weight explicitly in light of the hospitalization, adjusting it sequentially over two or more treatments while monitoring tolerance at each step, rather than treating the hypotension as an isolated hemodynamic problem to be managed with sodium profiling or ultrafiltration adjustment alone without addressing the underlying dry weight change.

Trap Logic: Post-hospitalization intradialytic hypotension can be managed symptomatically — slowing ultrafiltration, adjusting sodium profile — without recognizing that an outdated dry weight, no longer matching the patient's actual current euvolemic weight following the hospitalization, is the underlying driver requiring direct correction.

Response Anchor: A recent hospitalization with a documented weight change is a trigger for explicit dry weight reassessment, not simply a background detail to note in the chart.

DIALYSIS RECOGNITION & RESPONSE SYSTEM — Prescription Adjustment Arcs

Persistent Hyperkalemia Despite Reported Adherence: Review the dialysate potassium prescription and treatment adequacy before attributing the pattern to dietary nonadherence by default.

Unexplained Adequacy Shortfall: Evaluate for vascular access recirculation before escalating blood flow rate or treatment time further in response to a Kt/V or urea reduction ratio below target.

Post-Hospitalization Intradialytic Hypotension: Reassess dry weight explicitly and adjust it sequentially, rather than managing the hypotension symptomatically without addressing an outdated dry weight.

Summary and Key Concepts

A complete hemodialysis prescription integrates dialyzer selection, flow rates, treatment time, dialysate composition, anticoagulation, and ultrafiltration goal as interacting elements, documented alongside its clinical target rather than as an isolated checklist.

Dialysate potassium, calcium, bicarbonate, and temperature each involve genuine clinical trade-offs and should be individualized to a specific patient's risk profile rather than left at a single unit-wide default.

Treatment time, frequency, and ultrafiltration rate are interdependent; a shortened treatment time without a corresponding reduction in interdialytic weight gain forces a higher ultrafiltration rate with its own hemodynamic risks.

Prescription adjustment is best triggered by scheduled, periodic review rather than only by acute crisis, and multiple simultaneous changes should generally be avoided outside genuinely urgent situations to preserve diagnostic clarity about which change produced which effect.

Documented reasoning behind a prescription change, not merely the new parameter itself, supports safe continuity of care across covering clinicians and shifts.

CHAPTER 7: HEMODIALYSIS ADEQUACY: KT/V, UREA KINETICS, AND THEIR LIMITS

Learning Objectives

Explain the physiologic basis of Kt/V and distinguish single-pool from equilibrated Kt/V.

Calculate and interpret urea reduction ratio and recognize the common technical errors that distort adequacy measurement.

Identify what Kt/V does and does not capture about a patient's overall clinical status.

Interpret dose-escalation trial evidence and apply it to avoid over-reliance on Kt/V as a sole adequacy target.

Construct a whole-patient adequacy assessment that integrates Kt/V with residual kidney function, nutritional status, and clinical symptom burden.

Chapter Overview

Every prescription decision described in Chapter 6 is ultimately calibrated against a target, and for small-solute clearance that target has, for several decades, been Kt/V: a single dimensionless number intended to capture how effectively a treatment clears urea relative to the volume of body water it must clear it from. This chapter works through how Kt/V is derived and measured, why it is imperfect even on its own terms, and, most importantly, why an adequate Kt/V has never been sufficient by itself to confirm that a patient's overall dialysis prescription is truly adequate. The chapter's central argument, developed across all four sections, is that Kt/V is a necessary but insufficient adequacy metric, and that whole-patient assessment, not a single laboratory-derived number, is what adequacy actually requires. This argument matters practically, not merely as an academic qualification: a clinician who treats Kt/V as the entirety of adequacy will, over the course of a career, miss patients who are genuinely under-treated in ways a passing Kt/V cannot reveal, while a clinician who understands Kt/V's actual scope and limitations is positioned to catch exactly the kind of case developed later in this chapter, where a stable, at-target Kt/V coexists with a genuine and clinically significant decline in a patient's total adequacy.

Urea Kinetic Modeling and Kt/V Calculation

The Physiologic Basis of Kt/V

Kt/V expresses the clearance, K, achieved by the dialyzer over the treatment time, t, as a fraction of the patient's total urea distribution volume, V, which approximates total body water. Because urea distributes essentially throughout total body water rather than being confined to plasma or extracellular fluid alone, V is estimated using anthropometric formulas based on the patient's height, weight, age, and sex, and this estimation itself is a recognized source of variability in calculated Kt/V discussed later in this chapter, since two patients with identical dialyzer clearance and treatment time can have meaningfully different Kt/V values if their estimated V differs, independent of any actual difference in the adequacy of clearance delivered.

The urea kinetic model underlying Kt/V treats the body as a single, well-mixed compartment from which urea is removed at a rate proportional to the dialyzer's clearance, an assumption that holds reasonably well for the plasma-accessible fraction of body water but breaks down to some degree because urea equilibrates between intracellular and extracellular compartments more slowly than the treatment itself proceeds, a phenomenon addressed directly by the distinction between single-pool and equilibrated Kt/V developed in the next subsection.

The dimensionless nature of Kt/V, a ratio rather than an absolute clearance value expressed in volume-per-time units, is precisely what allows it to serve as a single comparable target across patients of different body sizes in the first place, but this same normalization is the root of the body-size and gender interpretive complications developed later in this chapter: because K and t are measured directly while V is estimated rather than measured, any systematic error in estimating a given patient's V propagates directly into their calculated Kt/V without any corresponding change in the actual clearance the treatment delivered, making V estimation accuracy just as consequential to a meaningful Kt/V value as accurate measurement of clearance and time themselves.

Single-Pool Versus Equilibrated Kt/V

Single-pool Kt/V, calculated directly from a blood urea nitrogen drawn immediately at the end of treatment, systematically overestimates true clearance because it is measured before intracellular urea has had time to re-equilibrate with the now-lower extracellular concentration achieved by dialysis; blood urea nitrogen drawn at this moment reflects only the more rapidly accessible extracellular pool, understating the total urea that remains to be cleared once the slower intracellular compartment redistributes into it over the following thirty to sixty minutes.

Equilibrated Kt/V corrects for this by either measuring blood urea nitrogen after allowing this redistribution to occur, typically thirty to sixty minutes post-treatment, or by applying a validated mathematical correction to the single-pool value that estimates what the equilibrated value would be without requiring the patient to remain for an additional blood draw after treatment ends. Because equilibrated Kt/V is consistently lower than single-pool Kt/V for the same treatment, the two are not interchangeable, and a target Kt/V value expressed in one framework should not be compared directly against a value calculated in the other without applying the appropriate conversion, a confusion that has historically led to inconsistent adequacy reporting across different centers and different eras of practice.

The magnitude of the difference between single-pool and equilibrated Kt/V is not constant across all patients and treatments but depends on factors including blood flow rate and treatment time, since a higher blood flow rate relative to a patient's cardiac output tends to produce a larger disequilibrium between the intracellular and extracellular urea pools at the moment treatment ends, and correspondingly a larger gap between the single-pool value measured at that moment and the equilibrated value measured after redistribution completes. This variability is one reason routine clinical practice in most centers has settled on consistent use of one framework, most commonly single-pool Kt/V with an applied correction factor to estimate the equilibrated value, rather than measuring both directly for every patient at every monitoring interval, balancing calculation consistency against the additional burden of a delayed post-treatment blood draw.

Practical Kt/V Calculation Methods

Formal urea kinetic modeling, solving the underlying differential equations that describe urea removal and generation over the course of treatment, produces the most rigorous single-pool Kt/V estimate but requires more detailed inputs — precise treatment time, ultrafiltration volume, and pre- and post-treatment blood urea nitrogen — than routine clinical practice always captures with full precision. Simplified formulas, developed to approximate the formal kinetic modeling result using only pre- and post-treatment blood urea nitrogen, treatment time, and estimated ultrafiltration volume, are in widespread clinical use because they are calculable directly from routinely available data without requiring iterative equation-solving, at a modest cost in precision relative to formal kinetic modeling.

Because these simplified formulas were derived and validated under the assumptions of standard thrice-weekly treatment, applying them without modification to markedly different treatment schedules, such as the more frequent regimens discussed in Chapter 20, introduces additional error beyond what the formula's inherent approximation already carries, and adequacy assessment for patients on non-standard schedules should use validated calculation approaches specific to that schedule rather than applying the standard formula unmodified and interpreting the result against thrice-weekly-derived targets.

Standardized Kt/V, a further metric developed specifically to allow comparison of dialysis dose across markedly different treatment frequencies by expressing weekly clearance in a manner equivalent to a continuous clearance process, addresses the specific problem that a given total weekly Kt/V delivered across three treatments is not clinically equivalent to the same total delivered across six, since the peak and trough urea concentrations experienced between treatments differ substantially between the two schedules even when cumulative weekly clearance is matched. This metric is most relevant to the home and intensive hemodialysis regimens discussed in Chapter 20, where treatment frequency departs from the standard thrice-weekly framework Kt/V and urea reduction ratio were originally developed to characterize, and its use allows a meaningful dose comparison across schedules that would otherwise be difficult to compare using conventional single-pool or equilibrated Kt/V alone.

Figure 7.1: Total Body Water Compartments and Urea Distribution

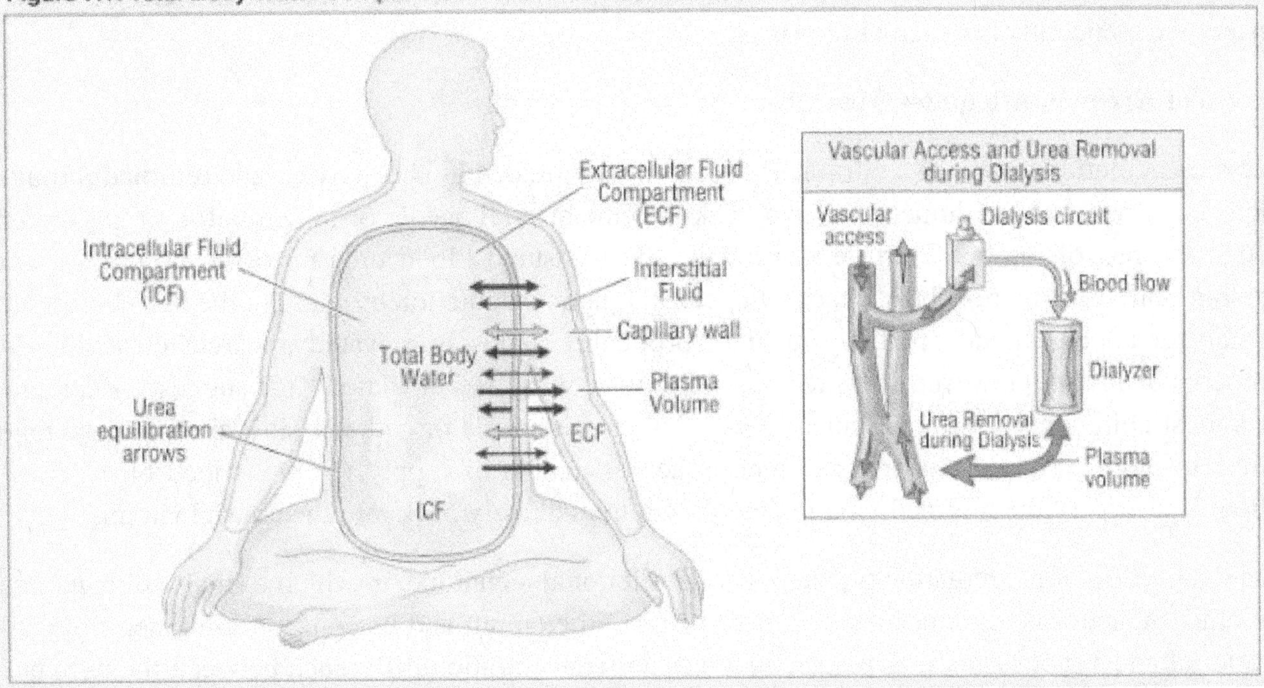

Urea Reduction Ratio and Practical Measurement

Calculating and Interpreting Urea Reduction Ratio

Urea reduction ratio, calculated simply as the fractional decline in blood urea nitrogen from the start to the end of a single treatment, is a considerably simpler calculation than Kt/V, requiring neither an estimate of urea distribution volume nor an accounting for ultrafiltration volume, and correlates reasonably well with Kt/V across most clinical scenarios, making it a useful, easily calculated adjunct or cross-check against a formally calculated Kt/V value.

Because urea reduction ratio does not account for ultrafiltration volume, however, it can diverge meaningfully from Kt/V in a patient undergoing a particularly large ultrafiltration volume during treatment, since convective urea removal accompanying substantial fluid removal contributes to the blood urea nitrogen decline captured by urea reduction ratio without being separately represented in the calculation the way it is implicitly reflected in a properly calculated Kt/V; this divergence is a recognized source of discrepancy when the two metrics are compared for the same treatment and should not automatically be assumed to reflect a calculation error in either figure.

Urea reduction ratio's simplicity makes it particularly useful as a rapid bedside cross-check against a formally calculated Kt/V that seems inconsistent with a patient's expected clearance, and as a metric readily understood by patients themselves, who can track their own urea reduction ratio trend over time as one accessible way of engaging with their own treatment adequacy without needing to understand the more technical urea kinetic modeling underlying formal Kt/V calculation. This accessibility has practical value in patient education contexts, including the home hemodialysis training discussed in Chapter 20, where patients managing their own treatment benefit from an adequacy metric they can calculate and interpret independently between clinic visits.

Sources of Error in Adequacy Measurement

Access recirculation, in which a portion of blood already treated by the dialyzer and returned through the venous needle or catheter lumen is drawn back into the arterial needle or lumen before it has circulated through the rest of the body, artificially lowers the measured blood urea nitrogen at both the arterial sampling point and, more subtly, distorts the entire kinetic calculation by making the blood presented to the dialyzer appear already partially cleared, producing a falsely elevated apparent clearance during treatment but a falsely low true delivered dose relative to what the calculated Kt/V suggests. Recirculation arises most commonly from a vascular access whose two needle or catheter sites are too close together relative to blood flow rate, or from a stenotic access unable to supply the prescribed blood flow rate without a portion of the returned blood being drawn immediately back into the arterial circuit.

Formal detection of recirculation typically uses a dilutional technique, in which a small volume of saline or another indicator is introduced at a defined point in the circuit and its concentration measured at both the arterial and venous sampling points; a significant concentration difference between the two, beyond what would be expected from dilution alone, confirms recirculation is occurring and, combined with vascular imaging of the access itself, helps localize whether the underlying cause is needle or catheter positioning versus a structural stenosis requiring intervention. Because recirculation of even a modest degree can meaningfully distort calculated Kt/V without necessarily being obvious from routine clinical examination of the access alone, a formal dilutional study, rather than physical examination findings by themselves, is the appropriate confirmatory test whenever recirculation is suspected as an explanation for an unexpectedly low Kt/V.

Sampling technique errors are a further, entirely avoidable source of adequacy measurement distortion: a post-treatment blood urea nitrogen drawn without first pausing or substantially slowing the blood pump captures blood that has been diluted by the access recirculation phenomenon described above even in an access without a true structural recirculation problem, since residual dialysate-side clearance continues to affect the sample drawn from a line still connected to a running circuit. Standardized post-treatment sampling protocols, which slow or stop the blood pump briefly before drawing the sample, reduce this artifact and are essential to obtaining a blood urea nitrogen value that genuinely reflects the patient's own circulating urea rather than blood still under the direct influence of the dialysis circuit at the moment of sampling.

A related but distinct sampling error arises from the timing of the pre-treatment blood draw relative to the patient's most recent meal or the start of the blood pump itself; a pre-treatment sample drawn after the blood pump has already been running for several minutes, rather than immediately before it starts, captures a blood urea nitrogen already modestly reduced by early treatment, artificially inflating the calculated urea reduction ratio and Kt/V by overstating the apparent decline from a starting point that was not truly the patient's pre-treatment baseline. Consistent, protocol-driven timing for both the pre-treatment and post-treatment sample, applied uniformly by all staff drawing these samples rather than varying by individual practice, removes this source of variability and ensures that trended Kt/V values across successive months are genuinely comparable to one another rather than reflecting inconsistent sampling timing from one month to the next.

A forty-four-year-old man on hemodialysis via an arteriovenous fistula has a Kt/V that has declined from consistently above target to modestly below target over two consecutive monthly measurements, despite no change in his prescribed blood flow rate, treatment time, or dialyzer. His nephrology team's initial impulse is to increase his prescribed treatment time to compensate, but before doing so, they review his sampling technique and confirm it has been performed correctly, then proceed to a dedicated recirculation study using a two-needle dilutional technique. The study confirms significant recirculation, and further evaluation reveals that his fistula's cannulation sites, adjusted somewhat closer together over recent treatments to accommodate a shorter usable segment of the vessel, are now positioned closely enough relative to his prescribed blood flow rate to produce clinically significant recirculation. Rather than extending his treatment time, which would not correct a problem rooted in access geometry, his team arranges vascular access imaging, which identifies a stenosis upstream of the venous needle site that has been progressively shortening his usable cannulation segment; the stenosis is treated with angioplasty, cannulation sites are repositioned appropriately, and his subsequent Kt/V returns to its prior above-target level without any change to his underlying prescription. This case illustrates directly why the framework's Response Anchor for this pattern specifies evaluating recirculation before escalating the prescription: extending his treatment time in the initial response would have added burden to the patient without addressing the actual, access-related cause of his declining measured dose. The broader lesson generalizes beyond this specific patient: whenever a previously reliable adequacy metric begins trending in an unexpected direction without a corresponding change in the prescription itself, the most productive first step is to ask what has changed in the measurement process or the access, not to assume the prescription itself has become inadequate and respond immediately by escalating it further.

KEY POINT: A low or inconsistent measured Kt/V should prompt evaluation for access recirculation and sampling technique error before the prescription itself is escalated in response to an apparently inadequate result.

DIALYSIS RECOGNITION & RESPONSE SYSTEM — Adequacy Assessment Arcs

The Pattern: A patient's measured Kt/V is unexpectedly and persistently low despite an apparently adequate prescription.

Stem Signature: A calculated Kt/V below target in a patient receiving blood and dialysate flow rates, treatment time, and dialyzer specification that would be expected to achieve an adequate dose, with no other clinical explanation for underdialysis apparent.

The Decision: Evaluate for access recirculation using a dedicated recirculation study and review the post-treatment sampling technique used, rather than escalating blood flow rate, treatment time, or dialyzer surface area in response to a Kt/V result that may reflect a measurement artifact rather than a true delivered-dose deficit.

Trap Logic: A low Kt/V is easily interpreted as straightforward evidence of an underpowered prescription, prompting escalation of flow rate or time that will not correct a result actually driven by recirculation or sampling error, and that in the case of recirculation may not even be achievable given the access's true delivery limit.

Response Anchor: An unexpectedly low Kt/V in a prescription that should otherwise be adequate warrants a recirculation and sampling-technique evaluation before the prescription itself is escalated.

Frequency of Adequacy Monitoring

Routine Kt/V or urea reduction ratio monitoring, typically performed monthly in stable patients, provides the regular surveillance needed to detect a gradual decline in delivered dose before it becomes clinically apparent through symptoms, while more frequent measurement is warranted following any change to the prescription itself, the vascular access, or the patient's body weight, since each of these changes can shift achieved Kt/V independent of any change in the underlying machine settings themselves.

A single Kt/V measurement reflects only the treatment on which it was drawn and can be affected by day-to-day variability in blood flow achieved, patient positioning, and other treatment-specific factors, so an isolated below-target result in an otherwise stable patient is often best interpreted in the context of the preceding trend rather than triggering an immediate prescription change on the strength of one measurement alone, provided the result is not so far below target as to warrant more urgent evaluation for recirculation or another acute cause.

Trending Kt/V results over several consecutive measurements, rather than reacting to any single value in isolation, also protects against a specific interpretive error: a Kt/V that fluctuates around target with no consistent directional drift generally reflects normal measurement variability and requires no prescription change, while a Kt/V that declines consistently across three or more consecutive measurements, even if each individual value remains within an acceptable range, reflects a genuine trend worth investigating proactively rather than waiting for the trend to cross below the numeric target before acting, since the whole-patient adequacy principle developed later in this chapter applies as much to catching an emerging decline early as it does to responding to an already-established deficit.

Limitations of Small-Solute Clearance Targets

What Kt/V Does Not Capture

As established in Chapter 4, Kt/V characterizes small-solute clearance specifically, and an adequate Kt/V provides no direct information about middle molecule clearance, which depends on convective volume rather than the flow-rate and time parameters Kt/V is calculated from, nor about protein-bound uremic toxin clearance, which depends on treatment time and frequency in ways only partially reflected in a Kt/V value calculated under the standard thrice-weekly framework. A patient can achieve a fully adequate Kt/V while remaining under-treated by either of these other clearance dimensions, This distinction develops the same principle established in Chapter 4 and revisited here specifically because Kt/V's prominence as the conventional adequacy metric can obscure how narrow its actual scope is.

Kt/V also captures nothing directly about volume status, nutritional status, anemia management, mineral and bone disorder control, or the broader symptom burden discussed throughout Part VII of this book, each of which contributes as much to a patient's overall clinical trajectory as small-solute clearance does, and each of which requires its own dedicated assessment rather than being inferred from an adequate Kt/V value.

This gap between small-solute adequacy and overall clinical adequacy is not a minor technical caveat but the central organizing insight of this entire chapter, and it explains a pattern familiar to any experienced nephrologist: a patient whose Kt/V trend looks entirely reassuring on a monthly summary report can nonetheless be declining clinically in ways that summary report gives no hint of, simply because the report reflects only the one dimension of adequacy Kt/V was ever designed to measure. Recognizing this gap explicitly, rather than treating a passing Kt/V as a general reassurance about a patient's overall trajectory, is what the whole-patient framework developed in the final section of this chapter is specifically designed to close.

The Body Size and Gender Paradoxes in Kt/V Interpretation

Because Kt/V normalizes clearance to estimated total body water rather than to body surface area or lean body mass, smaller-bodied patients, who tend to have a higher ratio of urea distribution volume to their actual muscle mass and metabolic urea generation rate, can achieve a numerically higher Kt/V for the same absolute dialyzer clearance than a larger-bodied patient would, without necessarily receiving a clearance that is truly more generous relative to their metabolic urea production. This body-size dependence has been proposed as a partial explanation for observed differences in outcomes across body size categories at ostensibly similar Kt/V targets, since a given Kt/V value may represent a meaningfully different absolute clearance relative to metabolic urea generation depending on the patient's body composition.

A related pattern, sometimes described as a gender paradox in Kt/V interpretation, arises because women, on average, have a higher ratio of total body water to muscle mass than men at a comparable body weight, which can produce a higher calculated Kt/V for women receiving what is, in absolute terms, a comparable or even lesser clearance relative to their actual urea generation rate. These patterns do not indicate that Kt/V should be abandoned as an adequacy metric, but they do argue against treating a single universal numeric Kt/V target as equally meaningful across every body size and composition without considering how that number was derived for the specific patient in front of the clinician.

Some proposed alternative or supplementary metrics attempt to address this limitation directly by normalizing clearance to a measure less dependent on total body water, such as body surface area or a standardized measure of metabolic rate, and while none of these alternatives has fully displaced Kt/V in routine clinical use, their existence reflects a broader recognition within the nephrology community that a single normalization approach cannot fully capture adequacy across the full range of body compositions a dialysis population presents. In practice, this means a clinician evaluating a Kt/V value for a notably small-bodied or notably large-bodied patient benefits from interpreting that value with some awareness of how body composition may be influencing the number, rather than treating every patient's Kt/V as equally comparable to a single population-derived target regardless of body habitus.

Muscle mass specifically, rather than total body weight alone, is the variable most directly relevant to this interpretive caution, since two patients of identical total body weight but markedly different muscle mass — a well-muscled, physically active patient compared with a sarcopenic, frail patient of the same weight — generate urea at meaningfully different rates and may warrant somewhat different interpretation of an identical calculated Kt/V, with the sarcopenic patient's numerically adequate Kt/V potentially reflecting a smaller absolute clearance burden than the same number would represent in the more muscular patient. This consideration connects directly to the nutritional assessment developed later in this chapter, since muscle mass and nutritional status are themselves closely related, meaning a thorough nutritional evaluation serves double duty by informing both adequacy interpretation and nutritional management simultaneously.

Evidence From Dose-Escalation Trials

Large randomized trials testing whether escalating Kt/V beyond standard adequacy targets improves clinical outcomes have generally failed to demonstrate additional benefit from higher small-solute clearance alone once a threshold adequacy level has been achieved, a finding that has been influential in shaping guideline recommendations away from progressively higher Kt/V targets and toward the whole-patient assessment framework developed in the final section of this chapter. This body of evidence parallels the finding, discussed in Chapter 18, that peritoneal dialysis adequacy assessment has undergone a similar evolution away from escalating a single small-solute clearance target and toward incorporating broader measures of patient-centered outcome.

The practical implication of this dose-escalation evidence is that a patient whose Kt/V already meets standard target should not be assumed to benefit from further escalation of blood flow rate, treatment time, or dialyzer surface area pursued solely to raise Kt/V further, and that persistent symptoms in such a patient are more productively addressed by investigating the other dimensions of adequacy — middle molecule clearance, volume status, nutrition, and the clinical markers discussed in the next section — than by continuing to escalate a metric that trial evidence suggests has already reached its point of diminishing clinical return.

These dose-escalation findings should be distinguished carefully from the hemodiafiltration mortality evidence discussed in Chapter 4, which found benefit specifically tied to convective volume rather than to small-solute Kt/V escalation; the two bodies of evidence are not in tension but instead reinforce the same underlying conclusion from different directions — escalating small-solute clearance alone, once an adequate threshold is reached, does not reliably improve outcomes, while escalating convective clearance specifically, a physiologically distinct intervention targeting a different molecular size range entirely, does show benefit in appropriately dosed patients. Conflating these two findings, or assuming that hemodiafiltration's benefit implies that pushing Kt/V still higher would produce a comparable benefit, misreads what each body of evidence actually supports.

The historical trajectory of Kt/V target-setting itself illustrates this dose-escalation evidence in practice: early adequacy guidelines set relatively modest Kt/V targets based largely on observational associations between dose and outcome, subsequent revisions raised these targets as further observational data suggested higher clearance correlated with better outcomes, and only later did dedicated randomized dose-escalation trials directly test whether prospectively raising Kt/V above the already-established target produced the anticipated additional benefit, generally finding that it did not. This sequence, from observational association to randomized disconfirmation of further escalation, is a pattern worth recognizing broadly in nephrology and in medicine more generally: an observed association between a higher dose of an intervention and better outcomes does not reliably predict that prospectively raising the dose further, once a reasonable threshold has already been reached, will replicate that same incremental benefit, since much of the original association may reflect selection effects — healthier patients tolerating and achieving higher doses in the first place — rather than a true causal dose-response relationship extending indefinitely upward.

Adequacy Dimension	What It Captures	What Kt/V Alone Misses
Small-Solute Clearance (Kt/V)	Urea and comparably sized solute removal per treatment	Provides the baseline metric but is the dimension already well characterized by Kt/V itself
Middle Molecule Clearance	Beta-2 microglobulin and comparable inflammatory mediators	Depends on convective volume, not flow rate or time — entirely unaddressed by Kt/V
Protein-Bound Toxin Clearance	Indoxyl sulfate, p-cresyl sulfate, and similar solutes	Depends on treatment time and frequency in ways only partially reflected in standard Kt/V
Volume Status	Interdialytic fluid accumulation and dry weight accuracy	Not assessed by Kt/V at all; requires dedicated clinical and objective evaluation
Nutritional Status	Protein-energy wasting and overall metabolic reserve	Not assessed by Kt/V, though undernutrition can artificially lower estimated urea generation and distort interpretation

Whole-Patient Assessment of Adequacy

Clinical Markers Beyond Kt/V

A patient's overall sense of well-being between and during treatments, their appetite and nutritional intake, their blood pressure and volume control, and their functional status all provide information about treatment adequacy that Kt/V cannot, and a clinician who reviews only the Kt/V trend at each monthly visit while overlooking these other markers risks missing a patient who is clinically under-treated despite a numerically adequate small-solute clearance value. Systematic review of these clinical markers at the same interval Kt/V is checked, rather than only when a patient spontaneously reports a new symptom, surfaces this kind of mismatch earlier.

Serum albumin, while influenced by inflammation and other non-nutritional factors and therefore an imperfect nutritional marker on its own, remains a useful component of this broader review when interpreted alongside dietary history and physical examination for evidence of muscle wasting, since a declining albumin trend in a patient with an adequate Kt/V should prompt nutritional assessment rather than reassurance that the patient's dialysis dose, having met its numeric target, requires no further attention.

Normalized protein catabolic rate, a calculated estimate of dietary protein intake derived from urea generation rate and used as a proxy for a patient's actual protein consumption between dialysis sessions, offers an additional nutritional data point that can be calculated from the same blood urea nitrogen values already collected for Kt/V determination, making it a relatively low-burden addition to routine adequacy monitoring. A declining trend in this calculated protein intake estimate, particularly when paired with a declining albumin and clinical evidence of muscle wasting, provides converging evidence of a nutritional problem that a Kt/V value in isolation would give no indication of whatsoever, reinforcing why a whole-patient review draws on several complementary data sources rather than any single one.

Integrating Residual Kidney Function Into Adequacy Assessment

Residual native kidney function, where present, contributes meaningfully to a patient's overall solute and fluid clearance and is not captured by a Kt/V calculation derived solely from the dialysis treatment itself, meaning two patients with identical dialysis-derived Kt/V but different residual kidney function have meaningfully different total clearance and, correspondingly, different actual adequacy despite an identical dialysis Kt/V value. This is the same principle developed in the peritoneal dialysis adequacy discussion in Chapter 18, where residual kidney function's contribution to total clearance is even more central to routine adequacy assessment, but it applies to hemodialysis as well and is sometimes underappreciated specifically because standard hemodialysis Kt/V reporting conventions do not routinely incorporate a residual function term the way peritoneal dialysis adequacy calculations do.

A patient with substantial residual kidney function may tolerate a dialysis-only Kt/V modestly below standard target without clinical consequence, since their total clearance, dialysis plus residual, remains adequate, while a patient with no residual function at all has no such margin and depends entirely on the dialysis-derived Kt/V to meet their total clearance need; recognizing which category a given patient falls into is part of interpreting their Kt/V value appropriately rather than applying an identical numeric target regardless of residual function status.

Because residual kidney function tends to decline progressively over the first one to two years of dialysis dependence, as introduced in Chapter 6's discussion of prescription adjustment, a patient's appropriate reliance on residual function as part of their total clearance picture is itself a moving target requiring periodic reassessment rather than a single determination made at dialysis initiation and assumed to remain valid indefinitely. Measuring residual function directly, typically through a timed urine collection assessing residual urea and creatinine clearance, provides more precise information than assuming a fixed rate of decline, though even where formal measurement is not performed routinely, attentiveness to urine output trends and the gradual emergence of interdialytic symptoms can serve as an indirect signal that residual function has diminished and that the dialysis-derived Kt/V now carries a larger share of the patient's total clearance burden than it did earlier in their treatment course, a signal worth building into the same structured, scheduled review this chapter recommends rather than leaving to incidental notice.

A Practical Framework for Adequacy Review

A structured monthly or quarterly adequacy review, integrating Kt/V trend, urea reduction ratio as a cross-check, residual kidney function where measured, nutritional markers including albumin and dietary history, volume status and interdialytic weight gain pattern, and the patient's own reported symptom burden, provides a more complete picture than any single metric reviewed in isolation, and is the practical embodiment of this chapter's central argument that adequacy is a multidimensional clinical judgment rather than a single passing or failing number.

Implementing this kind of structured review consistently, rather than as an occasional exercise reserved for patients who present with obvious symptoms, benefits from a standardized checklist or electronic template that prompts review of each dimension at the same interval Kt/V itself is checked, since without this structure the review predictably narrows over time to whichever single metric is most easily retrieved — typically Kt/V alone, given its prominence as the conventional adequacy target — even among clinicians who conceptually endorse the broader framework this chapter describes. This is, in effect, the same operational lesson developed for Life-Plan revision in Chapter 2 and goals-of-care review in Chapter 3: a sound clinical principle only reliably changes practice when it is built into a structured, repeatable workflow rather than left to individual clinician memory and intention, however genuine that intention may be.

A sixty-seven-year-old man on hemodialysis for four years has maintained a Kt/V consistently at or slightly above target for over a year, yet reports increasing fatigue and reduced appetite over the past two months, with a modest decline in serum albumin on routine monthly labs. Rather than reassuring the patient that his numerically adequate Kt/V rules out a dialysis-related explanation for his symptoms, his nephrology team pursues the broader review framework described above: his residual kidney function, previously measurable, is found to have declined to a negligible level over the preceding several months, meaning his total clearance has fallen even though his dialysis-derived Kt/V has not changed. His prescription is adjusted, extending treatment time modestly to compensate for the lost residual contribution, and a dietitian consultation addresses his declining appetite directly. His symptoms improve over the following month, illustrating that his numerically stable Kt/V had been masking a genuine decline in his total clearance that only the broader adequacy framework, incorporating residual function specifically, was positioned to catch, and reinforcing the chapter's recurring point that a passing number and genuine clinical adequacy are not the same thing.

CLINICAL PEARL: A stable Kt/V does not rule out declining total clearance; loss of residual kidney function can erode a patient's overall adequacy margin even while their dialysis-derived Kt/V remains unchanged.

Figure 7.2: **Blood Urea Nitrogen Decay and Post-Treatment Rebound.**

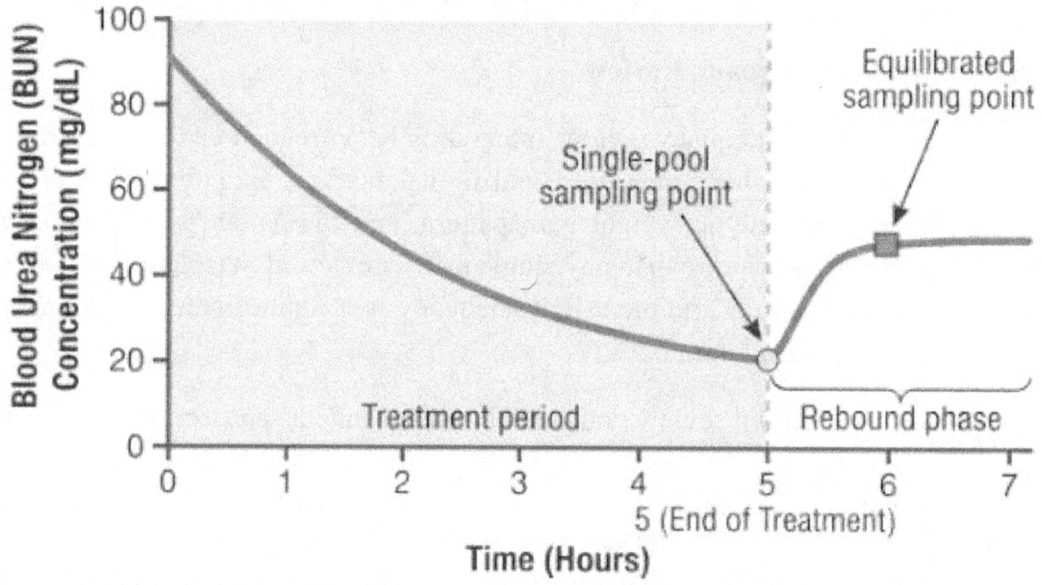

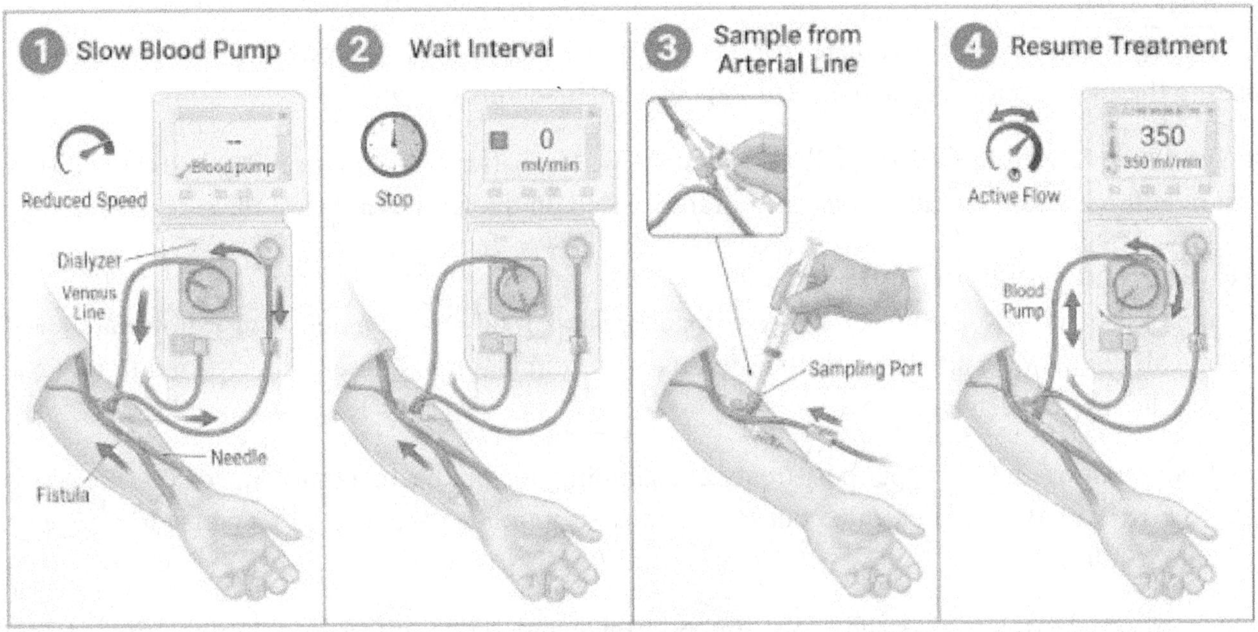

Figure 7.3: Proper Post-Treatment Sampling Technique to Avoid Recirculation Artifact

DIALYSIS RECOGNITION & RESPONSE SYSTEM — Adequacy Assessment Arcs

The Pattern: A patient with a stable, at-target Kt/V develops new fatigue, declining appetite, or a falling albumin trend.

Stem Signature: New or worsening constitutional symptoms and a declining nutritional marker in a patient whose Kt/V has remained at or above target throughout, with no change documented in the dialysis prescription itself.

The Decision: Pursue a whole-patient adequacy review — residual kidney function, nutritional assessment, volume status — rather than reassuring the patient that a numerically adequate Kt/V excludes a dialysis-related explanation for the new symptoms.

Trap Logic: An at-target Kt/V can be mistaken for confirmation that the dialysis prescription is fully adequate in every respect, when in fact Kt/V characterizes only small-solute clearance and says nothing directly about residual function, nutrition, or volume status.

Response Anchor: New symptoms despite a stable, at-target Kt/V warrant a whole-patient adequacy review, not reassurance based on the Kt/V number alone.

Unexpectedly Low Kt/V: Evaluate for access recirculation and sampling technique error before escalating the prescription in response to an apparently inadequate result.

New Symptoms Despite At-Target Kt/V: Pursue a whole-patient adequacy review — residual function, nutrition, volume status — rather than reassurance based on the Kt/V number alone.

Summary and Key Concepts

Kt/V expresses dialyzer clearance relative to estimated total body water, and equilibrated Kt/V is systematically lower than single-pool Kt/V because it accounts for post-treatment urea redistribution from the intracellular compartment.

Access recirculation and improper post-treatment sampling technique are common, correctable sources of falsely low Kt/V that should be ruled out before a prescription is escalated in response to an apparently inadequate result.

Kt/V captures small-solute clearance only, and body size and gender differences in the ratio of total body water to muscle mass mean a given Kt/V value can represent meaningfully different absolute clearance across different patients.

Dose-escalation trials have generally not shown additional benefit from raising Kt/V beyond standard target, shifting emphasis toward whole-patient adequacy assessment rather than progressively higher small-solute clearance targets.

A structured adequacy review integrating Kt/V, residual kidney function, nutritional markers, volume status, and patient-reported symptoms provides a more complete picture of adequacy than any single metric reviewed in isolation.

CHAPTER 8: ANTICOAGULATION IN HEMODIALYSIS

Learning Objectives

Explain why extracorporeal blood circulation requires anticoagulation and how standard heparin protocols achieve it.

Describe regional citrate anticoagulation and identify the patients for whom it offers a specific advantage.

Apply anticoagulation-free dialysis techniques for patients with an elevated bleeding risk.

Recognize and manage circuit clotting and bleeding complications related to anticoagulation choice.

Chapter Overview

Blood removed from the body and passed through an extracorporeal circuit encounters foreign surfaces — needle or catheter lumen, tubing, and the dialyzer membrane itself — that activate the clotting cascade far more readily than blood remaining within the patient's own endothelium-lined vasculature, and without some form of anticoagulation, the circuit would clot before a treatment could meaningfully proceed. This chapter surveys the anticoagulation approaches used to prevent this, from standard systemic heparin, appropriate for most patients, through regional citrate anticoagulation for patients requiring an anticoagulant effect confined to the circuit itself, to anticoagulation-free techniques for patients in whom any additional anticoagulant effect carries unacceptable bleeding risk.

Approach	Anticoagulant Scope	Best-Suited Patient	Key Monitoring Requirement
Unfractionated Heparin	Systemic, short half-life	Standard bleeding risk	Clotting time at initiation and dose changes
Low Molecular Weight Heparin	Systemic, longer half-life	Standard risk, dosing convenience preferred	Clinical bleeding surveillance; less frequent clotting time checks
Regional Citrate	Confined to circuit	Elevated systemic bleeding risk	Serial post-filter and systemic ionized calcium
Heparin-Coated Circuit	Localized to circuit surfaces	Moderate bleeding risk	Visual and pressure-trend circuit monitoring

Anticoagulation-Free (Saline Flush)	None	Highest bleeding risk	Frequent visual and pressure-trend circuit monitoring

Heparin Protocols and Monitoring

Standard Heparin Dosing Approaches

Standard hemodialysis anticoagulation typically uses unfractionated heparin, administered as an initial bolus at the start of treatment followed by a continuous infusion or intermittent additional boluses through the remainder of the session, calibrated to maintain adequate circuit anticoagulation while allowing the heparin effect to largely dissipate by treatment's end, minimizing the bleeding risk a patient carries once treatment concludes and needle sites are ready to be withdrawn. Because unfractionated heparin has a short half-life relative to a typical three-to-four-hour treatment, this dosing approach allows fine control over the anticoagulant effect within a single session, an advantage relative to longer-acting alternatives when the anticoagulation need is confined specifically to the treatment window itself, and a further advantage in the setting of an unplanned early treatment termination, where the anticoagulant effect of a still-infusing unfractionated heparin dose ends promptly once the infusion stops rather than persisting for hours afterward as a single large low molecular weight heparin dose administered at treatment start would.

Low molecular weight heparin, administered as a single dose at the start of treatment rather than requiring an infusion or repeated dosing through the session, offers a more convenient dosing profile and more predictable pharmacokinetics than unfractionated heparin, though its longer half-life means its anticoagulant effect persists further beyond treatment's end, a consideration relevant to patients in whom minimizing post-treatment bleeding risk from needle sites is a particular priority. Selection between unfractionated and low molecular weight heparin is therefore not simply a matter of convenience but involves weighing dosing simplicity against the more confined anticoagulant window unfractionated heparin's shorter half-life provides, a trade-off best made explicitly for each patient rather than defaulting to whichever agent a unit happens to stock as its routine choice.

Individual patient sensitivity to a given heparin dose varies considerably, and a weight-based starting dose, while a reasonable initial approach, should be understood as a starting point subject to verification rather than a precisely calibrated final answer for every patient at a given body weight, a distinction developed further in the case presented later in this chapter. Factors contributing to this variability include baseline antithrombin activity, concurrent medications affecting coagulation, and the degree of uremic platelet dysfunction discussed in Chapter 1, none of which a simple weight-based formula accounts for directly.

Heparin's mechanism, potentiating antithrombin's inhibitory effect on thrombin and factor Xa, depends on adequate baseline antithrombin activity to achieve its intended anticoagulant effect, and a patient with reduced antithrombin activity — whether from a congenital deficiency, a consumptive process, or severe hepatic synthetic dysfunction — may show an attenuated response to a standard heparin dose that a clotting time measurement, rather than the weight-based dose calculation alone, is positioned to reveal.

This is a further, specific illustration of why weight-based dosing functions best as a starting point for measurement-guided titration rather than as a definitive endpoint in itself, a principle that recurs throughout this book wherever a convenient starting formula must ultimately yield to individualized, measurement-guided adjustment.

Monitoring Anticoagulation Adequacy

Clotting time measurement, performed at the bedside using a point-of-care device, allows real-time assessment of whether a given heparin dose is achieving adequate circuit anticoagulation without requiring a formal laboratory coagulation panel, and is used most commonly when initiating a new patient on hemodialysis or when adjusting a dosing protocol, rather than as a routine measurement at every treatment for a patient whose established protocol has proven reliable over time. Visual inspection of the circuit itself — the dialyzer's fiber bundle and the drip chamber, both of which show visible clot formation before it becomes severe enough to compromise treatment — remains a practical, low-cost complementary check that experienced dialysis staff perform routinely throughout a treatment, independent of any formal clotting time measurement.

A circuit showing early signs of clotting, before frank occlusion develops, can sometimes be managed with a supplemental heparin bolus if this is safe given the patient's overall anticoagulation and bleeding risk profile, while an already substantially clotted circuit generally requires the affected dialyzer or line segment to be replaced rather than salvaged, since a heavily clotted circuit risks embolizing clot material to the patient if treatment continues rather than resolving safely on its own.

Beyond clotting time and visual inspection, the transmembrane pressure trend across a treatment provides a further, machine-derived indicator of circuit status, since a fiber bundle progressively occluding by clot formation presents increasing resistance to flow that manifests as a rising transmembrane pressure requirement to maintain the prescribed ultrafiltration rate, often before the clotting becomes visible to the naked eye on direct inspection of the dialyzer. Staff trained to recognize this pressure trend as an early clotting indicator, rather than only responding once clot is visually apparent, can intervene earlier in the process, when a supplemental anticoagulant bolus is more likely to salvage the circuit than it would be once clotting has progressed further.

Because transmembrane pressure also rises for reasons unrelated to clotting — an increase in prescribed ultrafiltration rate, a change in blood flow rate, or a dialyzer with inherently higher baseline resistance — interpreting a rising pressure trend as clotting-specific requires considering these alternative explanations as well, and staff who track each patient's typical baseline pressure trend for a given prescription are better positioned to recognize a genuine deviation from that patient's own normal pattern than staff relying solely on a generic, unit-wide expected pressure range that does not account for individual prescription differences across patients.

Establishing a reliable, patient-specific heparin protocol during a new patient's first several treatments, adjusting dose based on measured clotting time and observed circuit performance rather than continuing an unmodified starting dose regardless of how the first treatment actually performed, sets the foundation for the routine, lower-monitoring approach appropriate once that protocol has proven itself stable over subsequent sessions.

Catheter Lock Solutions Between Treatments

A central venous catheter not in active use between treatments requires its lumens filled with a lock solution to prevent clot formation within the catheter itself, distinct from the anticoagulation used during the treatment; heparin lock solutions, at a concentration considerably higher than any circulating systemic level the treatment itself would produce, are the traditional standard, though the small residual volume instilled means systemic absorption and effect remain limited in most patients despite the high local concentration within the catheter lumen.

Citrate-based lock solutions, and in some settings antimicrobial lock solutions combined with an anticoagulant, offer alternatives to standard heparin locks, particularly relevant for a patient with confirmed heparin-induced thrombocytopenia, for whom any heparin exposure, including a lock solution, must be avoided entirely, and for patients with recurrent catheter-related bloodstream infection, for whom an antimicrobial lock solution addresses a different, infection-prevention goal alongside the anticoagulant lock's patency-preservation purpose. Selection of lock solution, like every other anticoagulation decision in this chapter, should be documented explicitly in the patient's care plan and communicated clearly to any covering unit or provider, since an inadvertent reversion to a standard heparin lock in a patient with a documented heparin allergy or heparin-induced thrombocytopenia history represents exactly the kind of care-coordination failure discussed in Chapter 6's broader treatment of prescription communication across covering providers.

Lock solution volume must also be matched precisely to the specific catheter's documented internal lumen volume, since overfilling a lumen risks systemic infusion of the lock solution's concentrated contents directly into the patient's circulation at the start of the next treatment when blood is first aspirated from the line, an error with particular significance for a concentrated heparin lock and one that underscores why catheter lock volumes are drawn up and labeled according to the specific catheter's documented specifications rather than a generic volume applied uniformly across different catheter types and lumen sizes.

Heparin-Induced Thrombocytopenia and Alternative Anticoagulants

Heparin-induced thrombocytopenia, an immune-mediated reaction to heparin exposure that paradoxically produces a prothrombotic state despite the falling platelet count that gives the syndrome its name, is a recognized though uncommon complication of repeated heparin exposure and should be suspected in a hemodialysis patient who develops a substantial, otherwise unexplained platelet count decline, particularly one occurring five to ten days after initial heparin exposure or more rapidly in a patient with recent prior heparin exposure from another source such as a hospitalization. Because this diagnosis carries specific and serious implications — continued heparin exposure risks life-threatening thrombosis rather than merely an allergic-type reaction — a falling platelet count in a hemodialysis patient warrants active consideration of this diagnosis rather than being attributed reflexively to uremia-related thrombocytopenia or an unrelated cause without specific evaluation.

Confirmed or strongly suspected heparin-induced thrombocytopenia requires immediate discontinuation of all heparin exposure, including any low molecular weight heparin, heparin flushes used to maintain catheter patency between treatments, and heparin-coated circuit components discussed later in this chapter, since cross-reactivity among these heparin-derived products is common. Alternative anticoagulation for hemodialysis in this setting typically shifts to a non-heparin anticoagulant with a distinct mechanism, or to citrate-based or anticoagulation-free techniques discussed in the remainder of this chapter, and any heparin lock previously used to maintain a central venous catheter between treatments must also be changed to a heparin-free alternative, an easily overlooked detail given how routinely heparin locks are used for catheter maintenance outside the treatment itself.

Direct thrombin inhibitors, which act on the clotting cascade at a step downstream of and mechanistically distinct from heparin's antithrombin-potentiating effect, are the most commonly used non-heparin systemic anticoagulant option for hemodialysis in a patient with confirmed heparin-induced thrombocytopenia, since their mechanism carries no cross-reactivity with the heparin-dependent antibodies driving the syndrome. These agents require their own dedicated dosing and monitoring protocols distinct from standard heparin protocols, and units caring for patients with a history of heparin-induced thrombocytopenia benefit from having a defined alternative-anticoagulation protocol established in advance, rather than needing to develop one reactively once a case is identified, given the urgency with which heparin must be discontinued once the diagnosis is suspected.

Because the population of dialysis patients with a confirmed history of heparin-induced thrombocytopenia at any given unit is typically small, maintaining staff familiarity with the alternative protocol despite its infrequent use is a genuine practical challenge, and periodic simulation or refresher training on the alternative-anticoagulation protocol, similar in spirit to the alarm-response training discussed in Chapter 5, helps ensure that when a case does arise, staff execute the protocol correctly on the first attempt rather than needing to relearn it under the time pressure the diagnosis's urgency creates.

CAUTION: A substantial, otherwise unexplained platelet count decline in a hemodialysis patient warrants evaluation for heparin-induced thrombocytopenia; if confirmed or strongly suspected, discontinue all heparin exposure including catheter locks and coated circuit components, not only the dialysis treatment dose itself.

The Pattern: A hemodialysis patient develops a substantial, otherwise unexplained decline in platelet count.

Stem Signature: A platelet count decline of a magnitude and timing — typically five to ten days after heparin exposure, or sooner with recent prior exposure — consistent with an immune-mediated process, in a patient receiving routine heparin anticoagulation for dialysis and, often, heparin locks for catheter maintenance between treatments.

The Decision: Evaluate for heparin-induced thrombocytopenia specifically, and if confirmed or strongly suspected, discontinue all heparin exposure across every source — treatment dosing, catheter locks, and coated circuit components — transitioning to a non-heparin anticoagulant, citrate, or anticoagulation-free technique.

Trap Logic: A falling platelet count in a dialysis patient is easily attributed to uremia-related platelet effects or an unrelated cause, when heparin-induced thrombocytopenia's paradoxically prothrombotic nature makes it a specific, dangerous diagnosis that reflexive reassurance can miss.

Response Anchor: An unexplained platelet decline in a heparin-exposed dialysis patient is heparin-induced thrombocytopenia until evaluated otherwise — and confirmation requires eliminating heparin from every exposure source, not just the treatment dose.

KEY POINT: Unfractionated heparin's short half-life allows the anticoagulant effect to largely resolve by treatment's end; this confined window is an advantage specifically for patients in whom minimizing post-treatment bleeding risk from needle sites matters most.

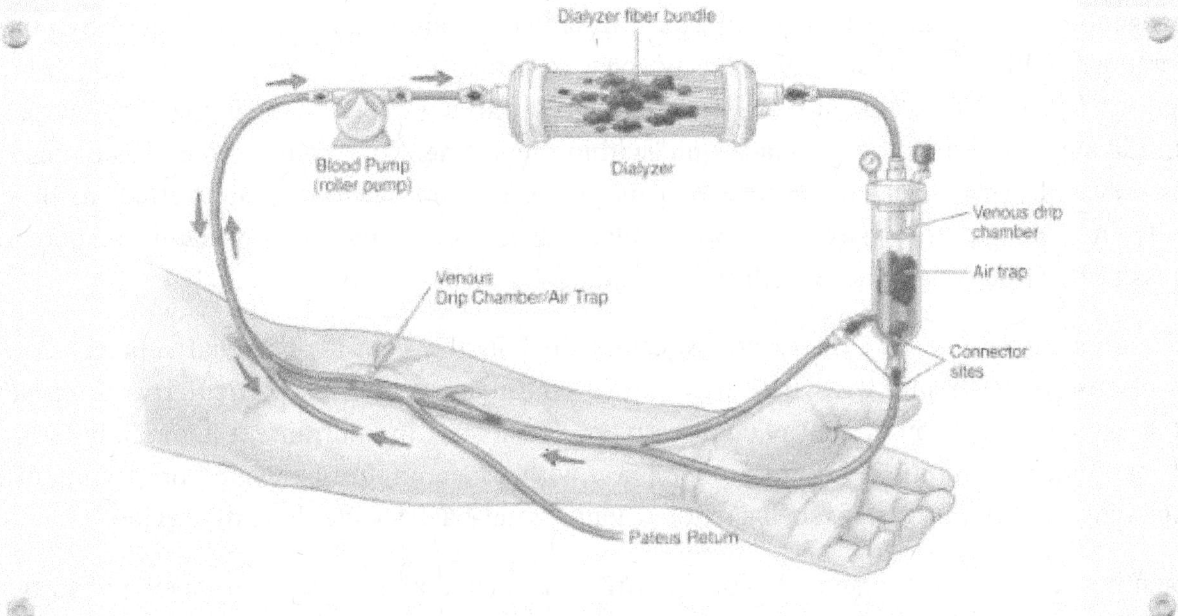

Figure 8.1: Extracorporeal Circuit Sites of Clot Formation

Citrate and Regional Anticoagulation

The Mechanism of Regional Citrate Anticoagulation

Regional citrate anticoagulation achieves anticoagulation confined specifically to the extracorporeal circuit by infusing citrate into the blood as it enters the circuit, where it chelates ionized calcium and thereby interrupts the calcium-dependent steps of the clotting cascade; calcium is then infused separately back into the returning blood line to restore the patient's own systemic ionized calcium before the blood re-enters the body, confining the anticoagulant effect to the circuit itself rather than producing systemic anticoagulation the way heparin does.

This regional confinement is citrate's principal clinical advantage: a patient with an elevated systemic bleeding risk, for whom heparin's systemic anticoagulant effect would be undesirable, can still receive effective circuit anticoagulation through citrate without the corresponding increase in bleeding risk elsewhere in the body, since citrate's calcium-chelating effect is substantially reversed by the calcium infusion before blood returns to the patient's systemic circulation.

Modern hemodialysis machines equipped for citrate anticoagulation typically automate much of the infusion calculation and delivery, adjusting citrate and calcium infusion rates in proportion to the prescribed blood flow rate so that the ratio of citrate delivered to blood volume presented to the circuit remains constant even as blood flow rate is adjusted during treatment, reducing the manual calculation burden that earlier, non-integrated citrate protocols placed on treating staff. This automation has contributed to citrate's expanding use in intermittent hemodialysis beyond its more established role in continuous renal replacement therapy, since much of the complexity that previously limited its practical adoption in a busy hemodialysis unit has been substantially reduced by integrated machine-based delivery.

Citrate's anticoagulant mechanism is distinct enough from heparin's that the two are not simply interchangeable choices along a single spectrum of anticoagulant intensity; heparin acts by potentiating antithrombin's inhibition of several clotting factors throughout the entire circulation wherever it distributes, while citrate acts locally and specifically by removing a cofactor, ionized calcium, required for multiple steps of the clotting cascade only within the segment of circuit where citrate concentration remains elevated. This mechanistic difference is precisely what allows citrate's effect to be confined regionally in a way that a systemically distributed heparin dose, by its very nature, cannot replicate regardless of how the heparin dose itself is adjusted.

Citrate anticoagulation is more extensively established in the continuous renal replacement therapy context discussed in Chapter 21, where its regional confinement offers a particularly strong advantage given the extended duration of continuous treatment, but its use in intermittent hemodialysis has grown as well, particularly in units caring for a population with a meaningfully elevated proportion of patients carrying significant bleeding risk, such as those in a hospital-based acute dialysis service.

Implementing citrate anticoagulation for intermittent hemodialysis requires machine software and consumable supplies specifically configured for citrate delivery and the associated calcium replacement, a more substantial infrastructure investment than the equipment adjustment required for a heparin dose change, and this investment is one practical reason citrate protocols have historically been more common in the continuous renal replacement therapy setting, where a smaller number of dedicated machines serve the entire program, than in a large outpatient hemodialysis unit running many machines simultaneously across a broad patient population with a lower average bleeding risk. Units considering wider adoption of citrate for intermittent hemodialysis weigh this infrastructure cost against the clinical benefit for their specific patient population's bleeding risk profile, a calculation that shifts meaningfully for a unit serving a hospital-based, higher-acuity population relative to a stable outpatient population.

Monitoring and Managing Citrate Anticoagulation

Citrate anticoagulation requires more intensive monitoring than standard heparin protocols, specifically serial measurement of ionized calcium at both the post-filter, pre-calcium-infusion point in the circuit and in the patient's own systemic circulation, since the two values are expected to differ substantially by design — low in the circuit itself, where citrate's chelating effect is intended, and normal systemically, where calcium replacement is intended to restore it — and monitoring both separately confirms the protocol is achieving its intended regional effect rather than either under- or over-correcting.

Citrate metabolism, occurring primarily in the liver, means patients with significant hepatic dysfunction may not clear infused citrate as effectively as patients with normal hepatic function, risking systemic citrate accumulation and a resulting metabolic alkalosis and hypocalcemia beyond what the protocol's calcium replacement is designed to correct; citrate protocols in patients with significant liver disease therefore require closer monitoring and, in some cases, dose adjustment relative to the standard protocol used in patients with normal hepatic function.

A rising total-to-ionized calcium ratio in the patient's systemic circulation, calculated from paired total and ionized calcium measurements, is a recognized early indicator of citrate accumulation before more overt metabolic derangement develops, and monitoring this ratio specifically in patients with any degree of hepatic impairment provides an earlier warning than waiting for systemic ionized calcium or acid-base status to drift outside their expected ranges.

A fifty-year-old man with cirrhosis and acute kidney injury requiring hemodialysis in an inpatient setting is placed on a standard citrate anticoagulation protocol given his elevated bleeding risk from underlying liver disease. Over the course of his second treatment, his systemic ionized calcium begins trending downward despite calcium infusion at the standard replacement rate, and his total-to-ionized calcium ratio is noted to be rising on serial monitoring. Recognizing these findings as early citrate accumulation related to his impaired hepatic citrate metabolism, his treating team increases his calcium infusion rate, reduces his citrate infusion rate modestly to lessen the total citrate load presented to his limited metabolic capacity, and monitors his ionized calcium and total-to-ionized ratio more frequently for the remainder of the treatment and subsequent sessions. His subsequent treatments proceed without further accumulation once this adjusted, more closely monitored protocol is in place. This case illustrates why standard citrate protocols, calibrated for patients with normal hepatic function, require proactive modification and closer monitoring in patients with significant liver disease rather than being applied unmodified and monitored only at the standard frequency.

Anticoagulation Considerations for Hemodiafiltration and High-Flux Therapies

Hemodiafiltration's substantial convective volume, discussed in Chapter 4, concentrates blood within the circuit to a greater degree than conventional diffusive hemodialysis, since a large volume of plasma water is continuously removed by ultrafiltration and replaced with substitution fluid, and this greater hemoconcentration within the circuit modestly elevates clotting risk relative to conventional hemodialysis at comparable blood flow rates, all else being equal. Anticoagulation protocols for patients on hemodiafiltration are therefore sometimes adjusted modestly upward relative to what the same patient would require on conventional hemodialysis, and units offering hemodiafiltration benefit from establishing this adjustment as a standard part of the hemodiafiltration order set rather than applying an unmodified conventional-hemodialysis anticoagulation dose and discovering the inadequacy only through recurrent circuit clotting that could have been anticipated from the outset.

The substitution fluid infusion point itself, whether pre-dilution, added to blood before it enters the dialyzer, or post-dilution, added after the dialyzer, also affects circuit clotting risk: post-dilution substitution, delivered after blood has already been maximally concentrated by ultrafiltration within the dialyzer, produces a higher degree of hemoconcentration at the point of highest filtration fraction than pre-dilution substitution does, and units using post-dilution hemodiafiltration should anticipate correspondingly higher anticoagulation requirements than the same patient would need on a pre-dilution protocol.

Filtration fraction, the proportion of plasma water entering the dialyzer that is ultimately removed by ultrafiltration over the course of the treatment, is a further parameter worth monitoring specifically in hemodiafiltration, since a filtration fraction pushed too high for a given blood flow rate concentrates the blood within the dialyzer to a degree that can precipitate clotting even with anticoagulation that would otherwise be entirely adequate for conventional hemodialysis at the same blood flow rate. Machine software on most contemporary hemodiafiltration platforms calculates and displays filtration fraction in real time and can be configured to alert staff if it approaches a threshold associated with elevated clotting risk, providing an additional layer of protection beyond anticoagulation dosing alone, and units newly adopting hemodiafiltration benefit from configuring and testing this alert threshold deliberately rather than relying on default settings that may not reflect the specific patient population and typical prescriptions the unit actually uses.

CAUTION: Citrate accumulation from impaired hepatic metabolism can produce systemic metabolic alkalosis and hypocalcemia beyond what standard calcium replacement corrects; monitor more closely in patients with significant liver disease.

DIALYSIS RECOGNITION & RESPONSE SYSTEM — Anticoagulation Decision Arcs

The Pattern: A patient with an elevated bleeding risk requires hemodialysis anticoagulation.

Stem Signature: A recent surgical procedure, active gastrointestinal bleeding, or another condition substantially elevating systemic bleeding risk in a patient who otherwise requires standard hemodialysis, with the treating team defaulting toward the unit's standard heparin protocol.

The Decision: Select regional citrate anticoagulation or an anticoagulation-free technique rather than standard systemic heparin, matching the anticoagulation approach to the patient's actual bleeding risk rather than applying the unit's default protocol uniformly.

Trap Logic: Standard heparin dosing is appropriate for most patients and can be applied by default without a deliberate check of the individual patient's bleeding risk profile, a check that becomes essential specifically in the subset of patients for whom systemic anticoagulation carries meaningfully elevated risk.

Response Anchor: An elevated bleeding risk is the trigger to select citrate or an anticoagulation-free approach — not a cue to proceed with the unit's standard heparin protocol by default.

Anticoagulation-Free Dialysis Techniques

Saline Flush Technique

Periodic saline flushes through the circuit, performed at intervals throughout treatment without any anticoagulant administered at all, dilute blood within the circuit and provide a visual check of early clot formation, offering a modest reduction in clotting risk relative to no intervention whatsoever, though at the cost of added fluid volume that must be accounted for in the patient's ultrafiltration goal and at a generally higher risk of circuit clotting than any pharmacologic anticoagulation approach.

This technique is most appropriate for patients with a very high bleeding risk in whom even citrate's regional, largely non-systemic effect is considered an unacceptable additional risk, and for treatments of shorter duration, since clotting risk accumulates progressively over the length of a treatment and a shorter session reduces the cumulative exposure during which clotting can develop without any anticoagulant protection at all.

Maximizing blood flow rate within what the patient's access safely tolerates, minimizing unnecessary interruptions to blood flow during treatment, and avoiding excessive ultrafiltration rates that concentrate blood within the circuit are additional supportive measures that reduce clotting risk during anticoagulation-free technique, none of which substitute for anticoagulation itself but each of which meaningfully reduces the residual clotting risk this technique otherwise carries.

Staff caring for a patient on anticoagulation-free technique benefit from explicit awareness that this approach carries a materially higher likelihood of requiring an unplanned circuit change mid-treatment than any anticoagulated approach, and should have a replacement dialyzer and circuit readily available before treatment begins rather than needing to source one reactively once clotting is already underway, since the time required to source a replacement circuit reactively adds to the total clotting exposure and can compound the very problem the anticoagulation-free approach was already accepting an elevated risk of.

Treatment duration itself is sometimes shortened deliberately for patients on anticoagulation-free technique, accepting a modest reduction in delivered Kt/V for a given session in exchange for a reduced cumulative clotting exposure window, a trade-off that is reasonable for the typically short-term circumstances in which anticoagulation-free technique is used — a brief period of severe bleeding risk expected to resolve — but that should be revisited and adjusted back toward standard treatment time once the patient's bleeding risk has sufficiently improved to permit a return to a more standard anticoagulation approach and, correspondingly, a more standard treatment duration without the same clotting-driven time constraint.

Heparin-Coated Circuit Components

Heparin-grafted or heparin-coated dialyzer membranes and circuit components, introduced in Chapter 5's discussion of specialized membrane surface modifications, provide localized anticoagulant activity along the blood-contacting surfaces of the circuit itself without requiring systemic heparin administration, offering an intermediate option between full anticoagulation-free technique and standard systemic heparin for patients whose bleeding risk is elevated but not so severe as to preclude any localized anticoagulant exposure whatsoever.

Because these surface-modified components reduce but do not eliminate clotting risk, they are frequently combined with the periodic saline flush technique described above for patients with the highest bleeding risk, rather than relied upon as a sole anticoagulation strategy, providing a layered approach that maximizes circuit patency within the constraints a given patient's bleeding risk imposes.

Selection among the anticoagulation-free and reduced-anticoagulation strategies described in this section — saline flush alone, heparin-coated components alone, or the two combined — is best guided by the specific reason a given patient's bleeding risk is elevated and by how that risk is expected to evolve, since a patient with a time-limited elevated risk, such as one recovering from a recent surgical procedure, may transition back to standard heparin once the acute risk period has passed, while a patient with a chronic, ongoing elevated bleeding risk requires a sustained strategy planned with that longer timeline in mind rather than treated as a temporary accommodation expected to resolve shortly.

Selection among the anticoagulation-free and minimal-anticoagulation options described in this section — saline flush alone, heparin-coated components alone, or the two combined — is best guided by the specific degree and nature of a given patient's bleeding risk rather than a uniform default applied to every patient whose risk is simply categorized as elevated: a patient with a moderate, time-limited elevation in bleeding risk, such as the perioperative scenario discussed later in this chapter, may be adequately served by heparin-coated components alone, while a patient with a severe, ongoing bleeding risk, such as active gastrointestinal hemorrhage, more often warrants the fullest combination of minimal-anticoagulation measures available.

Figure 8.2: Regional Citrate Anticoagulation Circuit Configuration

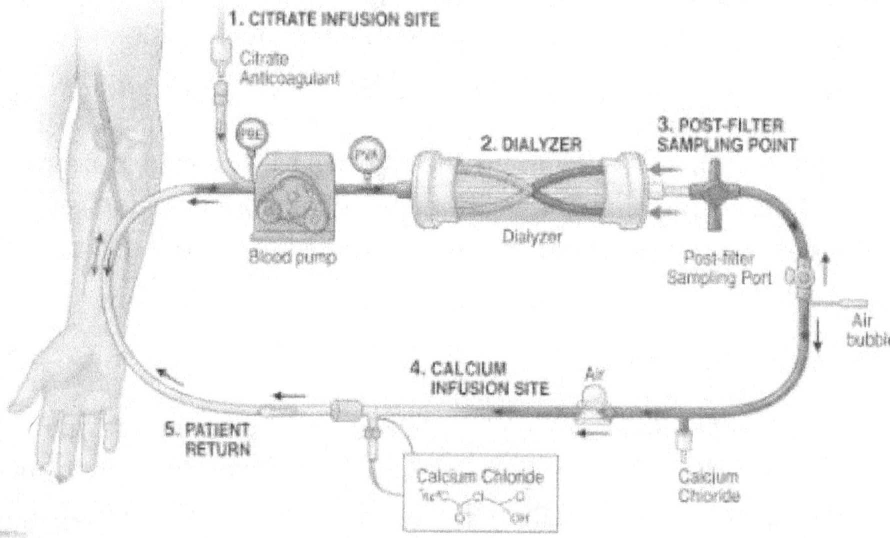

Managing Bleeding Risk and Clotting Complications

Recognizing and Responding to Circuit Clotting

Early circuit clotting typically presents as rising venous or pre-dialyzer pressure trends without an alternative explanation such as needle malposition, and recognizing this trend early, through the same pressure monitoring discussed in Chapter 5, allows intervention — a supplemental anticoagulant bolus where the patient's bleeding risk permits it, or planned early circuit replacement where it does not — before the circuit clots outright and treatment must be interrupted unexpectedly.

A circuit that clots despite appropriate anticoagulation warrants review of the anticoagulation protocol itself — whether dosing was adequate for the patient's individual heparin sensitivity, whether a citrate protocol's calcium and citrate infusion rates were properly calibrated — rather than simply replacing the circuit and continuing with an unmodified protocol that may clot again on the next treatment for the same underlying reason.

Repeated clotting despite an apparently adequate anticoagulation protocol should also prompt consideration of access-related contributors independent of anticoagulation itself, since a stenotic access delivering inadequate blood flow relative to the prescribed rate produces blood stasis within the circuit that can overwhelm even properly dosed anticoagulation, meaning the appropriate response to recurrent clotting is not always a change to the anticoagulation protocol but sometimes an evaluation of the access supplying the circuit in the first place.

A pattern of recurrent clotting confined to a specific dialyzer model or lot, occurring across multiple different patients rather than in a single patient specifically, points toward a manufacturing or membrane-related explanation rather than an anticoagulation or access issue in any individual patient, and recognizing this cross-patient pattern, in the same spirit as the water-treatment clustering discussed in Chapter 5, is what distinguishes a systemic equipment issue from an individual patient's anticoagulation or access problem. Units experiencing an unusual increase in circuit clotting across several patients within a short period should consider this possibility alongside the individual-patient causes discussed throughout this section.

Documentation of clotting episodes, including the specific dialyzer lot, the anticoagulation protocol and dose in use, and the point in treatment at which clotting was identified, supports exactly this kind of pattern recognition over time, allowing a unit's quality review process to distinguish an isolated, patient-specific event from a recurring pattern warranting broader investigation, whether that investigation ultimately points toward an equipment issue, a systematic gap in a particular anticoagulation protocol, or a training need among staff responsible for administering and monitoring anticoagulation across the unit.

A quarterly or similarly scheduled review of aggregated clotting episode data across a unit's full patient population, rather than reviewing each episode only in isolation as it occurs, surfaces patterns that would otherwise remain invisible at the level of any single patient's care — for example, a disproportionate clustering of clotting episodes among patients using a particular anticoagulation-free protocol, suggesting the protocol's supportive measures may need reinforcement, or among patients dialyzed on a specific machine, suggesting an equipment-specific issue worth investigating independent of any individual patient's clinical factors.

Managing Bleeding Complications

Excessive bleeding from needle or catheter sites following treatment, beyond what typically resolves with standard direct pressure over several minutes, should prompt reassessment of the anticoagulation approach used for that treatment, including whether heparin dosing was excessive relative to the patient's individual sensitivity or whether an underlying platelet dysfunction, discussed in Chapter 1 as a feature of the uremic milieu itself, is contributing independent of the anticoagulant technique chosen.

Bleeding risk assessment for anticoagulation purposes should be revisited at the same cadence as the broader prescription review described in Chapter 6, since a patient's bleeding risk is not a fixed, one-time determination made at dialysis initiation but a status that can change with a new medication affecting platelet function or coagulation, a new diagnosis such as a bleeding disorder or hepatic dysfunction, or a scheduled surgical procedure requiring temporary anticoagulation modification in the surrounding period. Coordinating anticoagulation adjustments around a planned surgical procedure specifically — often requiring a temporary shift to citrate or anticoagulation-free technique for the treatments immediately surrounding the procedure — is a common, foreseeable need that benefits from advance planning with the surgical team rather than being addressed reactively on the day of the procedure itself.

A sixty-three-year-old woman recently started on hemodialysis develops prolonged oozing from her catheter exit site after each of her first several treatments, well beyond the several minutes of direct pressure typically sufficient to achieve hemostasis. Reviewing her case, her nephrology team identifies that her standard weight-based heparin dose, while appropriate for most patients, has produced a clotting time indicating excessive anticoagulation for her specifically, likely reflecting individual heparin sensitivity rather than any protocol error. Her heparin dose is reduced and clotting time is rechecked to confirm adequate but not excessive anticoagulation at the lower dose; her post-treatment oozing resolves over her next several sessions. This case illustrates that standard weight-based heparin dosing, while a reasonable starting point, should be verified against measured clotting time and adjusted for individual sensitivity rather than assumed to be correctly calibrated for every patient at a given weight-based dose, echoing the same individualization principle this book has applied to dialysate composition in Chapter 6 and to dialysis prescription broadly throughout Part II.

A separate illustrative scenario involves a seventy-year-old man on standard heparin anticoagulation who is scheduled for an elective hernia repair in ten days. Rather than continuing his standard heparin protocol unmodified through the perioperative period, his nephrology team coordinates with the surgical service in advance, shifting his anticoagulation to an anticoagulation-free saline-flush technique for the treatment immediately preceding surgery and for the first treatment following it, then transitioning back to his standard heparin protocol once the surgical team confirms adequate wound healing and no ongoing bleeding concern. This advance coordination avoids both the risk of an unmodified heparin dose complicating perioperative hemostasis and the alternative failure mode of last-minute, poorly planned anticoagulation changes made reactively once the surgical team raises a concern shortly before the procedure. This case underscores a broader point applicable throughout this chapter: bleeding risk is not static, and anticoagulation planning benefits from anticipating foreseeable changes in that risk rather than only reacting once a complication has already occurred, a lesson that applies equally to the surgical scenario above and to the slower, more gradual changes in bleeding risk that accompany an evolving comorbidity profile over a patient's dialysis course.

Building a standing perioperative anticoagulation pathway into a unit's protocols — a checklist triggered automatically whenever a patient's chart is flagged for an upcoming procedure, specifying the anticipated anticoagulation adjustment and its timing relative to the procedure date — extends the same systemic, workflow-embedded approach this book has recommended for Life-Plan revision, goals-of-care review, and dialysis adequacy monitoring to the anticoagulation domain specifically, reinforcing the recurring principle that sound clinical judgment reliably changes practice only when built into a repeatable structure rather than left to individual recall in a busy clinical environment, rather than relying on any single clinician to remember every patient's upcoming procedure schedule unaided.

CLINICAL PEARL: Prolonged post-treatment bleeding despite standard heparin dosing should prompt clotting time verification and individualized dose adjustment rather than assuming the standard weight-based dose is correctly calibrated for every patient.

DIALYSIS RECOGNITION & RESPONSE SYSTEM — Anticoagulation Decision Arcs

---

The Pattern: A patient experiences recurrent circuit clotting or prolonged post-treatment bleeding despite an apparently standard anticoagulation protocol.

Stem Signature: Repeated early circuit clotting requiring dialyzer replacement, or prolonged oozing from needle or catheter sites beyond several minutes of direct pressure, in a patient receiving standard weight-based heparin dosing without individualized clotting time verification.

The Decision: Measure clotting time directly to assess whether the standard dose is under- or over-anticoagulating this specific patient, and adjust the dose based on that measurement rather than continuing an unmodified standard protocol or empirically guessing at an adjustment.

Trap Logic: Recurrent clotting or bleeding on a standard protocol can be attributed to the access, the circuit equipment, or chance, when individual variation in heparin sensitivity, which a standard weight-based dose does not account for, is a common and directly testable explanation.

Response Anchor: Recurrent clotting or bleeding on a standard heparin protocol warrants direct clotting time measurement and individualized dose adjustment, not an assumption that the standard dose must be correctly calibrated.

Elevated Bleeding Risk Requiring Dialysis: Select citrate or an anticoagulation-free technique matched to the patient's actual bleeding risk, rather than the unit's standard heparin protocol by default.

Unexplained Platelet Decline After Heparin Exposure: Evaluate for heparin-induced thrombocytopenia and, if confirmed or suspected, eliminate heparin from every exposure source, not only the treatment dose.

Recurrent Clotting or Bleeding on Standard Dosing: Measure clotting time directly and adjust for individual heparin sensitivity rather than assuming the standard weight-based dose is correctly calibrated.

Summary and Key Concepts

Standard hemodialysis anticoagulation uses unfractionated or low molecular weight heparin, each with a distinct half-life and dosing profile that should be matched to the patient's bleeding risk and treatment schedule, and verified against measured clotting time rather than assumed from weight-based dosing alone.

Regional citrate anticoagulation confines the anticoagulant effect to the extracorporeal circuit through calcium chelation and replacement, offering a specific advantage for patients with elevated systemic bleeding risk, though it requires more intensive monitoring and caution in hepatic dysfunction.

Anticoagulation-free techniques, including saline flushes and heparin-coated circuit components, carry higher clotting risk but are appropriate for patients whose bleeding risk precludes even citrate's largely regional effect.

Circuit clotting despite appropriate anticoagulation warrants review of the protocol itself and consideration of access-related contributors, rather than simple circuit replacement, and prolonged post-treatment bleeding warrants clotting time verification rather than an assumption that standard weight-based dosing is correctly calibrated for every patient.

CHAPTER 9: VASCULAR ACCESS PLANNING AND CREATION: FISTULA, GRAFT, AND CATHETER

Learning Objectives

Describe preoperative vessel mapping and how it informs vascular access selection.

Explain the physiology of arteriovenous fistula maturation and the timeline it requires.

Compare arteriovenous graft configurations and their role relative to fistulas.

Apply the ESKD Life-Plan framework from Chapter 2 to select an access type matched to an individual patient's trajectory.

Chapter Overview

Chapter 2 established the Life-Plan framework that determines which modality, and therefore which access, a given patient's trajectory should point toward. This chapter turns from that planning framework to the technical process of actually creating hemodialysis vascular access: how vessels are evaluated and selected preoperatively, how a fistula is constructed and matures into a usable access, how a graft differs from a fistula in construction and role, and how the choice among fistula, graft, and catheter should ultimately be reasoned through for an individual patient rather than defaulted to a single access type regardless of circumstance. The chapters that follow build directly on this foundation: Chapter 10 addresses how a matured access is actually cannulated and examined at the bedside, Chapter 11 addresses the complications that can develop in an established access over time, and Chapter 12 turns to the central venous catheter this chapter has repeatedly referenced as the option to be minimized wherever a durable surgical access is feasible. Read together, these four chapters trace a single access from initial vessel evaluation through years of clinical use, and the recurring emphasis on proactive surveillance and early intervention introduced here recurs, in modified form, throughout the remainder of Part III and, indeed, throughout this book as a whole.

Preoperative Vessel Mapping and Selection

Physical Examination and Duplex Ultrasound Mapping

Preoperative evaluation begins with physical examination of the candidate arm, assessing for adequate superficial veins by inspection and palpation, checking for a palpable radial and ulnar pulse confirming adequate arterial inflow, and performing an Allen test or equivalent assessment to confirm collateral hand perfusion will be preserved if the radial artery is used for a distal fistula configuration. While physical examination provides a useful initial impression, it is not sufficiently precise on its own to confirm adequate vessel caliber for surgical planning, particularly in patients with a higher body mass index in whom superficial veins may be present but not readily palpable.

Duplex ultrasound vessel mapping, performed as a dedicated preoperative study, measures vein diameter, patency, and continuity along the vessel's accessible length, and measures arterial diameter and flow characteristics at the anticipated anastomosis site, thereby providing the objective data needed to select both the specific vessel and the specific configuration — radiocephalic, brachiocephalic, or an alternative arrangement — most likely to mature successfully into a durable, long-term access. Minimum vein and artery diameter thresholds, established through outcome studies correlating preoperative vessel size with subsequent maturation success, guide this selection, though these thresholds function as general guidance informing surgical judgment rather than as an absolute cutoff applied mechanically without considering the full clinical picture.

Mapping also assesses the full length of the candidate vein rather than only the segment nearest the anticipated anastomosis, since an adequate diameter at the anastomosis site does not guarantee adequate diameter further along the vessel where cannulation will actually occur during treatment, and a vein that narrows unexpectedly partway along its accessible length may still mature adequately near the anastomosis while remaining unsuitable for cannulation at the segment where needles would actually need to be placed. This full-length assessment is part of why a dedicated mapping study, rather than a limited point-of-care ultrasound check at a single site, is the standard for adequate preoperative planning.

Central venous and arterial inflow assessment complements peripheral vessel mapping for patients with risk factors suggesting central pathology, including any history of central venous catheterization, cardiac device leads traversing the central veins, or symptoms suggesting arterial insufficiency such as claudication or a markedly diminished pulse on examination; identifying a central or inflow problem before peripheral access creation, rather than only after a peripherally well-planned access fails to function adequately, avoids the wasted procedural effort and delayed access availability that this sequencing error produces.

Cardiac implantable device leads deserve particular attention in this preoperative assessment, since a pacemaker or defibrillator lead traversing the subclavian and innominate veins on the same side as a planned access can produce central venous stenosis analogous to that caused by a prior dialysis catheter, and this device-related stenosis is sometimes overlooked specifically because it is not typically considered part of the standard vascular access history in the way prior catheter placement routinely is. Reviewing a patient's full device history, not only their dialysis and catheter history specifically, as part of preoperative central assessment closes this gap, and is best incorporated as a standard checklist item in the preoperative evaluation rather than left to be volunteered by the patient or discovered incidentally on imaging obtained for another purpose.

Selecting the Optimal Configuration and Site

Vessel selection follows a distal-to-proximal preference where anatomically feasible, favoring a wrist-level radiocephalic fistula as a first choice when vessel mapping supports it, both because a more distal access preserves more proximal vessels for a future access should the first one eventually fail, and because a successfully matured distal fistula generally carries a lower risk of the high-flow complications, discussed in Chapter 11, that can accompany a more proximal, larger-vessel configuration. Where distal vessels are inadequate on mapping, a more proximal brachiocephalic or brachiobasilic configuration is selected instead, accepting the trade-offs this proximal shift carries in exchange for the higher likelihood of successful maturation a larger-caliber vessel offers.

Site selection also accounts for the non-dominant arm being generally preferred over the dominant arm where vessel quality is comparable between the two, since a non-dominant-arm access interferes less with a patient's daily activities and self-care during the years of repeated cannulation that typically follow, and accounts for any prior central venous catheterization history in that arm, since central vein stenosis from a prior catheter, discussed further in Chapter 12, can compromise venous outflow from an otherwise well-selected peripheral access even when the peripheral vessels themselves appear adequate on mapping.

Because the most distal viable site is generally preferred specifically to preserve more proximal vessels for a future access, surgical planning for a patient's first access ideally considers the full sequence of future accesses that patient may eventually need over a multi-decade dialysis course, rather than optimizing only for the single access currently being created. This forward-looking approach, sometimes termed vessel preservation strategy in analogy to the interdialytic vein preservation principle introduced in Chapter 1, treats each access creation decision as one step in an anticipated sequence rather than an isolated procedure, a perspective particularly relevant for younger patients whose anticipated dialysis course, absent a successful transplant, may span several successive accesses over many years of ongoing treatment.

A brachiobasilic configuration, in which the basilic vein, running along the medial and posterior aspect of the upper arm rather than the more superficial and anteriorly located cephalic vein, is used for fistula creation, requires the vein to be surgically transposed to a more superficial position accessible for cannulation, since the basilic vein's native depth would otherwise make repeated needling impractical. This transposition adds surgical complexity relative to a standard cephalic-based fistula but extends fistula candidacy to patients whose cephalic vein is inadequate while their basilic vein remains suitable, illustrating that the fistula-versus-graft decision is not always a binary determined solely by cephalic vein quality.

Handling the Poor Candidate: When No Site Appears Adequate

A subset of patients present with bilateral upper extremity vessel mapping showing inadequate quality throughout, whether from longstanding diabetes-related vascular disease, extensive prior venous access history that has damaged multiple potential sites, or intrinsically small-caliber vessels unrelated to any specific damaging history, and this population requires a more extensive evaluation before an access plan can be finalized rather than a prompt default to catheter dependence. Lower extremity vessels, thigh-based fistula or graft configurations using the femoral vessels, and, less commonly, chest wall or other atypical configurations have all been described as options for this population, each carrying its own specific complication profile and requiring a surgical team experienced in these less common configurations.

Central venogram, evaluating the central veins for stenosis or occlusion from prior catheter use, is a necessary component of this extended evaluation, since even adequate peripheral vessels cannot support a functional access if central venous outflow is compromised, and identifying a central stenosis before attempting peripheral access creation avoids the frustrating and clinically costly scenario of a technically successful peripheral fistula or graft that fails to function adequately because of an unrecognized central outflow problem. For the small subset of patients in whom no surgical access option is ultimately feasible despite this extended evaluation, a well-managed, infection-minimized catheter approach, discussed fully in Chapter 12, becomes the necessary long-term access strategy rather than a temporary bridge, and this population's care benefits from the most rigorous possible application of the catheter-specific infection prevention measures that chapter describes.

Referral to a vascular access specialist or a dedicated multidisciplinary access planning clinic, where available, is particularly valuable for this poor-candidate population, since the range of atypical configurations and salvage techniques applicable to difficult vascular anatomy exceeds what a general surgical or nephrology practice encounters routinely enough to maintain deep familiarity with every option. Early referral to such specialized resources, before a patient has exhausted more conventional options through repeated failed attempts, generally yields better outcomes than referral only after standard approaches have already been tried and found unsuccessful, since some atypical configurations are more feasible when the patient's remaining vessel and central venous anatomy has not yet been further compromised by additional failed access attempts, and since the specialist team's experience with these less common configurations translates into a more efficient, better-planned procedure than a general surgical team encountering the same anatomy for the first time.

A multidisciplinary vascular access conference, bringing together nephrology, vascular or transplant surgery, and interventional radiology on a regular schedule to review upcoming and problematic access cases collectively rather than each discipline managing its portion of a given patient's access planning in isolation, has been adopted in a number of centers specifically to improve outcomes for this more complex population, mirroring the same multidisciplinary coordination principle this book has applied to Life-Plan construction in Chapter 2 and conservative care planning in Chapter 3. Such a conference allows the surgical team's assessment of technical feasibility, the interventional radiology team's assessment of salvage options for a failing access, and the nephrology team's assessment of the patient's overall trajectory and modality goals to inform a single, coordinated access plan rather than three separate, potentially inconsistent recommendations reaching the patient through different channels, a coordination benefit that becomes increasingly valuable as a patient's access history and vascular anatomy grow more complex over a longer dialysis course.

KEY POINT: Preoperative duplex ultrasound vessel mapping, not physical examination alone, provides the vessel diameter and patency data needed to select the access configuration most likely to mature successfully.

Figure 9.1: Preoperative Vessel Mapping for Fistula Planning

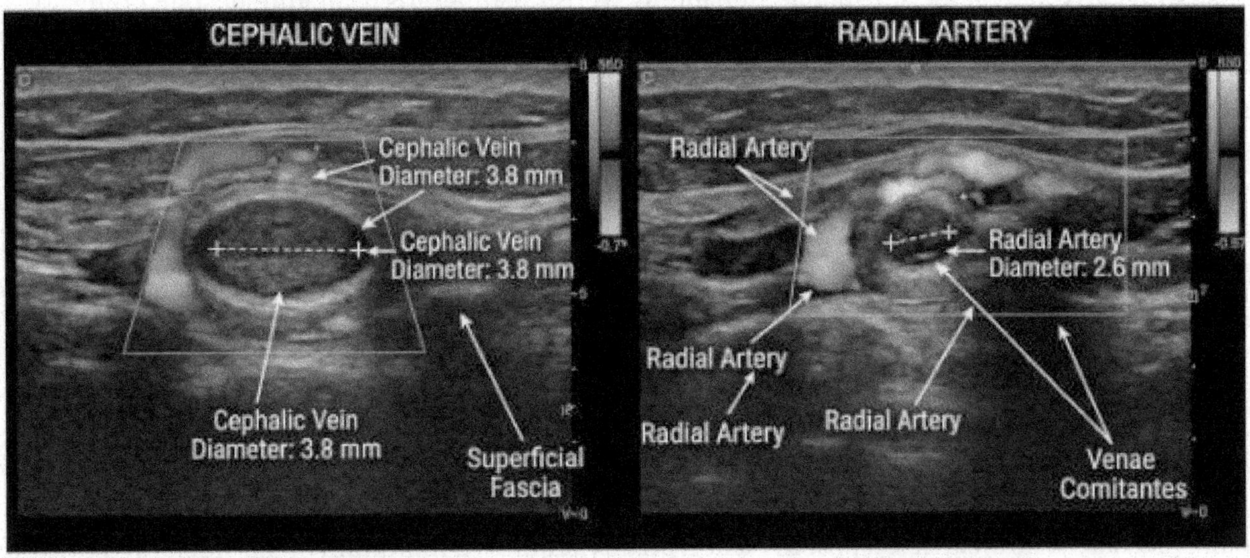

CEPHALIC VEIN RADIAL ARTERY

Arteriovenous Fistula Creation and Maturation

The Surgical Anastomosis and Early Postoperative Course

Fistula creation involves surgically joining the selected artery and vein directly, most commonly in a side-to-side or end-vein-to-side-artery configuration, allowing arterial blood to flow directly into the venous system without an intervening prosthetic conduit, and it is this direct arterial-to-venous connection, exposing the vein to arterial pressure and flow for the first time, that drives the maturation process discussed in the next subsection. The immediate postoperative period focuses on confirming a palpable thrill and audible bruit at the anastomosis, both indicating adequate flow through the newly created connection, and monitoring for early complications including bleeding, wound infection, and, in the distal hand, signs of the steal syndrome discussed further in Chapter 11.

Postoperative patient education at this stage, distinct from the cannulation-specific education addressed in Chapter 10, focuses on protecting the new access from external pressure, avoiding blood pressure measurement or blood draws on the affected arm, and recognizing early warning signs — loss of thrill, new pain, or swelling — that warrant prompt evaluation rather than being dismissed as expected postoperative discomfort.

Postoperative exercise, most commonly a simple regimen of intermittent hand-grip exercise performed with the affected arm, has been proposed and studied as a means of promoting more robust maturation by increasing flow through the developing fistula during the critical early weeks, though evidence for its independent benefit beyond standard postoperative care is mixed across available studies. Where recommended by the surgical team, this exercise is generally framed to patients as a low-risk, potentially beneficial adjunct rather than a guaranteed solution to maturation concerns, since attributing too much weight to an intervention with uncertain independent benefit risks both false reassurance in patients who exercise diligently and undue self-blame in patients whose fistula fails to mature despite doing so.

The choice of anesthesia for fistula creation, most commonly regional block anesthesia rather than general anesthesia, carries a secondary physiologic benefit beyond its primary role in surgical pain control: the sympathetic blockade accompanying a regional block produces vasodilation in the operated limb that may modestly enhance early postoperative flow through the newly created fistula relative to what would be achieved under general anesthesia alone, a consideration that has informed anesthesia selection for fistula creation procedures in centers where regional block technique is routinely available and the patient's overall clinical status permits its use.

Physiology of Maturation

Maturation describes the vein's physiologic adaptation to arterial flow and pressure over the weeks following creation: the vein wall thickens and the vessel dilates in response to the markedly increased flow and pressure it now carries, a process that typically requires a minimum of six weeks and often longer before the vessel reaches a caliber and wall thickness adequate to tolerate repeated cannulation, though the exact timeline varies considerably based on the patient's underlying vessel quality, the configuration created, and individual healing characteristics.

The commonly cited "rule of sixes" — a fistula reaching approximately six millimeters in diameter, located no more than six millimeters below the skin surface, with a flow rate of approximately six hundred milliliters per minute, roughly six weeks after creation — offers a useful mnemonic framework for assessing maturation adequacy, though these figures function as general benchmarks informing clinical judgment rather than precise thresholds that must be met exactly before an access can be safely used. Maturation assessment combining physical examination with a follow-up ultrasound to confirm diameter, depth, and flow provides a more reliable basis for the decision to proceed with cannulation than physical examination alone.

The physiologic driver of this dilation and wall thickening is the markedly increased wall shear stress the vein experiences once arterialized, a hemodynamic stimulus that triggers endothelial and smooth muscle remodeling analogous, though distinct in its specific mechanisms, to the vascular remodeling seen in other high-flow physiologic states; a vein that fails to experience adequate shear stress, whether from inadequate arterial inflow, a downstream outflow obstruction, or diversion of flow through an accessory branch, will correspondingly fail to remodel adequately, which is precisely why the maturation failure discussed in the next subsection so often traces back to one of these specific, identifiable flow-limiting causes rather than to an unexplained general failure of the maturation process.

This shear-stress-driven remodeling also explains why a fistula's favorable characteristics tend to continue improving somewhat even after the initial maturation period has passed and the access has already been in successful clinical use for some time, since ongoing exposure to arterial flow continues to exert the same remodeling stimulus, within limits, that drove the initial maturation process; this is part of why an established, well-functioning fistula used for years is generally considered a more robust and reliable access than one only recently matured to the minimum threshold needed for initial cannulation, a distinction relevant when weighing the relative durability of an existing older fistula against a newly matured alternative in a patient requiring a second or subsequent access over the course of a long dialysis history.

Managing Maturation Failure

A meaningful proportion of newly created fistulas, across all surgical series and patient populations reported in the literature, fail to mature adequately for cannulation despite an apparently well-performed surgical creation, most commonly due to a juxta-anastomotic stenosis, a focal narrowing near the surgical connection itself that limits the flow needed to drive full maturation of the vessel, or due to accessory vein branches diverting flow away from the intended cannulation segment before it has the chance to dilate adequately over time. Recognizing maturation failure early, through the scheduled follow-up assessment described above rather than only once cannulation is attempted and found unsuccessful, allows for a corrective intervention — angioplasty of a juxta-anastomotic stenosis or ligation of a diverting accessory branch — that can salvage the existing fistula rather than requiring an entirely new access creation procedure.

A patient whose fistula has not matured adequately by ten to twelve weeks after creation, without an identified and correctable cause, is generally referred back for further vascular evaluation and, where salvage is not feasible, for creation of an alternative access rather than continuing to wait indefinitely for a maturation process that has already extended well beyond the typical expected timeline, since prolonged waiting without intervention delays the point at which the patient has a usable access and may unnecessarily prolong reliance on a central venous catheter in the interim, a delay with its own attendant infection and complication risks that must be weighed against the possibility, however uncertain, that further waiting alone might eventually yield a usable fistula.

Salvage success rates for a correctable maturation failure — angioplasty of a focal stenosis or ligation of a single diverting branch — are generally favorable when the underlying cause is identified and addressed within this ten-to-twelve-week window, but decline the longer intervention is delayed, since a chronically underdeveloped vein subjected to prolonged inadequate flow can undergo secondary changes that make it a poorer surgical or endovascular candidate even once the original flow-limiting lesion is corrected. This time-sensitivity is a further reason scheduled maturation assessment, rather than assessment only once cannulation is attempted, matters practically rather than merely as a procedural formality.

A twenty-nine-year-old woman with a radiocephalic fistula created eight weeks earlier presents for scheduled maturation assessment with a palpable thrill but a vein diameter on ultrasound modestly below the expected threshold and flow measured at approximately three hundred milliliters per minute, well below the anticipated range for a fistula of this age. Rather than proceeding to attempt cannulation despite these borderline findings, or waiting further without evaluation, her team obtains a fistulogram, which identifies a discrete juxta-anastomotic stenosis narrowing the vessel immediately downstream of the surgical connection. Angioplasty of this stenosis is performed the same week, and repeat assessment two weeks later shows the fistula now meeting standard maturation criteria, with flow increased to approximately seven hundred milliliters per minute and vein diameter now adequate for cannulation. She proceeds to successful cannulation and use of the fistula without further complication. This case illustrates the salvage pathway this chapter recommends: identifying a discrete, correctable lesion promptly at scheduled assessment, rather than waiting to see whether an already-borderline fistula might improve on its own, converted what could have become a maturation failure requiring an entirely new access into a successfully salvaged, usable fistula within a matter of weeks.

DIALYSIS RECOGNITION & RESPONSE SYSTEM — Access Creation Arcs

The Pattern: A fistula fails to show adequate maturation at the scheduled six-week assessment.

Stem Signature: A fistula that, at scheduled follow-up assessment approximately six weeks after creation, lacks the expected diameter, depth, or flow characteristics despite an apparently uncomplicated surgical creation and early postoperative course.

The Decision: Pursue targeted vascular imaging to identify a correctable cause — juxta-anastomotic stenosis or a diverting accessory branch — and intervene to salvage the fistula, rather than waiting further in the hope that maturation will proceed on its own or proceeding directly to an entirely new access creation without first evaluating for a salvageable cause.

Trap Logic: Delayed maturation can be mistaken for a fistula simply needing more time, when a correctable structural cause is present in a substantial proportion of cases and becomes progressively less salvageable the longer intervention is delayed.

Response Anchor: Inadequate maturation at the scheduled assessment warrants targeted imaging for a correctable cause before further waiting or before abandoning the fistula for a new access creation.

Arteriovenous Graft Placement and Configuration

Graft Material and Configuration Options

An arteriovenous graft uses a prosthetic conduit, most commonly constructed from expanded polytetrafluoroethylene, to connect an artery and vein where the patient's own vessels are unsuitable for a direct fistula connection, most often due to inadequate vein caliber or quality on preoperative mapping. Because the graft material itself, rather than a maturing native vein, is what is cannulated during treatment, a graft can typically be used sooner after creation than a fistula, once postoperative swelling has resolved and the graft has incorporated adequately into surrounding tissue, generally within two to four weeks rather than the six or more weeks a fistula requires.

Graft configurations vary in shape — straight, curved, or looped — chosen based on the specific vessels available and the geometry needed to connect them without excessive tension or kinking, and in some centers grafts incorporating self-sealing material designed to tolerate earlier cannulation, sometimes within hours of placement, are used specifically for patients requiring more urgent access than even the standard graft timeline allows, though these specialized grafts carry their own cost and availability considerations relative to standard graft material.

Graft diameter is generally more uniform and predictable than the variable caliber of a maturing native vein, which can simplify cannulation technique once the graft is ready for use, though this same uniformity means a graft's total cannulation surface is fixed at the time of placement rather than capable of the further favorable remodeling a native fistula can continue to undergo over months to years of use, a distinction relevant to long-term access planning for a patient anticipated to require dialysis access for an extended period.

Biologic graft materials, derived from processed human or animal tissue rather than synthetic polymer, have also been used in select circumstances, particularly where infection risk or prior graft infection makes a fully synthetic material less desirable, though these materials carry their own cost, availability, and durability trade-offs relative to standard synthetic grafts and are generally reserved for specific clinical scenarios rather than used as a routine first-line alternative to synthetic material.

Grafts Relative to Fistulas: Trade-offs

Grafts generally carry a higher risk of both infection and thrombosis compared to a mature native fistula, reflecting the foreign material's greater susceptibility to bacterial colonization and the graft-vein anastomosis's tendency to develop venous stenosis from the intimal hyperplasia response the prosthetic-to-native-vessel junction provokes, a mechanism discussed further in Chapter 11's treatment of vascular access complications, and one that distinguishes the graft-specific complication profile from the complication profile of a mature fistula in ways clinicians should recognize when counseling a patient about to undergo graft rather than fistula creation. These considerations are precisely why the vessel mapping and configuration selection described earlier in this chapter favor a native fistula wherever vessel quality permits, reserving grafts specifically for patients whose vessels do not support a viable fistula option.

Registry data comparing fistula and graft outcomes consistently shows fistulas achieving longer functional patency and requiring fewer interventions per year of use than grafts, though this aggregate comparison should be interpreted with the same caution applied to modality comparisons in Chapter 2: fistulas and grafts are not typically created in identical patient populations, since grafts are disproportionately placed in patients whose vessel quality was already assessed as poorer, meaning some, though likely not all, of the observed outcome difference reflects underlying patient and vessel characteristics rather than an intrinsic property of the graft material itself. This caveat does not undermine the general preference for fistula creation where feasible, but it does argue against over-interpreting the absolute magnitude of the fistula-graft outcome gap as evidence of graft material inferiority in isolation from the population differences that accompany real-world graft placement patterns.

Despite these trade-offs, a graft remains a considerably better option than prolonged reliance on a central venous catheter for a patient whose vessels genuinely do not support fistula creation, since even a graft's elevated infection and thrombosis risk relative to a fistula remains substantially lower than a catheter's risk profile, discussed in full in Chapter 12, making the graft-versus-catheter comparison, rather than the graft-versus-fistula comparison alone, the more clinically relevant framing for a patient who has already been assessed as a poor fistula candidate.

CLINICAL PEARL: For a patient without adequate vessels for a fistula, the clinically relevant comparison is graft versus catheter, not graft versus fistula — a graft's elevated risk relative to a fistula remains considerably lower than a catheter's risk profile.

Graft Surveillance and Early Revision

Because a graft's thrombosis risk is driven predominantly by venous anastomotic stenosis developing progressively over the graft's lifespan, routine surveillance — combining physical examination for changes in thrill character and venous pressure trends observed during dialysis, discussed in Chapter 5, with periodic formal imaging in some protocols — aims to detect a developing stenosis before it progresses to outright thrombosis, since a stenosis identified and treated with angioplasty while the graft remains patent carries a considerably better prognosis than an already-thrombosed graft requiring thrombectomy or replacement.

A graft that has already thrombosed can sometimes be salvaged through mechanical or pharmacomechanical thrombectomy combined with angioplasty of the underlying stenosis that precipitated the clot, restoring graft function without requiring an entirely new access creation procedure, though repeated thrombosis episodes in the same graft eventually favor consideration of a new access rather than continued salvage attempts, since each thrombosis and subsequent intervention carries its own cumulative risk and progressively narrows the graft's remaining useful lifespan. The threshold for shifting from repeated salvage toward new access creation is a matter of clinical judgment weighing the specific stenosis pattern, the patient's remaining vessel options, and the practical burden repeated interventions place on the patient, rather than a fixed number of permitted salvage attempts applied uniformly.

Documenting each surveillance finding and intervention in a manner accessible across the full treating team, rather than only in the interventionalist's own procedural notes, allows the pattern of a given graft's stenosis recurrence and intervention history to inform the salvage-versus-replacement judgment described above; a graft with a well-documented history of recurring stenosis at the same anatomic site despite repeated angioplasty presents a different clinical picture, and a different threshold for considering replacement, than one with an isolated single stenosis successfully treated without recurrence.

Figure 9.2: Arteriovenous Graft Configurations

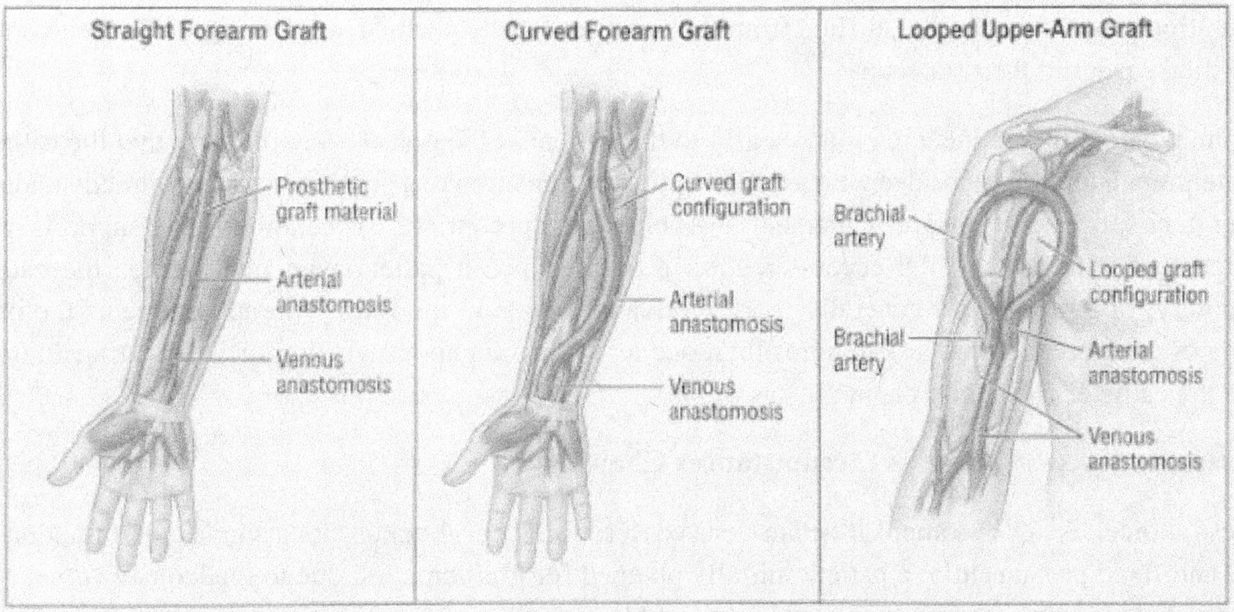

Choosing Access Type Within the Life-Plan

Matching Access Creation Timing to the Life-Plan

The choice among fistula, graft, and catheter, and the timing of whichever access creation procedure is pursued, follows directly from the Life-Plan framework established in Chapter 2 rather than from vessel mapping results alone: a patient with excellent vessel quality but a near-term preemptive transplant already scheduled may reasonably defer any access creation, as discussed in Chapter 2's worked example, while a patient with equally excellent vessel quality but no transplant prospect proceeds to fistula creation timed to the trajectory established in Chapter 1.

A patient whose Life-Plan anticipates a multi-year hemodialysis course without a near-term transplant prospect is the clearest candidate for prioritizing fistula creation and accepting the longer maturation timeline this requires, since the fistula's superior long-term infection and thrombosis profile relative to a graft or catheter compounds in value the longer the anticipated duration of use, while a patient with a shorter anticipated hemodialysis course, such as one bridging to an already-scheduled transplant, may reasonably accept a graft's faster availability or, in the shortest-bridge scenarios discussed in Chapter 2, a catheter, if the anticipated duration of use is too brief for a fistula's maturation timeline to be worthwhile.

This timing calculus also interacts with the late-referred patient scenario discussed in Chapter 2: a patient identified with advanced kidney disease only shortly before dialysis becomes necessary, with no runway for fistula maturation before treatment must begin, requires an initial catheter as a bridge regardless of otherwise-excellent vessel quality, with fistula or graft creation pursued in parallel once the immediate need for dialysis has been addressed, rather than delaying dialysis initiation itself to await fistula maturation in a patient whose clinical status does not permit that delay. The access type ultimately used for long-term treatment in this scenario still follows the same vessel-quality-driven selection process described throughout this chapter; only the sequencing, catheter first while fistula or graft creation and maturation proceed in parallel, differs from the unhurried, well-planned sequencing available to a patient identified earlier in their trajectory.

Communicating this sequencing plan clearly to the patient at the outset — explaining that the catheter is an intentional, temporary bridge with a defined plan for transition to a permanent access already underway, rather than an open-ended arrangement — helps set appropriate expectations and supports patient engagement with the parallel access-creation process, since a patient who understands the catheter's temporary, bridging role is generally more motivated to attend the follow-up appointments the parallel fistula or graft creation process requires than one left uncertain about whether or when a transition away from the catheter is actually planned.

Reassessing Access Choice as Circumstances Change

Access choice, like every other Life-Plan-derived decision in this book, is not a single determination made once and fixed permanently: a patient initially planned for graft creation due to inadequate vessel quality on an initial mapping study may, following weight loss or other physiologic change, warrant repeat vessel mapping to determine whether a fistula has become feasible, and a patient initially bridging toward an anticipated near-term transplant with a catheter, whose transplant timeline is subsequently delayed substantially, may warrant reconsideration of a more durable access as the anticipated duration of dialysis dependence extends beyond what was originally planned.

Building this reassessment into the same structured, trigger-based review infrastructure recommended throughout this book for the Life-Plan itself, prescription review, and adequacy monitoring — rather than relying on an individual clinician to separately remember to reconsider access choice on their own initiative — is what makes this kind of proactive reassessment reliably occur across a full patient population rather than only in the occasional case where a particularly attentive clinician happens to notice the mismatch. A vascular access registry or chart flag that surfaces whenever a patient's Life-Plan is formally revised, prompting an explicit access-choice reconsideration at the same time, extends this book's recurring systemic-workflow principle to the vascular access domain specifically.

A thirty-nine-year-old man with polycystic kidney disease and a GFR of fourteen milliliters per minute is evaluated for access creation with an initial vessel mapping study showing marginal forearm vein quality, bilaterally, attributed in part to his elevated body mass index. Rather than proceeding directly to graft creation on the basis of this single mapping study, his surgical and nephrology team recommend a structured weight-management program over several months, given his trajectory suggests he has adequate time before reaching kidney failure, followed by repeat vessel mapping once meaningful weight loss has been achieved. The repeat mapping study, performed four months later following an eighteen-pound weight loss, identifies a cephalic vein now meeting standard diameter criteria for fistula creation, and he proceeds to a successful radiocephalic fistula rather than the graft that would have been created based on his initial mapping alone. This case illustrates that access choice, particularly when initial vessel mapping is marginal rather than clearly inadequate, benefits from considering whether a correctable factor might shift the assessment before defaulting to the next-best access option, provided the patient's trajectory allows the necessary time for that factor to be addressed.

KEY POINT: Marginal, rather than clearly inadequate, vessel mapping results warrant considering whether a correctable factor — weight, timing, vein preservation — might shift a patient from graft to fistula candidacy before defaulting to the graft option, provided the trajectory allows the necessary time.

DIALYSIS RECOGNITION & RESPONSE SYSTEM — Access Creation Arcs

The Pattern: A patient's Life-Plan trajectory changes after an access type has already been chosen based on the original plan.

Stem Signature: A patient originally planned for a shorter-duration access, such as a catheter bridging to an anticipated near-term transplant, whose transplant timeline is subsequently delayed substantially beyond what was originally anticipated.

The Decision: Reassess access choice against the revised trajectory, considering whether a more durable access — fistula or graft — is now warranted given the extended anticipated duration of dialysis dependence, rather than continuing the original shorter-duration access plan unexamined.

Trap Logic: An access choice made appropriately under the original Life-Plan can continue by inertia even after the trajectory that justified it has changed, in the same way an unrevised dialysis prescription or goals-of-care document can persist past the point it remains appropriate.

Response Anchor: A materially changed trajectory is the trigger to reassess access choice, not merely dialysis prescription or goals of care — access decisions require the same active revision discipline established throughout this book.

DIALYSIS RECOGNITION & RESPONSE SYSTEM — Access Creation Arcs

The Pattern: A patient with bilaterally poor peripheral vessel mapping and a history of prior central venous catheterization is being evaluated for access creation.

Stem Signature: Inadequate vein caliber on peripheral mapping in both arms, combined with a history of one or more prior central venous catheters, in a patient being considered for graft creation based on the peripheral mapping findings alone.

The Decision: Obtain a central venogram before proceeding to graft creation, since central venous stenosis from the prior catheter history could compromise outflow from an otherwise technically adequate graft regardless of peripheral vessel quality.

Trap Logic: Peripheral vessel mapping alone can appear to fully answer the access-planning question, but a history of prior central catheterization specifically raises the likelihood of a central stenosis that peripheral mapping cannot detect and that would compromise any peripheral access created without first evaluating for it.

Response Anchor: A history of prior central venous catheterization in a patient being evaluated for a new access is the trigger to obtain a central venogram before proceeding — not to rely on peripheral mapping findings alone.

DIALYSIS RECOGNITION & RESPONSE SYSTEM — Access Creation Arcs

Inadequate Maturation at Scheduled Assessment: Pursue targeted imaging for a correctable cause — juxta-anastomotic stenosis or a diverting branch — before further waiting or abandoning the fistula for a new access.

Prior Central Catheterization With Poor Peripheral Mapping: Obtain a central venogram before proceeding to graft creation, since central stenosis can compromise outflow regardless of peripheral vessel quality.

A Changed Trajectory After Access Choice: Reassess access choice against the revised trajectory rather than continuing an access plan made under circumstances that no longer apply.

Summary and Key Concepts

Preoperative duplex ultrasound vessel mapping, rather than physical examination alone, provides the objective vessel diameter and patency data needed to select the access configuration most likely to mature successfully, and should assess the vessel's full accessible length and, where risk factors suggest it, central inflow and outflow as well.

Fistula maturation is a physiologic adaptation to arterial flow, driven by wall shear stress, requiring a minimum of roughly six weeks, and inadequate maturation at scheduled assessment warrants targeted evaluation for a correctable cause before further waiting or abandoning the access.

Grafts can be used sooner after creation than fistulas but carry higher infection and thrombosis risk, primarily from venous anastomotic stenosis; for a patient without adequate vessels for a fistula, the clinically relevant comparison is graft versus catheter, not graft versus fistula.

Patients with bilaterally inadequate vessels warrant extended evaluation, including central venogram and consideration of atypical configurations, ideally through early referral to a dedicated vascular access specialist, before defaulting to long-term catheter dependence.

Access type and creation timing should follow directly from the patient's Life-Plan established in Chapter 2, and should be reassessed whenever that trajectory changes materially rather than continued unexamined from the original plan.

CHAPTER 10: CANNULATION TECHNIQUE AND VASCULAR ACCESS PHYSICAL EXAMINATION

Learning Objectives

Compare rope-ladder, area, and buttonhole cannulation techniques and identify the risks and candidacy considerations specific to each.

Perform and interpret inspection, palpation, and auscultation of a vascular access as a structured physical examination.

Distinguish a maturing access from one ready for safe cannulation using bedside findings.

Educate patients in daily access self-care and in recognizing warning signs that require prompt evaluation.

Chapter Overview

Chapter 9 established how a vascular access is planned, created, and matured. This chapter addresses what happens once that access is actually put to use: the specific needling techniques used to cannulate it treatment after treatment, the structured physical examination that confirms an access remains healthy before each use, the bedside judgment needed to distinguish a still-maturing access from one genuinely ready for cannulation, and the daily self-care patients themselves are responsible for between treatments. Every one of these skills is exercised far more frequently than the creation and maturation process discussed in the previous chapter, since a single access is cannulated hundreds of times over its working life, and the cumulative quality of that repeated cannulation and examination does as much to determine an access's eventual longevity as the original surgical creation did. The complications that can result when these bedside skills are applied inconsistently — aneurysm, stenosis, thrombosis, and infection — are developed in full in Chapter 11, but their prevention begins here, in the routine, repeated practices this chapter describes.

Rope-Ladder, Area, and Buttonhole Cannulation

Rope-Ladder Cannulation Technique

Rope-ladder cannulation systematically rotates needle placement along the full cannulation length of the vascular access itself, moving progressively from one end of the usable segment to the other before beginning again at the first site, so that no single site is punctured more frequently than any other over a defined cycle of treatments. This systematic rotation is the technique most strongly associated with preserving long-term access integrity, since distributing the cumulative trauma of repeated needling across the vessel's full length avoids concentrating wall injury, scarring, and the aneurysmal degeneration discussed in Chapter 11 at any single, overused site.

Successful rope-ladder technique depends on the access having an adequately long cannulation segment to rotate across in the first place, and depends on cannulating staff, or a patient performing self-cannulation for home hemodialysis, consistently following the rotation pattern rather than defaulting to whichever site seems easiest to access on a given treatment day; a rotation pattern abandoned under time pressure or staff inexperience effectively converts rope-ladder technique into the area cannulation pattern discussed next, with the complications that pattern carries.

Documenting the specific sites used at each treatment, whether through a simple diagram marked in the patient's chart or a more structured electronic tracking system, supports consistent rotation across a team of rotating staff members who might otherwise have no way of knowing which sites were used at the patient's prior treatments, a particular risk in a busy unit where a given patient may be cannulated by a different staff member at each session.

Some units have adopted a numbered-site mapping system, in which each patient's access has a documented series of designated cannulation sites labeled sequentially, with staff simply advancing to the next numbered site at each treatment and cycling back to the first once the full sequence has been used; this kind of explicit, low-effort system removes the burden of remembering or reconstructing a rotation pattern from memory or from reviewing prior chart entries, and has been associated with more consistent rotation adherence than relying on general staff education about the importance of rotation without a concrete, easy-to-follow tracking mechanism.

Area Cannulation and Its Risks

Area cannulation, in which the same one or two sites are punctured repeatedly at every treatment rather than rotating across the access's full length, was historically common largely because it is technically easier for cannulating staff, who become familiar with a specific site's anatomy and needling angle through repeated use, but it concentrates cumulative vessel wall trauma at those specific sites in a manner now recognized to predispose strongly to aneurysm formation and to focal stenosis immediately adjacent to the overused segment.

Because these risks are now well established, area cannulation is generally discouraged as a routine technique in contemporary practice, reserved as an unavoidable fallback only when an access's usable cannulation length is too short to support rope-ladder rotation, or during the period immediately following creation when only a limited segment has matured sufficiently for use. Where area cannulation is unavoidable for these reasons, closer surveillance for the aneurysmal and stenotic complications this pattern predisposes to, discussed further in Chapter 11, is warranted relative to a rope-ladder-cannulated access.

A unit identifying that a patient has been managed with area cannulation, whether due to prior staffing inconsistency or an access with genuinely limited usable length, benefits from an explicit, planned transition toward rope-ladder technique where the access's length actually permits it, rather than continuing area cannulation indefinitely simply because it has become the established pattern for that patient. This transition is best undertaken gradually, introducing one or two additional rotation sites at a time rather than abruptly switching to a fully unfamiliar rotation pattern, allowing both the vessel and the patient to adapt progressively rather than facing an abrupt change in a well-established routine.

CAUTION: Area cannulation, repeatedly puncturing the same one or two sites, predisposes strongly to aneurysm formation and focal stenosis; reserve it only for accesses whose usable length genuinely cannot support rope-ladder rotation.

Buttonhole Cannulation Technique and Candidacy

Buttonhole cannulation uses the same two exact puncture sites at every treatment, similarly to area cannulation, but differs fundamentally in that the needle is inserted along the identical tract and at the identical angle each time, allowing a mature, epithelialized tunnel track to form over a period of repeated consistent use, through which a blunt needle can eventually be passed rather than the sharp needle required for a fresh puncture at a new site each time. This established tract is intended to reduce the pain of cannulation once fully formed, and, because the same soft-tissue tract is reused rather than a new puncture created at each treatment session, has been associated in some studies with reduced aneurysm formation relative to area cannulation, despite superficially resembling area cannulation in its use of fixed sites.

Establishing a buttonhole tract requires an initial period, typically eight to twelve sessions, during which a sharp needle is used at the exact same site and angle at every treatment to create the tract, before transitioning to a blunt needle once the tract has formed adequately; this establishment period requires considerably more consistency in staffing and technique than either rope-ladder or area cannulation, since even a modest deviation in angle or site during tract formation can produce a poorly formed or false tract that fails to support reliable blunt-needle cannulation later.

A false tract, in which the needle during the establishment phase deviates even slightly from the exact prior path, creates a secondary channel alongside the intended tract rather than reinforcing a single consistent path, and once a false tract has formed, subsequent blunt-needle attempts may enter either the true or the false channel unpredictably, risking infiltration or vessel injury; recognizing early signs of tract inconsistency during the establishment phase, and correcting technique promptly rather than continuing an already-deviating pattern, prevents this false-tract complication from developing into a persistent problem that can compromise the buttonhole site's long-term usability.

Some units address the risk of inconsistent tract formation by designating a small, fixed group of staff members responsible for establishing every new buttonhole tract at that unit, rather than allowing the establishment phase to be performed by whichever staff member happens to be available on a given day, since concentrating this specific, technique-sensitive task among a smaller group of practiced staff reduces the inter-examiner variability that most often produces a false tract during the establishment period.

Buttonhole technique carries a specific and clinically significant infection risk distinct from the other techniques: the soft, non-scarred tissue tract, while easier to cannulate once established, appears to carry a higher risk of localized infection, including a specific concern regarding Staphylococcus aureus colonization of the tract itself, than the scar-tissue-lined tracts that develop with rope-ladder technique, and this risk has led some centers to recommend buttonhole technique cautiously, reserved for patients specifically suited to it — notably those performing self-cannulation for home hemodialysis, where the technique's reduced pain and easier needle placement offer a particular advantage — rather than adopting it as the routine default technique across a general in-center dialysis population.

Meticulous antiseptic technique at each buttonhole cannulation, including removal of the scab that forms over the tract between treatments using a dedicated sterile technique rather than simply pushing the needle through it, is essential to mitigating this elevated infection risk, and units offering buttonhole cannulation should have a specific, written protocol for this scab removal and site preparation process distinct from their standard rope-ladder site preparation protocol, since applying the standard protocol unmodified to a buttonhole site does not adequately address the tract's specific infection risk profile.

Technique	Site Pattern	Key Advantage	Key Risk
Rope-Ladder	Systematic rotation across full length	Best long-term vessel preservation	Requires adequate cannulation length and consistent staff adherence
Area	Same one or two sites repeatedly	Technically easier for inexperienced staff	Strongly predisposes to aneurysm and focal stenosis
Buttonhole	Same exact tract and angle repeatedly	Reduced cannulation pain once tract established; suited to self-cannulation	Elevated localized infection risk, including Staphylococcus aureus

Figure 10.1: Rope-Ladder Versus Buttonhole Cannulation Site Patterns

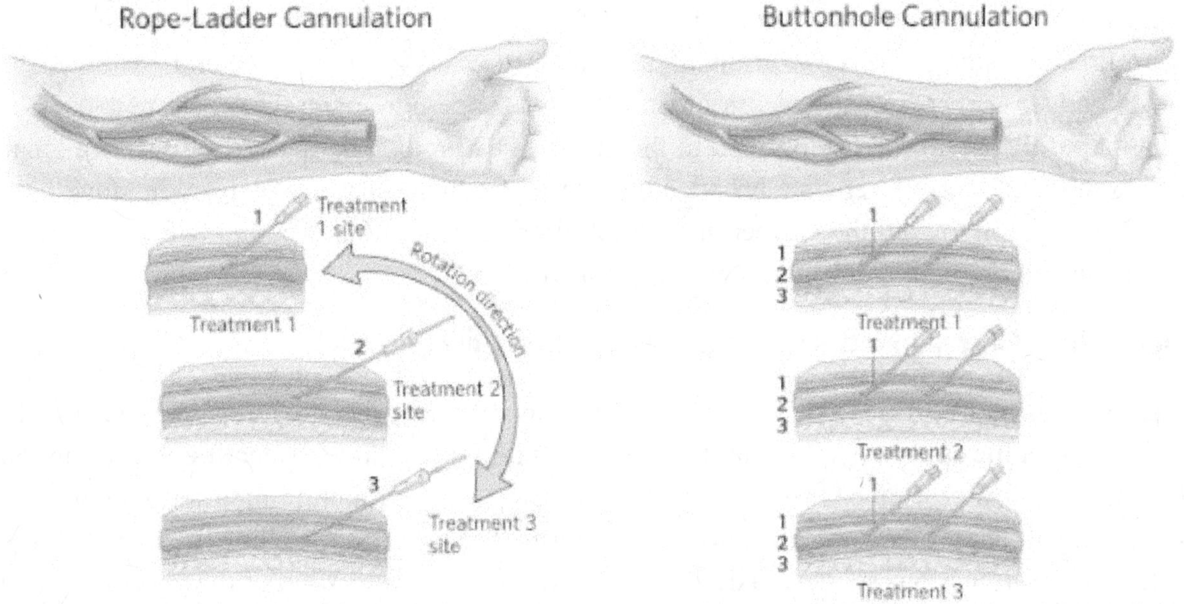

Physical Examination: Inspection, Palpation, and Auscultation

Inspection Findings and Their Significance

Visual inspection of a vascular access begins before the hands ever touch the patient's arm: assessing overall limb color and swelling for signs of venous outflow obstruction, examining the skin overlying the access for erythema, warmth, or drainage suggesting infection, and looking specifically for aneurysmal dilation, defined as a focal, ballooning outpouching of the vessel wall, which is most often found at previously overused cannulation sites and represents a segment of vessel wall weakened by repeated trauma.

Skin overlying an aneurysmal segment deserves particular attention for thinning, shine, or a bluish discoloration, since these findings suggest the overlying skin itself has become compromised and carries an elevated risk of spontaneous rupture, a vascular access emergency discussed in Chapter 11 that inspection at this stage is specifically intended to catch before it progresses to that point. Any patient reporting spontaneous pain, throbbing, or a sensation of pressure over an existing aneurysmal segment, even without an obviously alarming visual change on that day's examination, warrants the same urgency of evaluation as a visually concerning finding, since symptoms can precede visible skin compromise by a meaningful margin in some patients. Comparing current appearance against prior examination findings, ideally documented with photographs or a structured description in the chart at prior visits, allows a gradually enlarging aneurysm or gradually thinning overlying skin to be recognized as a concerning trend rather than assessed only against the examiner's general impression of what a concerning aneurysm looks like in isolation.

Inspection also assesses the surrounding limb for signs suggesting a broader circulatory problem rather than a finding isolated to the access itself: unilateral hand or finger discoloration, coolness, or pain distal to the access raises concern for the steal syndrome discussed in Chapter 11, in which the fistula or graft diverts a clinically significant proportion of arterial inflow away from the hand, while diffuse limb swelling extending well beyond the access site itself raises concern for central venous stenosis or occlusion rather than a purely local process confined to the access. Distinguishing these patterns — a local finding confined to the access itself versus a broader limb-level finding — at the inspection stage helps direct subsequent evaluation toward the correct underlying process rather than treating every abnormal finding as a generic access problem requiring identical evaluation.

Palpation: Thrill Characteristics and Pulse Augmentation Test

A normal fistula or graft thrill is a continuous, low-frequency vibration palpable along the vessel's length, present throughout the cardiac cycle rather than confined to systole alone, reflecting the continuous, high-volume, relatively low-resistance flow that characterizes a properly functioning arteriovenous connection over time. A thrill that has become discontinuous, confined to systole, or notably diminished in intensity relative to prior examinations suggests a developing outflow stenosis restricting the previously continuous flow pattern, and this qualitative change in thrill character is often detectable before flow has declined enough to produce more overt symptoms or alarm-triggering pressure changes during actual treatment.

The augmentation test, performed by briefly occluding the access with a finger at a point proximal to where the thrill is being assessed and observing whether the thrill augments, or strengthens, distal to the occlusion, helps localize a suspected stenosis: normal augmentation with occlusion at a given point suggests the segment being palpated, distal to the occlusion, has adequate inflow, while a segment that fails to augment despite proximal occlusion suggests a stenosis between the occlusion point and the segment being examined. This test is a simple, no-equipment bedside maneuver that experienced examiners use to build an initial impression of stenosis location before, where warranted, confirming with formal imaging.

The augmentation test's interpretation requires some caution in a very early, still-maturing fistula, since a vessel not yet fully matured may show a less robust augmentation response even in the absence of true pathologic stenosis, simply reflecting its still-developing flow characteristics rather than an acquired stenotic lesion; applying this test with the same interpretive threshold used for a long-established, fully mature fistula risks over-diagnosing stenosis in a vessel that is, in fact, still within its normal maturation trajectory, which is one further reason the maturation-stage assessment discussed later in this chapter should inform how physical examination findings, including augmentation testing, are interpreted for any given access.

Elevation of the arm, observing whether a distended, poorly collapsing access falls promptly with elevation, provides a further bedside assessment of outflow: a normally functioning access collapses substantially with arm elevation as gravity assists venous drainage, while an access with significant downstream outflow obstruction remains distended even with the arm elevated, since the obstruction, not gravity, is what is limiting drainage in that scenario. This elevation finding, performed alongside the augmentation test, adds a further data point to the bedside stenosis localization process without requiring any additional equipment beyond the examiner's own observation.

Consistency in how and where palpation is performed matters as much as the technique itself: examining the same points along the access at every visit, using comparable pressure, and documenting findings in comparable terms across different examiners allows a meaningful comparison against the patient's own established baseline rather than each examination standing alone as an isolated, unanchored snapshot subject to inter-examiner variation in technique and terminology. Structured examination templates, prompting the examiner to assess and document specific, defined points along the access rather than recording only a general impression, support this consistency across a team of rotating staff members examining the same patient at different visits. Such templates also facilitate meaningful trend review during periodic chart audits, allowing a unit's quality team to identify whether a given patient's access findings have been drifting gradually in a concerning direction across several months even when no single visit's finding was, by itself, alarming enough to prompt individual clinician concern.

Auscultation: Bruit Characteristics

A normal bruit, auscultated with a stethoscope along the access length, is a low-pitched, continuous sound present through both systole and diastole, mirroring the continuous nature of the thrill described above and reflecting the same underlying continuous, relatively low-resistance flow pattern. A bruit that has become high-pitched, discontinuous, or confined predominantly to systole suggests the same developing stenosis that a discontinuous thrill on palpation would suggest, and auscultation performed alongside palpation provides a complementary confirmation of the same underlying finding through an independent sensory modality, increasing the examiner's confidence in a suspected abnormality detected through either technique alone.

Auscultation at multiple points along the access length, rather than only at a single site, helps localize the level at which a bruit's character changes from normal to abnormal, since a stenosis produces its characteristic high-pitched, turbulent sound specifically at and just downstream of the narrowed segment, while segments upstream of the stenosis retain the normal continuous low-pitched bruit; systematically auscultating from the arterial anastomosis progressively along the vessel's length toward the venous outflow allows this transition point to be identified with reasonable precision at the bedside.

New staff training in vascular access examination benefits substantially from direct, hands-on supervision by an experienced examiner over a series of real patient examinations, since thrill and bruit characteristics, while describable in words, are ultimately tactile and auditory skills that develop through guided repeated practice rather than through reading a description alone; a structured competency assessment, confirming a new staff member can reliably distinguish a normal from an abnormal finding under direct observation, is a reasonable and worthwhile investment before that staff member is relied upon to perform this examination independently.

KEY POINT: A discontinuous, systolic-only thrill or bruit, in contrast to the normal continuous, low-pitched finding, is the single most reliable bedside indicator of a developing outflow stenosis and warrants further evaluation.

DIALYSIS RECOGNITION & RESPONSE SYSTEM — Access Surveillance Arcs

The Pattern: Routine pre-treatment physical examination reveals a change in thrill or bruit character from a patient's established baseline.

Stem Signature: A thrill that has become discontinuous or confined to systole, or a bruit that has become high-pitched and turbulent rather than the patient's usual continuous, low-pitched finding, identified on routine examination before cannulation for that day's treatment.

The Decision: Perform the augmentation and elevation tests to localize the suspected stenosis, document the finding and its comparison against the patient's baseline examination, and refer for formal vascular imaging rather than proceeding with cannulation and treatment as though the examination were unremarkable.

Trap Logic: A subtle change in thrill or bruit character can be dismissed as normal day-to-day variation, particularly by staff unfamiliar with the specific patient's own baseline examination findings, when it in fact represents the earliest detectable sign of a developing stenosis well before more overt symptoms or pressure alarms would appear during treatment.

Response Anchor: A change in thrill or bruit character from a patient's own established baseline warrants augmentation testing and imaging referral — not reassurance that the access remains grossly functional.

Recognizing the Maturing Versus Mature Access

Distinguishing Maturation Stages at the Bedside

A fistula in the early weeks after creation typically shows a palpable thrill and audible bruit confirming basic patency, but lacks the visible dilation, adequate depth, and cannulation-length development that define true maturation as discussed in Chapter 9; recognizing this distinction at the bedside, rather than treating any palpable thrill as sufficient justification to attempt cannulation, is what prevents the premature cannulation attempts that themselves risk damaging a fistula still in the vulnerable early stages of its remodeling process.

A genuinely mature fistula shows visible, not merely palpable, dilation along a cannulation-length segment, sits at a depth from the skin surface shallow enough for reliable needle placement, and demonstrates the flow characteristics discussed in Chapter 9's rule-of-sixes framework; the combination of these findings, rather than any single one considered in isolation, supports a confident bedside determination that an access is ready for its first cannulation attempt.

A common bedside error is treating a strong, easily palpable thrill as sufficient evidence of maturation on its own, without separately confirming adequate visible dilation and depth; a fistula can develop a robust thrill relatively early after creation, reflecting adequate basic patency and flow, while still lacking the wall thickening and dilation that true maturation requires, and attempting cannulation on the basis of thrill alone risks infiltration, vessel wall injury, or hematoma formation in a vessel not yet structurally ready to tolerate repeated needling despite its reassuring flow characteristics, a distinction the following case illustrates concretely.

A thirty-three-year-old woman with a radiocephalic fistula created seven weeks earlier is brought to the dialysis unit for her scheduled first cannulation. Palpation confirms a strong, continuous thrill, and the referring note describes the fistula as "ready." The experienced access nurse performing the assessment, however, notes on inspection that the vessel, while patent, shows only modest visible dilation and remains somewhat deep to the skin surface at the intended cannulation site, findings inconsistent with full maturation despite the reassuring thrill. Rather than proceeding with cannulation on the strength of the thrill alone, she defers cannulation and arranges a follow-up ultrasound, which confirms the vessel has not yet reached adequate diameter, and recommends an additional two to three weeks before reattempting cannulation. This deferral, while requiring the patient to continue on her bridging catheter briefly longer than originally planned, avoided a premature cannulation attempt on a vessel not yet structurally ready to tolerate it, illustrating why thrill alone, however reassuring, should never substitute for the fuller maturation assessment this chapter and Chapter 9 both describe.

CAUTION: A strong, easily palpable thrill reflects adequate flow but does not by itself confirm adequate vessel dilation and depth; assess all three maturation criteria together before proceeding with a first cannulation attempt.

Special Considerations for Graft Physical Examination

Physical examination of a graft follows the same inspection, palpation, and auscultation framework applied to a fistula, but interpretation differs in several respects reflecting the graft's distinct construction: a graft's thrill and bruit are typically somewhat more localized and less variable in intensity along its length than a native fistula's, since the uniform prosthetic conduit does not show the same degree of natural caliber variation a native vessel does, and a graft's most common site of developing stenosis, the venous anastomosis where prosthetic material meets native vein, deserves particular auscultation and palpation attention distinct from the fistula's more common juxta-anastomotic stenosis pattern discussed in Chapter 9.

Aneurysmal degeneration in a graft, termed pseudoaneurysm formation since it involves a defect in the graft wall itself rather than a true aneurysmal dilation of native vessel tissue, tends to present more abruptly and can progress more rapidly than native fistula aneurysm formation, making inspection for this finding at every single examination particularly important as part of graft-specific surveillance practice, and a pseudoaneurysm identified on examination generally warrants more urgent evaluation than an equivalent-appearing native fistula aneurysm, given the underlying prosthetic material's different failure characteristics.

Graft surveillance protocols in many units incorporate periodic recirculation testing and, in some programs, scheduled duplex ultrasound at defined intervals in addition to the routine physical examination performed at every treatment, reflecting the generally higher and more rapidly progressive stenosis risk grafts carry relative to native fistulas discussed in Chapter 9; this more intensive surveillance schedule for grafts, layered on top of the same physical examination framework applied to fistulas, is a further practical expression of the general principle that access surveillance intensity should match the specific access type's known risk profile rather than applying an identical monitoring schedule uniformly across every access type a unit's patient population uses.

The specific surveillance interval and imaging modality used varies across units and is influenced by available resources and local practice patterns as much as by any single universally agreed standard, but the underlying principle — that a graft's known higher and more rapidly progressive stenosis risk justifies a more proactive surveillance posture than a native fistula typically requires — is broadly consistent across the variation in specific protocols different units have adopted to operationalize it.

When to Begin Cannulation

The first cannulation attempt on a newly matured access is best performed by the most experienced available staff member, using a single-needle approach at reduced blood flow rate for the first one to several sessions before progressing to standard two-needle cannulation at full prescribed flow, an approach that allows the vessel's response to initial cannulation to be assessed under lower-stress conditions before committing to the full demands of standard treatment. A poor first cannulation experience, whether from technical difficulty, infiltration, or patient anxiety, can undermine both the vessel's physical integrity and the patient's confidence in the access going forward, making this initial cannulation a moment deserving particular care rather than being treated as routine simply because the access has technically met maturation criteria on paper.

A twenty-two-year-old man with a brachiocephalic fistula created ten weeks earlier is scheduled for his first cannulation and initiation of hemodialysis, having previously been maintained on a bridging catheter. Rather than proceeding directly to standard two-needle cannulation at full prescribed blood flow, his team's most experienced access nurse performs the first cannulation using a single needle at a reduced blood flow rate, closely monitoring for infiltration or excessive discomfort. The fistula tolerates this initial reduced-intensity approach well, and over his following three treatments blood flow rate is progressively increased and a second needle is introduced, reaching his full standard prescription by his fourth treatment. This graduated approach, rather than immediately subjecting a newly matured fistula to full-intensity two-needle cannulation, allowed early problems, had they arisen, to be identified and addressed at lower stakes, and gave both the vessel and the patient time to adapt to the demands of regular cannulation before the full treatment prescription was applied.

This graduated cannulation approach also serves an important psychological function alongside its physiologic rationale: a patient's confidence in a new access, particularly one that has already required a lengthy wait through creation and maturation before finally becoming usable, benefits from an initial cannulation experience that goes smoothly, and a difficult or painful first attempt can create lasting anxiety around subsequent cannulations that persists well beyond what the initial technical difficulty alone would predict. Framing the graduated approach to patients explicitly, as a deliberate strategy to ensure a smooth transition rather than an indication that something about their particular access is especially fragile or concerning, helps set appropriate expectations for what is, in fact, a standard and recommended practice for every newly matured access.

CLINICAL PEARL: The first cannulation of a newly matured access is best performed by the most experienced available staff member, using a single-needle, reduced-flow approach for the first several sessions before progressing to standard two-needle cannulation at full prescribed flow.

Patient Self-Care and Access Protection

Patient Education for Daily Access Care

Patients bear substantial responsibility for their own access's day-to-day protection between treatments, and structured education covering this responsibility, delivered explicitly rather than assumed to be self-evident, includes checking for a palpable thrill at least once daily, keeping the access site clean and observing standard hygiene around it, and avoiding activities that place direct pressure on the access, including sleeping with the access arm underneath the body, wearing tight clothing or jewelry over the site, or allowing blood pressure cuffs, tourniquets, or blood draws to be performed on the access arm.

This education is most effective when delivered repeatedly across multiple encounters rather than as a single dense information session at access creation, since the volume of information involved, similar to the modality education discussed in Chapter 2, exceeds what most patients retain fully from a single delivery, and since specific elements of this education — particularly the instruction to prevent any blood pressure measurement or blood draw on the access arm — benefit from being reinforced at every subsequent healthcare encounter the patient has, including those unrelated to their dialysis care specifically, given how easily a well-meaning but uninformed clinician elsewhere in the healthcare system might otherwise use the access arm for a routine blood pressure check.

A wearable medical alert bracelet or similar identifier specifying the access arm and instructing against blood pressure measurement or venipuncture on that specific limb provides a practical safeguard extending beyond what verbal patient education alone can guarantee, particularly relevant for a patient who might present to an emergency department or an unfamiliar healthcare setting unable to communicate this instruction themselves, whether due to the acuity of their presenting complaint or a temporary alteration in their ability to communicate clearly, such as a patient who arrives unconscious, confused, or otherwise unable to advocate for their own access protection at the exact moment it matters most.

Patients pursuing self-cannulation for home hemodialysis, discussed further in Chapter 20, require a more extensive skills-based education program beyond the general protective measures described above, including hands-on training in sterile technique, needle insertion, and recognition of complications requiring the patient to seek help rather than continue self-treatment, and this training is generally conducted over an extended period with direct supervision and graduated independence rather than compressed into a brief instructional session, reflecting the meaningfully higher stakes and skill demands of self-cannulation relative to the general protective self-care education applicable to every access patient.

Buttonhole technique, discussed earlier in this chapter, is particularly relevant to this self-cannulation population, since the reduced pain and simplified needle placement it offers once a tract is established make it an appealing option for a patient cannulating their own access without the assistance of a trained clinician; the elevated infection risk this technique carries, however, requires that self-cannulating patients receive training in tract care and scab removal at least as rigorous as the training provided to clinical staff performing buttonhole cannulation in-center, since a patient inconsistently or improperly maintaining their own buttonhole tract faces the same infection risk this chapter has already described, without a supervising clinician present to catch a developing problem early.

Home hemodialysis training programs that incorporate a structured, competency-based buttonhole curriculum specifically, rather than treating tract care as a minor addendum to broader self-cannulation training, report better outcomes with respect to buttonhole-related infection than programs providing only general guidance, reinforcing that the same specific, protocol-driven approach this chapter recommends for in-center buttonhole care applies with equal or greater force once the responsibility for maintaining tract hygiene shifts entirely to the patient themselves, who no longer has a supervising clinician present at every treatment to catch an early lapse in technique before it produces a clinically significant infection.

Recognizing Warning Signs Requiring Prompt Evaluation

Patient education for self-monitoring parallels the structured physical examination taught to clinical staff earlier in this chapter, translated into terms a patient without formal medical training can reliably apply: checking for the presence of a thrill, described to patients as a buzzing or vibrating sensation rather than using clinical terminology, at the same time each day; watching for new swelling, redness, warmth, or drainage at the access site; and recognizing that a sudden loss of the previously palpable buzzing sensation, whether or not accompanied by pain, constitutes an urgent finding requiring same-day evaluation rather than a routine concern that can wait until the next scheduled dialysis session.

Distinguishing genuinely urgent warning signs from more minor, expected findings is a further component of thorough patient education: mild, transient bruising after a cannulation is common and expected, while a rapidly expanding hematoma or an actively bleeding puncture site that does not respond to direct pressure within several minutes is not, and patients benefit from explicit guidance on this distinction so that education emphasizing vigilance does not inadvertently produce excessive anxiety or unnecessary emergency department visits for findings that are, in fact, a normal part of living with a cannulated access.

Providing patients with a written, one-page reference summarizing these distinctions — what is expected and self-limited versus what requires prompt evaluation — supports retention of this nuanced guidance better than verbal instruction alone, and a reference the patient can consult at home during an actual episode of concern is generally more useful in the moment than relying entirely on memory of a conversation that may have occurred months earlier at a very different point in their dialysis course.

Structured teach-back, in which the patient demonstrates their own thrill-checking technique and describes in their own words what would prompt them to seek urgent evaluation, confirms genuine understanding more reliably than simply asking whether the patient has questions, since a patient who nods along to verbal instruction without actually internalizing the specific warning signs may not recognize a genuine problem when it eventually arises, weeks or months after the original education was delivered.

Repeating this teach-back assessment periodically, rather than only at the time of initial education, guards against the natural fading of retained detail that occurs over months and years even after an initially successful teach-back demonstration, and provides a further opportunity to reinforce any updated guidance, such as a change in the patient's specific access type or cannulation technique that would modify what warning signs are most relevant to their particular situation, or a change in the patient's own cognitive or functional status that might affect their ability to reliably self-monitor going forward.

A fifty-five-year-old woman with a well-established fistula of three years' duration calls her dialysis unit on a non-treatment day reporting that she noticed the buzzing sensation over her fistula felt different that morning compared to how it usually feels, though she is otherwise asymptomatic and the arm appears normal to her. Rather than being told to simply monitor it and mention it at her next scheduled treatment two days later, she is instructed to come in for same-day evaluation given the specific, if subtle, change she has described. Examination confirms a discontinuous thrill and a physical examination pattern consistent with a new stenosis, subsequently confirmed on imaging and successfully treated with angioplasty before the access progressed to thrombosis. This case illustrates why patient-reported subjective changes in thrill character, even when vague or difficult for the patient to articulate precisely, warrant the same urgency as a clinically identified abnormal finding, since patients who have lived with their access for years often develop a reliable, if informally described, sense for their own baseline that is itself a valid clinical data point.

KEY POINT: A patient's own report of a subjectively altered thrill sensation, even if vague or difficult to describe precisely, warrants same-day evaluation rather than deferral to the next scheduled treatment.

DIALYSIS RECOGNITION & RESPONSE SYSTEM — Access Surveillance Arcs

---

The Pattern: A patient reports a subjective change in their access's sensation between scheduled treatments.

Stem Signature: A patient calling on a non-treatment day to report that their fistula or graft feels different than usual, often vaguely described, without other symptoms such as pain, swelling, or fever, and without the patient scheduled to be seen again for a day or more.

The Decision: Arrange same-day evaluation rather than deferring assessment to the next scheduled treatment, since a patient's own longstanding familiarity with their access's baseline sensation is a valid clinical signal even when they cannot articulate the change in precise clinical terms.

Trap Logic: A vague, subjectively described symptom without other objective findings can be deprioritized as unlikely to represent a genuine problem, when in fact a patient's years of daily familiarity with their own access often allows them to detect a subtle change before it would be obvious to an examiner seeing the access for the first time at a delayed visit.

Response Anchor: A patient-reported change in access sensation warrants same-day evaluation, not deferral to the next scheduled treatment, regardless of how imprecisely the patient can describe the change.

DIALYSIS RECOGNITION & RESPONSE SYSTEM — Access Surveillance Arcs

A Change in Thrill or Bruit Character on Examination: Perform augmentation and elevation testing and refer for imaging rather than proceeding with treatment as though the examination were unremarkable.

A Patient-Reported Change in Access Sensation: Arrange same-day evaluation rather than deferring to the next scheduled treatment, regardless of how imprecisely the change is described.

Summary and Key Concepts

Rope-ladder cannulation, systematically rotating sites across the vessel's full length, best preserves long-term access integrity; area cannulation predisposes strongly to aneurysm and stenosis and should be reserved for accesses whose length cannot support rotation.

Buttonhole cannulation offers reduced cannulation pain once an established tract forms but carries an elevated localized infection risk requiring a dedicated antiseptic protocol distinct from standard site preparation.

A normal thrill and bruit are continuous through the cardiac cycle; a discontinuous, systolic-only finding is the most reliable bedside indicator of a developing stenosis and warrants augmentation testing and imaging referral.

A genuinely mature access shows visible dilation, adequate depth, and sufficient flow along a cannulation-length segment, and the first cannulation of a newly matured access is best performed by experienced staff using a graduated, reduced-intensity approach.

Patient self-care education, reinforced repeatedly and confirmed through teach-back, should treat any patient-reported change in access sensation as warranting prompt evaluation rather than deferral to the next scheduled treatment.

CHAPTER 11: VASCULAR ACCESS COMPLICATIONS: STENOSIS, THROMBOSIS, AND INFECTION

Learning Objectives

Explain the pathophysiology of vascular access stenosis and apply surveillance methods to detect it before thrombosis occurs.

Recognize acute access thrombosis and select an appropriate salvage strategy.

Diagnose and manage vascular access infection and aneurysmal or pseudoaneurysmal degeneration.

Recognize dialysis access steal syndrome and high-output cardiac failure as distinct, access-attributable complications requiring specific management.

Chapter Overview

Chapters 9 and 10 addressed how an access is created, matured, cannulated, and examined. This chapter addresses what goes wrong: the four major complication categories that threaten an established access's function and, in some cases, the patient's safety more broadly. Stenosis, thrombosis, infection, and the less common but clinically significant steal syndrome and high-output cardiac failure are not equally likely, equally urgent, or equally managed, and this chapter works through each in turn, building directly on the surveillance and physical examination foundation Chapter 10 established. A recurring theme across all four complications is that early detection through the routine surveillance already described consistently outperforms late detection through overt symptoms or treatment-disrupting emergencies, and each section below returns to this theme in the specific context of the complication it addresses. This chapter closes Part III's treatment of hemodialysis access with catheters specifically, and the central venous catheter discussed throughout this chapter as the access type most consistently minimized in favor of a durable surgical alternative receives its own dedicated treatment in Chapter 12.

Stenosis Detection and Surveillance

Pathophysiology of Access Stenosis

Venous outflow stenosis, the most common lesion threatening both fistulas and grafts, arises predominantly from intimal hyperplasia, a proliferative response of the vessel wall's inner lining to the mechanical and hemodynamic stresses the access imposes: turbulent flow at the anastomosis, repeated cannulation trauma along the cannulation segment, and, in grafts specifically, the foreign-body response at the prosthetic-to-native-vein junction all provoke this same underlying proliferative process, which progressively narrows the vessel lumen over months to years of access use. In a native fistula, stenosis develops most commonly at the juxta-anastomotic segment, immediately downstream of the surgical connection, reflecting the concentrated turbulence this specific location experiences; in a graft, stenosis develops most commonly at the venous anastomosis, where the mechanical mismatch between prosthetic and native tissue is most pronounced.

Because intimal hyperplasia is a gradual, progressive process rather than a sudden event, a stenosis typically narrows the vessel lumen over an extended period before flow becomes critically compromised, providing a window during which surveillance, described in the next subsection, can detect the developing lesion and direct intervention before the access progresses to the acute thrombosis discussed later in this chapter. This gradual timeline is precisely what makes proactive surveillance so much more valuable than reactive management in this specific complication: a stenosis caught at fifty percent luminal narrowing is a straightforward outpatient angioplasty, while the same stenosis, left undetected until it progresses to complete thrombosis, requires a more complex and higher-risk thrombectomy procedure with a meaningfully worse subsequent patency prognosis.

Arterial inflow stenosis, considerably less common than venous outflow stenosis but clinically important when it occurs, limits the volume of blood actually delivered to the access regardless of how favorable the venous outflow segment appears, and produces a distinct examination pattern — a weak or absent thrill even at the arterial anastomosis itself, rather than the more distally located diminished thrill pattern venous outflow stenosis typically produces. Recognizing this distinction at the bedside directs subsequent imaging toward the arterial inflow specifically rather than defaulting to an evaluation focused solely on the venous outflow segment where stenosis is statistically more common but not, in this specific presentation, where the actual lesion is most likely located.

Arterial inflow stenosis is also worth considering specifically in a patient whose venous outflow has already been evaluated and found unremarkable despite persistent examination or performance abnormalities, since a clinician who stops the diagnostic evaluation once venous outflow has been cleared, without considering the less common but still clinically important arterial inflow possibility, may fail to identify the actual lesion responsible for a patient's ongoing access dysfunction.

The molecular and cellular drivers of intimal hyperplasia — growth factor signaling triggered by mechanical shear stress and vessel wall injury, smooth muscle cell migration and proliferation into the vessel's inner lining, and extracellular matrix deposition that further narrows the effective lumen — have been studied extensively in an effort to identify a pharmacologic intervention capable of preventing or slowing this process, but no such intervention has yet achieved reliable clinical benefit sufficient to become standard practice, leaving surveillance and timely mechanical intervention, discussed throughout this section, as the primary tools available for managing this essentially inevitable biological response to the mechanical demands vascular access imposes on the vessels involved.

Surveillance Methods and Their Comparative Value

Physical examination, as detailed comprehensively in Chapter 10, remains the foundation of routine stenosis surveillance, performed at every single treatment by cannulating staff and requiring no specialized equipment beyond trained hands and ears; a discontinuous thrill, a high-pitched bruit, and an abnormal augmentation or elevation test each provide evidence of a developing stenosis using only the routine pre-cannulation assessment already built into standard practice. Static and dynamic venous pressure monitoring during treatment, tracking the pressure required to achieve the prescribed blood flow rate and how that pressure trends across successive treatments, provides a complementary, machine-derived surveillance signal that can detect a developing stenosis even when physical examination findings remain subtle or ambiguous.

Access blood flow measurement, performed using dilutional techniques similar to the recirculation testing discussed in Chapter 7, tracks the actual volume of blood flowing through the access over time, and a declining flow trend, even one that remains numerically above an absolute threshold, often precedes a threshold-crossing decline by weeks to months, making trend analysis considerably more valuable than any single flow measurement interpreted in isolation. Duplex ultrasound surveillance, performed at defined intervals in many surveillance protocols, directly visualizes the stenotic segment and quantifies its severity, offering the most detailed anatomic information among these methods but at a greater resource and scheduling cost than physical examination or pressure monitoring, which is why most surveillance programs layer these methods rather than relying on ultrasound alone as a first-line, routine screening tool.

Comparative studies evaluating which surveillance combination most effectively reduces thrombosis rates have produced somewhat inconsistent results across different patient populations and practice settings, reflecting real variation in access type distribution, baseline stenosis prevalence, and the specific technical execution of each surveillance method across different studies; this inconsistency in the comparative literature is itself a reason most guideline bodies recommend a combined, layered approach rather than endorsing any single method as demonstrably superior, since the available evidence does not clearly support choosing one method over the others as a sole strategy.

No single surveillance method has been shown to be unambiguously superior to a combination approach in reducing thrombosis rates across the full range of comparative studies, and most contemporary vascular access programs therefore combine routine physical examination at every treatment, periodic flow or pressure trend review on a monthly or quarterly cycle, and dedicated ultrasound imaging triggered by an abnormal finding from either of the first two methods, rather than committing to any single surveillance modality as sufficient on its own. This layered approach reflects the same general principle this book has applied throughout Part I to Life-Plan revision, goals-of-care review, and dialysis adequacy assessment: a structured, multi-source review process reliably catches more than any single metric or method applied in isolation.

Implementing this layered surveillance consistently across an entire dialysis unit's patient population requires the same systemic, workflow-embedded infrastructure this book has recommended repeatedly for other structured review processes: a defined schedule for flow measurement and pressure trend review, a clear escalation pathway specifying when an abnormal finding triggers ultrasound referral, and a mechanism for tracking each patient's surveillance status so that a due or overdue assessment is flagged automatically rather than depending on an individual clinician remembering each patient's specific surveillance schedule amid the many other responsibilities a busy dialysis unit demands.

Intervening on a Detected Stenosis

A hemodynamically significant stenosis, generally defined as a narrowing exceeding fifty percent of the luminal diameter accompanied by a corroborating clinical or hemodynamic abnormality such as an abnormal physical examination, declining access flow, or rising venous pressure, warrants intervention, most commonly percutaneous transluminal angioplasty performed by an interventional radiologist or vascular surgeon, restoring luminal diameter and flow without requiring open surgical revision in the substantial majority of cases. Angioplasty's effect, however, is not permanent: intimal hyperplasia frequently recurs at the same site over subsequent months, and a meaningful proportion of angioplastied lesions require repeat intervention within a year, a pattern that should be anticipated and discussed with patients as an expected feature of long-term access maintenance rather than a sign that the original intervention failed or was performed incorrectly. Framing recurrence in these terms during the initial post-angioplasty discussion helps patients interpret a future recurrence, should one occur, as an anticipated part of ongoing access maintenance rather than as evidence their access has begun failing outright, reducing unnecessary anxiety at the point recurrence is eventually detected on routine surveillance.

Repeated, rapidly recurring stenosis at the same site despite appropriately performed angioplasty may warrant consideration of a stent placement across the lesion, providing more durable patency than angioplasty alone in this specific recurring-stenosis scenario, though stents carry their own considerations, including cost and the theoretical, though generally modest in practice, concern for complicating any future surgical revision at that same site should one eventually become necessary. Surgical revision, creating a new anastomosis or otherwise bypassing the stenotic segment surgically rather than treating it endovascularly, is generally reserved for lesions that fail repeated angioplasty or stenting, or for lesions in an anatomic location poorly suited to an endovascular approach in the first place.

Timing of intervention relative to the next scheduled dialysis treatment matters practically: a stenosis identified well before the access becomes critically compromised allows angioplasty to be scheduled electively, coordinated around the patient's treatment calendar without disrupting their regular dialysis schedule, while a stenosis identified only once flow has declined to a level threatening imminent thrombosis requires more urgent intervention, potentially disrupting the patient's regular treatment schedule and requiring temporary catheter placement if the access cannot be safely used before the corrective procedure can be performed. This timing difference is a further practical argument, beyond the purely clinical considerations already discussed, for proactive surveillance over reactive management: elective, well-scheduled intervention is simply easier on the patient and the treating unit's workflow than urgent, disruptive intervention forced by a late-detected lesion.

Surveillance Method	What It Detects	Frequency	Key Limitation
Physical Examination	Thrill, bruit, and augmentation abnormalities	Every treatment	Requires trained, consistent examiner technique
Venous Pressure Trend	Rising resistance to prescribed blood flow	Every treatment, reviewed periodically	Can be affected by needle position and technique
Access Flow Measurement	Declining volumetric flow trend	Monthly to quarterly	Requires dedicated equipment and technique
Duplex Ultrasound	Direct anatomic visualization and severity grading	Triggered by abnormal finding, or scheduled in some protocols	Higher resource and scheduling cost

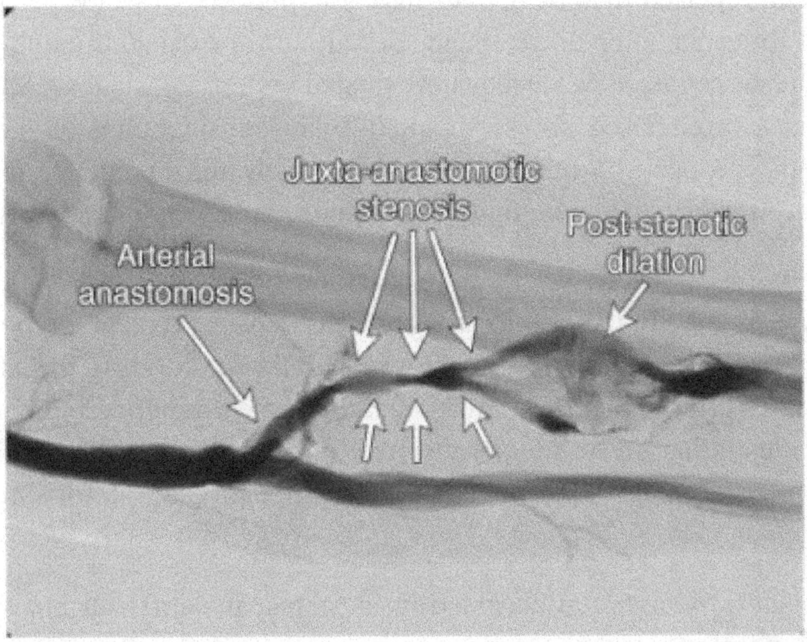

Figure 11.1: Venous Outflow Stenosis at the Juxta-Anastomotic Segment

DIALYSIS RECOGNITION & RESPONSE SYSTEM — Access Complication Arcs

The Pattern: Access flow trend or venous pressure trend shows a gradual decline or rise over several consecutive treatments without a single dramatic threshold-crossing value.

Stem Signature: A monthly access flow measurement or venous pressure reading that has moved consistently in a concerning direction over three or more consecutive measurements, with each individual value still falling within a technically acceptable range when considered alone.

The Decision: Treat the consistent trend itself as the actionable finding and refer for duplex ultrasound evaluation, rather than waiting for any single measurement to cross an absolute numeric threshold before acting.

Trap Logic: Each individual measurement in a slowly worsening trend can appear reassuring in isolation, and a clinician reviewing only the most recent value rather than the trend across several measurements can miss a developing stenosis that trend analysis would have flagged considerably earlier.

Response Anchor: A consistent multi-measurement trend, not any single value, is the actionable surveillance signal — refer for imaging based on the trend rather than waiting for a threshold crossing.

Thrombosis Recognition and Salvage

Recognizing Acute Access Thrombosis

Acute thrombosis presents unmistakably once fully established: the previously palpable thrill and audible bruit are entirely absent, replaced by a firm, cord-like, non-pulsatile vessel on palpation, and the access can no longer be used for cannulation or treatment. Because thrombosis this complete typically develops on a background of an unrecognized or inadequately treated underlying stenosis, as discussed throughout the preceding section, a thrombosed access should prompt consideration of the vascular lesion that permitted the thrombosis to occur in the first place, not solely the immediate mechanical problem of restoring patency, since restoring flow without addressing the underlying stenosis frequently results in rapid rethrombosis.

Patients themselves are frequently the first to recognize thrombosis, typically reporting that their access "stopped buzzing" or feels different in a way consistent with the loss of thrill this chapter and Chapter 10 have both emphasized as a critical, urgent warning sign; this patient-reported finding, exactly as discussed in Chapter 10's case illustrating the value of subjective patient reports, warrants immediate evaluation rather than deferral, since the window during which salvage remains straightforward narrows the longer a thrombosed access goes unaddressed.

Distinguishing a genuinely thrombosed access from a technically difficult but still-patent access can occasionally be less straightforward than the classic presentation described above suggests, particularly in a heavily scarred or aneurysmal access where palpation is inherently more difficult to interpret; bedside Doppler ultrasound, where available, can quickly confirm the absence of flow in an ambiguous case, avoiding either an unnecessary urgent thrombectomy referral for an access that is, in fact, still patent, or a delayed referral for one that has genuinely thrombosed but was initially misjudged as merely difficult to palpate.

Salvage Techniques: Thrombectomy and Angioplasty

Mechanical thrombectomy, using specialized catheter-based devices to macerate and aspirate thrombus from within the access, combined with angioplasty of the underlying stenosis that precipitated the clot, is the standard salvage approach for a thrombosed fistula or graft presenting within a reasonable window, typically considered most successful when performed within the first day or so after thrombosis is recognized, though successful salvage beyond this window remains possible and should not be assumed futile without attempting evaluation. Pharmacomechanical approaches, combining mechanical thrombectomy with a locally infused thrombolytic agent to assist clot dissolution, are used in some centers and clinical scenarios as an alternative or adjunct to mechanical thrombectomy alone, with selection between approaches generally guided by local expertise, equipment availability, and the specific characteristics of the thrombosed segment.

Successful salvage restores both patency and, critically, addresses the underlying stenosis through angioplasty performed at the same procedural setting, since thrombectomy alone, without treating the causative lesion, predictably results in early rethrombosis; a salvage procedure that restores flow without identifying and treating an underlying stenosis has not actually solved the problem that caused the thrombosis in the first place; and post-procedure surveillance following any thrombosis and salvage episode should proceed on a heightened schedule relative to the routine surveillance described in the previous section, since a thrombosed and salvaged access carries a demonstrably higher subsequent thrombosis risk than one with no thrombosis history.

The decision between mechanical thrombectomy and a pharmacomechanical approach incorporating a thrombolytic agent is also influenced by the estimated age of the thrombus, since a more organized, longer-standing clot generally responds less readily to thrombolytic dissolution than a fresh clot does, making mechanical maceration and aspiration the more reliable primary approach once thrombus age is uncertain or likely to exceed the window in which thrombolytics remain most effective; this consideration is one further reason prompt recognition and referral, discussed at the start of this section, matters beyond simply preserving the option of salvage at all, since it also preserves the option of the full range of salvage techniques rather than narrowing the choice to mechanical approaches alone by the time the patient is actually evaluated.

When Salvage Is Not Feasible

Extensive thrombus burden, a chronically diseased vessel with limited remaining usable segments, or a patient whose overall clinical status makes a salvage procedure higher-risk than the benefit it would offer are each reasonable grounds to forgo salvage in favor of proceeding directly to a new access, following the same vessel evaluation and creation process detailed in Chapter 9; this decision should weigh the specific salvage prospects for the thrombosed access itself against the patient's remaining vessel options for a new access, rather than defaulting reflexively to either salvage or new creation without this individualized comparison.

A patient facing this decision benefits from the same kind of explicit, collaborative conversation this book has recommended for other major access decisions throughout Part III: weighing the interventional radiology or vascular surgery team's technical assessment of salvage feasibility against the patient's remaining vessel options and the practical burden either path imposes, including the temporary catheter dependence a new access creation would require during its maturation period versus the more immediate, if less certain, restoration a salvage attempt might offer. Neither path is universally preferable, and the individualized weighing this decision requires echoes the same access-choice reasoning developed at length in Chapter 9.

A fifty-one-year-old man on hemodialysis via a brachiocephalic fistula for two years presents to the dialysis unit reporting that his fistula "stopped working" the previous evening. Examination confirms a firm, non-pulsatile, thrombosed vessel with no palpable thrill along its length. He is referred urgently for thrombectomy, performed the same day, which successfully restores patency and identifies and treats an underlying venous outflow stenosis with angioplasty at the same setting. His access resumes normal function, and given his recent thrombosis history, his surveillance schedule is intensified to monthly access flow measurement for the following six months rather than his prior quarterly schedule, a modification made explicitly because his thrombosis episode places him at demonstrably higher risk of recurrence than a patient with no such history. This case illustrates both the standard combined thrombectomy-and-angioplasty salvage approach and the appropriate post-salvage surveillance intensification this chapter recommends.

Reviewing this case at his unit's subsequent quality meeting, the team also identifies that his pre-thrombosis surveillance data, reviewed retrospectively, had in fact shown a gradually declining access flow trend over the preceding two months that had not triggered an imaging referral under the unit's existing protocol threshold; this retrospective finding prompts the unit to revise its own internal escalation threshold to trigger imaging referral somewhat earlier in a declining trend, illustrating how individual complication cases, reviewed systematically rather than treated as isolated events, can improve a unit's surveillance protocol for the entire patient population going forward.

CLINICAL PEARL: Successful thrombosis salvage requires treating the underlying stenosis, not merely restoring flow, and should be followed by intensified surveillance given the demonstrably higher subsequent thrombosis risk a prior thrombosis episode confers.

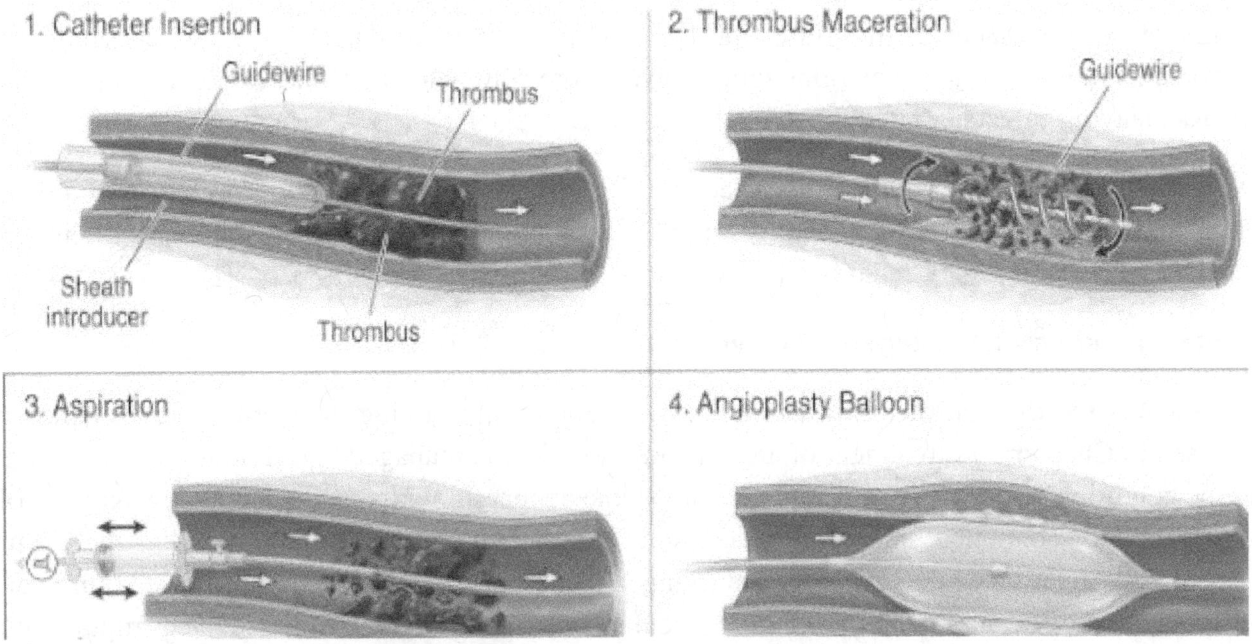

Access Infection and Aneurysmal Degeneration

Recognizing and Managing Access Infection

Native fistula infection is uncommon relative to graft or catheter infection, reflecting the fistula's use of the patient's own endothelium-lined tissue rather than foreign material, but when it occurs typically presents with localized erythema, warmth, tenderness, and sometimes purulent drainage at a cannulation site, and, in more advanced cases, with systemic signs of bacteremia including fever and rigors. Graft infection, considerably more common given the foreign prosthetic material's greater susceptibility to bacterial colonization discussed in Chapter 9, presents similarly at the local level but carries a higher risk of extending along the graft's length and of associated bacteremia, given the graft material's propensity to harbor infection resistant to antibiotic penetration alone.

Blood cultures, obtained before initiating empiric antibiotic therapy wherever the patient's clinical stability permits the brief delay this requires, guide antibiotic selection and duration and help distinguish a localized, superficial infection from a more serious bacteremic process requiring more aggressive management, including graft excision in severe or refractory cases. A graft infection that fails to respond to appropriate antibiotic therapy within an expected timeframe, or that presents with extensive involvement along the graft's length rather than a localized segment, generally requires surgical excision of the infected segment rather than continued antibiotic therapy alone, since infected prosthetic material, unlike a localized soft-tissue infection, does not reliably clear with antibiotics alone regardless of how appropriately those antibiotics are selected and dosed.

Partial graft excision, removing only the clearly infected segment while preserving the remainder for continued use where technically feasible, is preferred over complete graft removal where the infection remains anatomically confined, since preserving any usable portion of an existing access reduces the need for immediate creation of an entirely new access; however, this partial approach requires confident intraoperative assessment that the infection has not spread beyond the visibly affected segment, and a surgeon uncertain of adequate margins should favor more complete excision over an incomplete resection that risks leaving infected material behind.

CAUTION: Extensive graft infection or bacteremia that fails to respond to appropriate antibiotic therapy within an expected timeframe generally requires surgical excision of the infected segment; infected prosthetic material does not reliably clear with antibiotics alone.

Aneurysm and Pseudoaneurysm Management

True aneurysmal dilation of a native fistula, most commonly arising at overused cannulation sites as discussed in Chapter 10's treatment of area cannulation risk, is managed based on its size, rate of growth, and the condition of the overlying skin: a small, stable aneurysm with healthy overlying skin can often be monitored with continued surveillance and modified cannulation technique avoiding the aneurysmal segment specifically, while a rapidly enlarging aneurysm or one with compromised, thin, or shiny overlying skin warrants surgical or endovascular intervention given the elevated rupture risk this presentation carries.

Pseudoaneurysm in a graft, representing an actual defect in the graft wall rather than a true dilation of intact vessel tissue, is generally considered to warrant a lower threshold for intervention than an equivalent-appearing native fistula aneurysm, given the underlying structural defect's less predictable and potentially more rapidly progressive failure characteristics discussed in Chapter 10; a pseudoaneurysm identified on routine examination should prompt vascular surgical evaluation rather than the more conservative monitoring approach that might be reasonable for a comparably sized, stable native fistula aneurysm with healthy overlying skin.

Modified cannulation technique for a patient with an established, monitored aneurysm — explicitly avoiding needle placement within the aneurysmal segment itself and instead cannulating adjacent, non-aneurysmal portions of the vessel — both protects the weakened aneurysmal wall from additional direct trauma and helps prevent the aneurysm from expanding further under continued cannulation pressure; this modification requires explicit communication to every staff member who might cannulate the patient, since a staff member unaware of the aneurysm's location and the modified technique it requires could inadvertently cannulate directly within the compromised segment.

The Pattern: A patient with a vascular access graft develops localized erythema and tenderness at a cannulation site.

Stem Signature: New warmth, erythema, tenderness, or drainage at a graft cannulation site, with or without accompanying systemic symptoms such as fever, in a patient whose graft has otherwise been functioning normally.

The Decision: Obtain blood cultures before initiating empiric antibiotic therapy where clinical stability permits, and monitor closely for response; extensive involvement or failure to respond within the expected timeframe warrants surgical evaluation for possible graft excision rather than continued antibiotic therapy alone.

Trap Logic: A localized-appearing infection can be treated with antibiotics alone under the assumption that it will resolve as a typical soft-tissue infection would, without recognizing that infected prosthetic graft material carries a materially different, less antibiotic-responsive natural history than infection in native, non-prosthetic tissue.

Response Anchor: Graft infection that is extensive or fails to respond to appropriate antibiotics within the expected timeframe requires surgical evaluation for excision — not continued antibiotic therapy alone.

Steal Syndrome and High-Output Cardiac Effects

Recognizing Dialysis Access Steal Syndrome

Steal syndrome occurs when a fistula or graft diverts a clinically significant proportion of arterial inflow away from the distal hand, since the low-resistance pathway the access provides preferentially draws blood away from the higher-resistance distal arterial bed, producing distal ischemia in the hand supplied by the same artery feeding the access. Presentation ranges from mild, exercise-induced coolness or tingling in the fingers, often noticed only during dialysis treatment itself when access flow is highest, to severe, rest-pain ischemia with digital ulceration or tissue loss in advanced, untreated cases, and this range of severity is why every new access patient should be specifically asked about hand symptoms rather than relying on the patient to spontaneously volunteer symptoms they may not recognize as connected to their vascular access.

The onset of steal syndrome relative to access creation also varies meaningfully: some patients develop symptoms almost immediately after creation, reflecting a particularly pronounced diversion effect from the outset, while others develop symptoms only months or years later as the access matures further and its flow increases progressively over time, meaning a patient's hand symptoms should be reassessed at every visit throughout the access's working life rather than considered a concern relevant only to the immediate postoperative period this chapter and Chapter 9 both discuss.

Risk factors for steal syndrome include diabetes and peripheral arterial disease, both of which compromise the distal arterial bed's own baseline perfusion and its capacity to compensate for the additional diversion the access imposes, and a more proximal access configuration, which diverts flow from a larger, higher-flow arterial segment than a distal configuration does; these risk factors are precisely why preoperative evaluation, discussed in Chapter 9, assesses distal perfusion specifically before committing to a configuration, particularly a proximal one, in a patient carrying these risk factors.

Because steal syndrome symptoms are often most apparent specifically during dialysis treatment, when access flow reaches its peak, a patient may report symptoms only when directly asked about hand sensation during treatment rather than volunteering them spontaneously, particularly if the symptoms are mild and the patient has not connected them to their vascular access; routine, structured questioning about hand symptoms during treatment, rather than relying on spontaneous patient reporting, is therefore an important component of ongoing access surveillance specifically for this complication, complementing the physical examination and flow-based surveillance described earlier in this chapter that primarily target stenosis and thrombosis rather than steal syndrome specifically.

Management of confirmed, symptomatic steal syndrome ranges from conservative measures for mild cases, including simple monitoring and patient reassurance where symptoms are minor and non-progressive, through surgical banding procedures that narrow the fistula's outflow to reduce the diversion effect while preserving adequate flow for dialysis, to, in the most severe cases threatening tissue viability, ligation of the access entirely, accepting the loss of the access to preserve the hand's viability. This range of management options underscores why prompt recognition matters clinically: a mild case caught early may respond to a less invasive intervention, while delayed recognition risks progression to a severity requiring the access's complete sacrifice.

A sixty-year-old woman with diabetes and a brachiocephalic fistula created four months earlier reports coldness and tingling in her fingers specifically during her dialysis treatments, though her hand feels normal between sessions. Examination during treatment confirms diminished capillary refill and coolness in the fingers of the access hand, improving somewhat when the access is briefly, temporarily occluded, consistent with mild-to-moderate steal syndrome. Given her diabetes and the proximal configuration of her fistula, both recognized risk factors, and given her symptoms remain confined to treatment sessions without rest pain or tissue changes between them, her vascular surgery team elects a period of close monitoring with hand-warming measures during treatment rather than proceeding directly to a surgical banding procedure, reasoning that her presentation remains in the milder range of the syndrome's spectrum. Over the following months her symptoms remain stable without progression to rest pain or tissue compromise, and continued monitoring, rather than intervention, remains appropriate for her specific presentation. This case illustrates that steal syndrome management is calibrated to symptom severity and progression rather than triggering surgical intervention reflexively at first recognition, provided the presentation remains genuinely mild and non-progressive on continued monitoring.

Her team documents a specific plan for reassessment, including defined criteria — development of rest pain, any visible skin or tissue change, or symptom progression beyond the treatment-only pattern she currently exhibits — that would prompt escalation to surgical evaluation, rather than leaving the decision to continue monitoring open-ended without a defined trigger for reconsidering that approach; this explicit criteria-based plan mirrors the same structured, trigger-based reassessment principle this book has applied to the Life-Plan, goals of care, and dialysis adequacy throughout its earlier chapters, now extended to the specific context of monitoring a mild, non-progressive access complication.

KEY POINT: Steal syndrome severity ranges from mild, treatment-only symptoms to severe, tissue-threatening ischemia; management is calibrated to this severity spectrum rather than defaulting to surgical intervention at first recognition of any hand symptom.

High-Output Cardiac Failure From Vascular Access

A mature, high-flow fistula, particularly a proximal, large-caliber configuration, can carry a flow volume substantial enough to impose a meaningful additional workload on the heart, since the heart must pump this additional shunted volume on top of its normal systemic circulatory demand; in most patients with otherwise adequate cardiac reserve, this additional workload is well tolerated indefinitely, but in a patient with limited underlying cardiac reserve, whether from preexisting heart failure, valvular disease, or other structural cardiac pathology, this added burden can precipitate or worsen high-output cardiac failure, a distinct clinical entity from the more common volume-overload heart failure discussed in Chapter 24.

Recognizing access-attributable high-output cardiac failure requires specifically considering the access as a contributing factor when a dialysis patient develops new or worsening heart failure symptoms, rather than attributing the presentation solely to the more common volume-related and structural cardiac causes discussed elsewhere in this book; a formal access flow measurement, demonstrating a flow volume disproportionate to what the patient's cardiac output can accommodate without strain, supports this diagnosis and distinguishes it from heart failure driven primarily by interdialytic volume accumulation or intrinsic cardiac disease unrelated to the access.

Management of confirmed access-attributable high-output cardiac failure centers on reducing access flow to a level the patient's cardiac reserve can accommodate, most commonly through a surgical flow-reduction banding procedure similar in principle to the steal-syndrome banding procedure discussed above but targeting excessive total flow rather than distal arterial diversion specifically, or, in the most severe cases where flow reduction alone is insufficient or not technically feasible, ligation of the access and creation of an alternative, lower-flow configuration. As with steal syndrome, this decision weighs the access's ongoing value against the cardiac risk it now poses, and is made collaboratively between nephrology, cardiology, and vascular surgery rather than by any single discipline acting in isolation, given the genuinely multidisciplinary nature of the trade-off involved.

Screening for this complication proactively in patients carrying elevated risk — those with known cardiac disease at the time of access creation, or those whose access has been noted on examination to carry an unusually vigorous, high-volume thrill and bruit relative to typical findings — through periodic cardiac assessment alongside routine access surveillance allows access-attributable high-output cardiac failure to be identified and addressed before it progresses to overt, symptomatic heart failure, mirroring the same proactive-versus-reactive principle this chapter has applied throughout its treatment of stenosis, thrombosis, and steal syndrome alike.

CLINICAL PEARL: New or worsening heart failure in a dialysis patient with a large-caliber, high-flow fistula should prompt consideration of access-attributable high-output cardiac failure, confirmed with formal access flow measurement, alongside the more common volume- and cardiac-driven causes.

Figure 11.3: Hand Ischemia From Dialysis Access Steal Syndrome

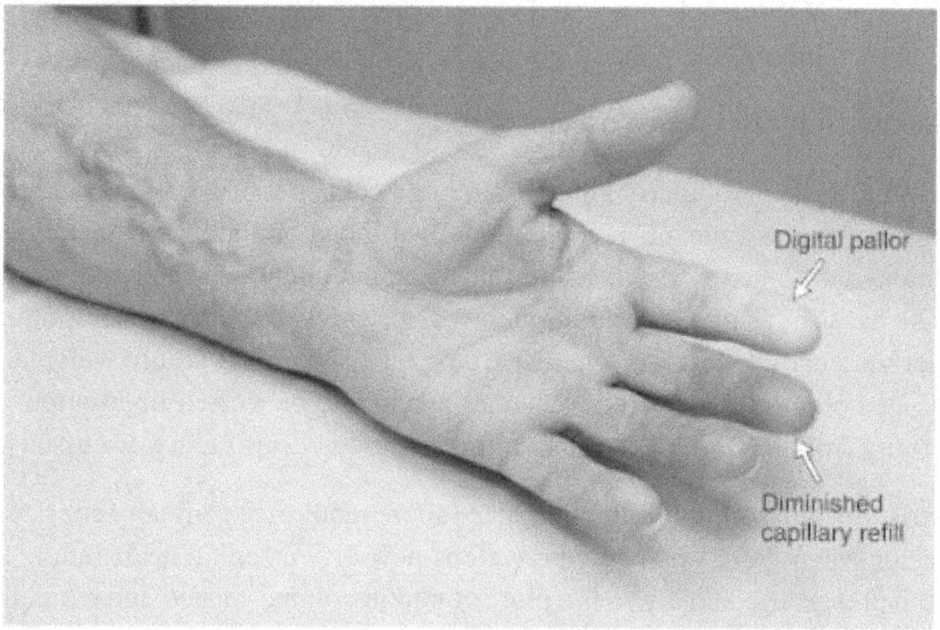

DIALYSIS RECOGNITION & RESPONSE SYSTEM — Access Complication Arcs

The Pattern: A dialysis patient with a large-caliber, proximal fistula develops new or worsening heart failure symptoms.

Stem Signature: New dyspnea, fatigue, or other heart failure symptoms in a patient with a high-flow, proximal configuration fistula, where the presentation is being attributed solely to volume overload or intrinsic cardiac disease without consideration of the access itself as a contributing factor.

The Decision: Consider access-attributable high-output cardiac failure specifically, obtain formal access flow measurement, and involve vascular surgery for possible flow-reduction banding if the access is confirmed as a meaningful contributor, rather than managing the heart failure through volume and cardiac-directed therapy alone.

Trap Logic: Heart failure symptoms in a dialysis patient are reflexively attributed to volume status or intrinsic cardiac disease, both far more common explanations, causing the access's contribution to be overlooked specifically in the patient population — those with large-caliber, high-flow, proximal configurations — where it is most likely to be clinically relevant.

Response Anchor: New heart failure in a patient with a large-caliber, high-flow fistula warrants formal access flow measurement to evaluate for an access-attributable contribution, not management directed solely at volume and cardiac causes.

DIALYSIS RECOGNITION & RESPONSE SYSTEM — Access Complication Arcs

---

A Gradual Multi-Measurement Surveillance Trend: Refer for imaging based on the trend itself rather than waiting for any single measurement to cross an absolute threshold.

Graft Infection Not Responding to Antibiotics: Pursue surgical evaluation for possible excision rather than continuing antibiotic therapy alone against infected prosthetic material.

New Heart Failure With a High-Flow Fistula: Obtain formal access flow measurement to evaluate for an access-attributable contribution rather than managing solely with volume and cardiac-directed therapy.

Summary and Key Concepts

Venous outflow stenosis, driven by intimal hyperplasia, is the most common lesion threatening both fistulas and grafts, and layered surveillance combining physical examination, pressure or flow trends, and triggered ultrasound consistently outperforms any single surveillance method used alone.

Successful thrombosis salvage requires treating the underlying stenosis alongside restoring patency, and warrants intensified post-salvage surveillance given the demonstrably higher subsequent thrombosis risk a prior episode confers.

Graft infection, unlike native fistula infection, involves foreign prosthetic material that does not reliably clear with antibiotics alone; extensive or non-responsive infection generally requires surgical excision.

Pseudoaneurysm in a graft warrants a lower threshold for intervention than an equivalent-appearing native fistula aneurysm, given its less predictable structural failure characteristics.

Steal syndrome and access-attributable high-output cardiac failure are distinct, access-specific complications requiring specific recognition and a management approach calibrated to severity, ranging from monitoring through flow-reduction procedures to, in the most severe cases, access ligation.

CHAPTER 12: CENTRAL VENOUS CATHETERS: PLACEMENT, CARE, AND CATHETER-RELATED BLOODSTREAM INFECTION

Learning Objectives

Compare tunneled and non-tunneled central venous catheters and select the appropriate type and insertion site for a given clinical circumstance.

Describe ultrasound-guided insertion technique and confirm appropriate catheter tip position.

Classify catheter dysfunction and apply locking solutions and other interventions to restore adequate function.

Diagnose catheter-related bloodstream infection and select between antibiotic lock salvage and catheter removal.

Chapter Overview

Every chapter in Part III to this point has treated the central venous catheter as the access type to be minimized: a bridge while a fistula matures, a last resort when no vessel supports a surgical access, an urgent stopgap for the late-referred patient. This final chapter of Part III gives the catheter the dedicated, detailed treatment its continued clinical necessity demands, because even in a unit that has fully internalized every principle in the preceding three chapters, some patients will need a catheter, sometimes for a period of weeks and sometimes, for the small population genuinely without a surgical access option, indefinitely. A catheter used well, with disciplined insertion technique, meticulous locking protocol, and prompt recognition of dysfunction and infection, carries meaningfully lower risk than a catheter managed inconsistently, and the difference between these two outcomes lies almost entirely in the practices this chapter describes rather than in any inherent, unmodifiable property of catheters as an access category. This chapter closes Part III of this book; Part IV turns to the intradialytic complications that can arise regardless of access type, building on the access-specific foundation these four chapters have established.

Tunneled Versus Non-Tunneled Catheter Selection

Catheter Construction and the Tunneling Principle

A non-tunneled catheter passes directly from the skin insertion site into the central vein, with no subcutaneous course between the skin and the vessel entry point, making it quick to place but also more prone to dislodgement and, because the skin-to-vein path is short and direct, more vulnerable to organisms migrating along the catheter's external surface into the bloodstream. A tunneled catheter, by contrast, is threaded through a subcutaneous tunnel of several centimeters between a separate skin exit site and the point where it actually enters the vein, and this tunnel serves two distinct protective functions: it creates a longer, indirect path that organisms must traverse to reach the bloodstream, and it allows a Dacron cuff positioned within the tunnel to become incorporated by surrounding fibrous tissue over several weeks, anchoring the catheter securely and providing a further physical barrier to organism migration along the catheter's outer surface.

This constructional difference translates directly into differing infection rates and differing appropriate durations of use: non-tunneled catheters are intended for short-term use, generally days to at most a few weeks, reflecting both their higher infection risk with prolonged dwell time and their greater susceptibility to dislodgement without the anchoring cuff a tunneled catheter provides, while tunneled catheters, once the cuff has become fully incorporated, are suitable for weeks to months of continued use and are the standard choice whenever a catheter is anticipated to be needed beyond the immediate, days-long window a non-tunneled catheter is designed for.

The tunnel itself requires several weeks to fully incorporate the cuff, and during this incorporation period a tunneled catheter carries an intermediate risk profile, more secure than a non-tunneled catheter from the moment of placement but not yet benefiting from the full protective effect the mature, incorporated tunnel eventually provides; this incorporation window is a further reason a newly placed tunneled catheter deserves particularly careful exit-site care and monitoring in its first several weeks, before the tunnel has had the chance to mature into its full protective configuration.

Catheter material and surface coating have also been studied as further modifiable factors in infection risk, with some catheters incorporating antimicrobial or antithrombogenic surface treatments intended to reduce bacterial colonization or thrombus formation along the catheter's external and internal surfaces respectively; while these modified catheters have shown some benefit in individual studies, the underlying tunneling principle and the disciplined care practices detailed throughout this chapter remain the dominant determinants of a given catheter's actual infection and dysfunction risk, with surface modification functioning as a modest additional layer of protection rather than a substitute for meticulous insertion technique and locking protocol.

Selecting Site: Internal Jugular, Subclavian, and Femoral

The right internal jugular vein is the preferred site for both tunneled and non-tunneled catheter placement in the substantial majority of clinical circumstances, offering a relatively direct, low-resistance path to the right atrium, a lower rate of central venous stenosis than the subclavian site, and a technically straightforward approach under ultrasound guidance; the left internal jugular vein is an acceptable alternative when the right is unavailable, though it requires the catheter to traverse a longer and more circuitous path to reach the same central position, a consideration relevant to tip position confirmation discussed later in this chapter.

The subclavian vein, though anatomically accessible and historically commonly used, is now actively avoided wherever an alternative site is feasible, because subclavian catheterization carries a substantially higher rate of subsequent central venous stenosis than internal jugular placement, and a stenotic subclavian vein on the same side as a planned or existing arm vascular access can compromise that access's venous outflow entirely, precisely the central-vein complication discussed in Chapter 9's treatment of preoperative vessel mapping. Because this stenosis risk is specifically relevant to any patient who may eventually need or already has an arm-based fistula or graft, essentially the entire hemodialysis population by definition, subclavian catheterization is reserved for circumstances in which both internal jugular sites are genuinely unavailable rather than used as a routine alternative site.

The femoral vein is used primarily for short-term, non-tunneled access in an urgent or acute setting, including the acute kidney injury and continuous renal replacement therapy circumstances discussed in Chapter 21, but carries a higher infection risk than internal jugular placement given its proximity to the perineum and the practical difficulty of maintaining an immaculate exit site in this anatomic location, and is poorly suited to a patient who is ambulatory or expected to remain catheterized for any extended period, given the mobility restriction a femoral catheter imposes and the elevated risk profile a prolonged femoral dwell carries relative to the internal jugular alternative.

A patient's overall body habitus and neck anatomy also factor into site and, occasionally, technique selection: a patient with a particularly short neck or a history of prior neck surgery or radiation may present technical challenges to standard internal jugular access that warrant additional imaging planning or a more experienced operator, and recognizing these anatomic considerations before attempting insertion, rather than discovering them only during a difficult procedure already underway, allows appropriate additional planning or operator selection in advance.

KEY POINT: The right internal jugular vein is the preferred site for essentially all central venous catheter placements; the subclavian vein is reserved for circumstances in which both internal jugular sites are genuinely unavailable, given its disproportionate central stenosis risk.

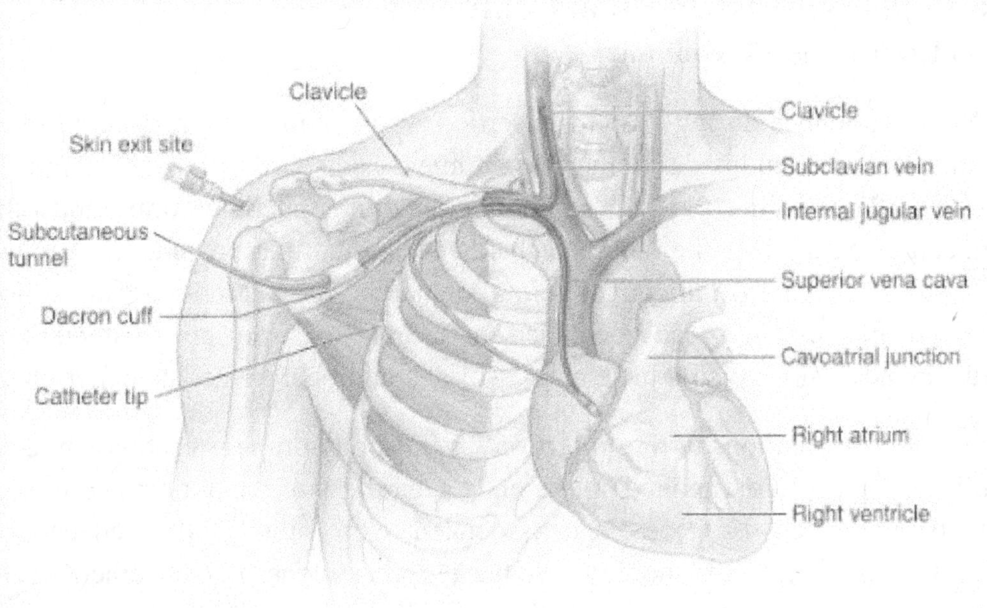

Figure 12.1: Tunneled Catheter Anatomy and Subcutaneous Course

Matching Catheter Type to Clinical Circumstance

A patient requiring urgent dialysis with no time to arrange tunneled placement receives a non-tunneled catheter as an immediate bridge, with conversion to a tunneled catheter, or to a surgical access per the Life-Plan framework established in Chapter 2, planned as soon as the clinical circumstance allows; continuing a non-tunneled catheter well beyond its intended short-term window, simply because the patient has stabilized and the more urgent original indication has passed, exposes the patient to elevated infection and dislodgement risk that a timely conversion to a tunneled catheter, or to a definitive surgical access, would have avoided.

For the population discussed in Chapter 9 whose vessels genuinely do not support any surgical access after thorough evaluation, a tunneled catheter becomes the necessary long-term access strategy rather than a bridge, and this population deserves the most rigorous possible application of every technique this chapter describes — careful site selection, meticulous locking protocol, and vigilant infection surveillance — precisely because they lack the option of transitioning away from catheter dependence that most other patients eventually have available to them.

A patient's own preferences and circumstances also factor into this matching process in select cases: a patient with a strong, well-founded preference for peritoneal dialysis who is temporarily bridging on hemodialysis while their peritoneal catheter heals, for example, may reasonably use a tunneled hemodialysis catheter for this defined, time-limited bridging period rather than pursuing a permanent hemodialysis access that the patient's overall Life-Plan does not anticipate needing beyond this transition, echoing the individualized, trajectory-driven access reasoning developed at length in Chapters 2 and 9.

Insertion Technique and Tip Position Confirmation

Ultrasound-Guided Insertion Technique

Real-time ultrasound guidance during catheter insertion, visualizing the target vein directly rather than relying on external anatomic landmarks alone, has become the standard of care for central venous catheter placement, substantially reducing the rate of arterial puncture, pneumothorax, and other mechanical insertion complications relative to the landmark-based technique that preceded it; ultrasound guidance also allows the operator to confirm the target vein's patency before attempting cannulation, avoiding an attempted placement into a vein already occluded or thrombosed from prior catheterization, a finding landmark-based technique alone would have no way of detecting before needle insertion.

Maximal sterile barrier precautions during insertion — full-body drape, sterile gown and gloves, mask, and cap for the inserting operator, applied consistently regardless of the anticipated urgency or duration of the catheter being placed — have been associated with substantially reduced catheter-related bloodstream infection rates relative to more limited barrier precautions, and this practice should be applied uniformly to every central venous catheter insertion, tunneled or non-tunneled, urgent or elective, rather than reserved selectively for circumstances judged to carry higher perceived infection risk, since the infection-reduction benefit of full barrier precautions has been demonstrated across insertion circumstances generally rather than only in a specific higher-risk subset.

For a tunneled catheter specifically, the subcutaneous tunnel is created after venous access has already been secured with a guidewire, with the catheter then passed through the tunnel from a separate exit site incision before final passage into the vein over the guidewire; meticulous technique in creating this tunnel, avoiding excessive tension or a path that kinks the catheter within the subcutaneous tissue, supports both a favorable cosmetic and functional outcome and the tunnel's eventual proper incorporation of the Dacron cuff discussed earlier in this chapter.

Exit-site positioning also deserves deliberate planning rather than being treated as an incidental byproduct of the tunnel's course: an exit site positioned on the anterior chest wall, below the clavicle and away from skin folds or areas of friction from clothing, generally supports easier patient self-care and dressing maintenance than one positioned in a less accessible or more friction-prone location, and this positioning consideration should be discussed with the patient before the procedure where feasible, since the patient will be responsible for exit-site care for as long as the catheter remains in place.

Confirming Tip Position

The catheter tip should terminate at or near the cavoatrial junction, the point where the superior vena cava meets the right atrium, a position that provides both adequate blood flow for the high flow rates hemodialysis requires and appropriate positioning to minimize the risk of central vein or atrial wall irritation and the arrhythmia this irritation can provoke if the tip is positioned too deeply within the atrium itself; a tip positioned too proximally within the superior vena cava, well short of the cavoatrial junction, risks inadequate flow and a higher rate of the dysfunction discussed later in this chapter, since a more proximal position sits within a segment of vein with comparatively lower flow than the cavoatrial junction provides.

A post-insertion chest radiograph remains the standard method for confirming tip position and for excluding pneumothorax after an internal jugular or subclavian insertion, though intraprocedural fluoroscopy, where available, allows tip position to be confirmed and adjusted in real time during the same procedure rather than requiring a separate confirmatory study and a potential return trip to correct a malpositioned tip identified only afterward. Some centers have adopted electrocardiographic guidance, using the characteristic change in the intracardiac electrocardiogram's P-wave morphology as the catheter tip approaches the cavoatrial junction, as a further real-time confirmation method that, combined with fluoroscopy or used as a standalone technique in centers with the appropriate equipment and expertise, can reduce reliance on a separate post-procedure radiograph.

Tip position should also be reassessed, not merely confirmed once at insertion, whenever a catheter's function changes unexpectedly or whenever a patient reports new symptoms such as arrhythmia or chest discomfort during treatment, since a catheter's tip position can migrate over time, particularly with vigorous patient activity or coughing, and a tip that has migrated from its original appropriate position may explain a new pattern of dysfunction or symptoms that would otherwise be attributed to one of the other mechanisms discussed later in this chapter.

CAUTION: A catheter tip positioned too deeply within the right atrium risks arrhythmia and cardiac perforation; confirm tip position at or near the cavoatrial junction with radiograph, fluoroscopy, or electrocardiographic guidance before relying on the catheter for treatment.

Immediate Post-Insertion Complications

Pneumothorax, arterial puncture, and hemothorax, though each meaningfully reduced by the ultrasound-guided technique discussed above relative to landmark-based insertion, remain possible complications of internal jugular and especially subclavian catheterization, and post-insertion assessment, including the confirmatory radiograph already recommended for tip position, should specifically screen for these complications before the catheter is used for treatment, since initiating dialysis through a catheter associated with an undetected pneumothorax or significant arterial injury compounds an already serious complication with the additional physiologic stress dialysis treatment itself imposes.

Cardiac arrhythmia during insertion, most commonly related to guidewire or catheter tip contact with the right atrial wall or the conduction system during passage, is generally transient and resolves with guidewire or catheter withdrawal, but should prompt immediate attention and a pause in the insertion procedure until the rhythm has normalized, rather than continuing to advance the guidewire or catheter through a sustained arrhythmia in the hope that it will resolve on its own once final position is reached.

A thirty-eight-year-old woman requiring urgent dialysis initiation for a uremic emergency, discussed in Chapter 1, undergoes ultrasound-guided right internal jugular non-tunneled catheter placement. During guidewire passage, the cardiac monitor shows a brief run of ventricular ectopy, and the inserting physician immediately withdraws the guidewire several centimeters, resolving the arrhythmia before re-advancing more cautiously to the appropriate depth. Post-insertion chest radiograph confirms appropriate tip position at the cavoatrial junction without pneumothorax, and dialysis is initiated without further complication. This case illustrates the appropriate response to an intraprocedural arrhythmia: immediate recognition, guidewire withdrawal, and confirmation of rhythm normalization before proceeding, rather than pushing through a concerning intraprocedural finding under the pressure of an urgent clinical situation.

Continuous cardiac monitoring throughout catheter insertion, not merely intermittent spot-checking, is what allowed this arrhythmia to be recognized promptly in this case, and units performing catheter insertions outside a monitored procedural suite, such as at bedside in an inpatient unit, should ensure equivalent continuous monitoring capability is available before the procedure begins rather than relying on intermittent vital sign checks that could miss a transient arrhythmia occurring between checks.

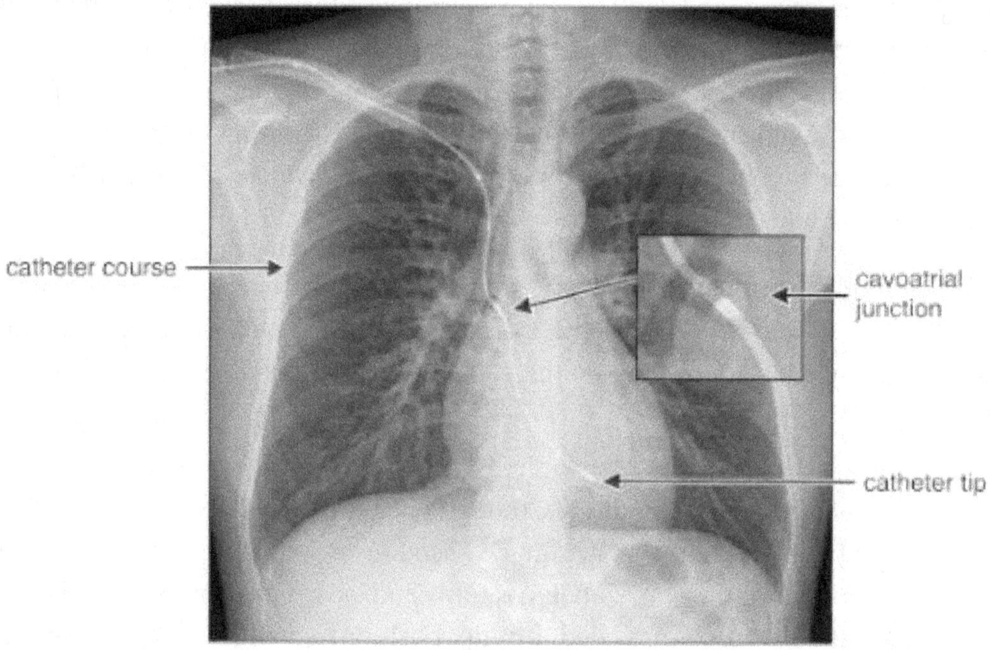

Figure 12.2: Confirming Central Venous Catheter Tip Position

Catheter Dysfunction and Locking Solutions

Recognizing and Classifying Catheter Dysfunction

Catheter dysfunction, most commonly manifesting as an inability to achieve the prescribed blood flow rate or as excessive pre-pump arterial pressure alarms during treatment, arises from several distinct mechanisms that require different corrective approaches: intraluminal thrombus obstructing the catheter lumen itself, a fibrin sheath enveloping the catheter's external surface and creating a one-way valve effect that permits infusion but not aspiration, or catheter tip malposition against the vessel wall, each producing a similar clinical picture of inadequate flow but requiring a distinct diagnostic and management approach to resolve effectively.

A fibrin sheath, developing gradually over the weeks to months following insertion as the body's normal response to a foreign intraluminal device, is distinguished from acute intraluminal thrombus by its more gradual onset and by a characteristic pattern in which the catheter can still infuse fluid relatively easily but cannot aspirate blood adequately, reflecting the sheath's tendency to collapse against the catheter's side holes during aspiration while permitting forward flow during infusion; this distinctive pattern, easily elicited by simply attempting to both infuse and aspirate through the catheter during assessment, helps distinguish a fibrin sheath from acute thrombus, which typically impairs both infusion and aspiration more symmetrically.

Recirculation, discussed in Chapter 7 in the context of vascular access adequacy assessment, is also relevant to catheter function specifically: a catheter whose arterial and venous lumens have become reversed in function, whether from tip malposition or from the fibrin sheath partially obstructing one lumen preferentially, can produce clinically significant recirculation even when overall blood flow appears adequate on superficial assessment, underscoring why formal recirculation testing, not merely a visual assessment of achieved blood flow rate, remains a relevant component of catheter function evaluation alongside the direct dysfunction assessment this section primarily addresses.

Locking Solutions and Their Purpose

Between treatments, each catheter lumen is filled with a locking solution intended to prevent thrombus formation within the lumen during the interdialytic interval when no blood is flowing through the catheter; standard heparin locking solution, instilled at the end of each treatment and aspirated before the next, has long been the conventional approach, though its systemic absorption, even at the small volumes involved, carries some bleeding risk in a patient with an elevated bleeding tendency, and its efficacy in reducing catheter dysfunction and infection relative to alternative locking solutions has been questioned in some comparative studies.

Citrate locking solution, distinct from the systemic citrate anticoagulation discussed in Chapter 8 but sharing citrate's calcium-chelating anticoagulant mechanism, has been adopted as an alternative or preferred locking solution in many centers, offering an anticoagulant effect confined to the catheter lumen itself with minimal systemic absorption at the concentrations typically used for locking rather than systemic anticoagulation, and some studies suggest citrate locking solution also carries antimicrobial properties that may contribute to reduced catheter-related infection rates relative to standard heparin locking, though this comparative infection benefit is not uniformly demonstrated across all available studies.

The specific concentration and volume of locking solution instilled must match the catheter's own documented internal lumen volume, printed on the catheter's packaging or documented in the insertion record, since underfilling the lumen leaves a portion of its length without protective locking solution coverage, while overfilling risks systemic infusion of the locking solution's full concentration directly into the patient's circulation as the lock is instilled, a distinction particularly relevant for citrate and antibiotic-containing locks where systemic infusion of the full locking concentration could produce clinically significant effects beyond what the intended catheter-confined dose is designed to achieve.

Antibiotic-containing locking solutions, incorporating a low-concentration antibiotic alongside the anticoagulant component, have been studied specifically for infection prevention in patients with recurrent catheter-related bloodstream infection, and while not universally adopted as a first-line locking approach given concerns about promoting antibiotic resistance with widespread prophylactic use, represent a targeted option for the specific population who have already experienced recurrent catheter infection despite standard locking solution and infection prevention practices otherwise being followed correctly.

Managing Persistent Dysfunction

A catheter with suspected intraluminal thrombus can often be restored to function with a thrombolytic instillation, most commonly a brief dwell of a tissue plasminogen activator preparation within the affected lumen, dissolving the obstructing clot without requiring catheter exchange or replacement; this is typically the first-line intervention for a dysfunctional catheter given its relative simplicity and low risk profile compared to the mechanical interventions discussed below, and many units maintain a standing protocol for thrombolytic instillation that dialysis staff can initiate directly when catheter dysfunction is identified, without requiring a separate physician order for each individual occurrence.

A fibrin sheath, less responsive to thrombolytic instillation than acute intraluminal thrombus given its location along the catheter's external surface rather than confined to the lumen itself, often requires a more mechanical intervention: catheter exchange over a guidewire, in which the dysfunctional catheter is removed and a new catheter placed through the same tract over a retained guidewire, disrupts the fibrin sheath's attachment and frequently restores adequate function without requiring an entirely new insertion at a different site. Fibrin sheath disruption using a specialized balloon or snare device, performed under fluoroscopic guidance without necessarily exchanging the catheter itself, is a further option in some centers, avoiding catheter exchange altogether where the sheath can be adequately disrupted through this less invasive approach.

Recurring dysfunction despite repeated thrombolytic instillation or a single guidewire exchange should prompt broader reconsideration rather than continued repetition of the same intervention: repeated fibrin sheath formation at the same catheter may reflect a particularly reactive tissue response in that specific patient, in which case a new insertion at a different site, allowing a fresh start away from the previously affected tissue, may ultimately prove more durable than continuing to cycle through repeated exchanges and disruption attempts at the same location.

Catheter tip malposition, identified through the imaging techniques discussed earlier in this chapter, generally requires catheter repositioning or exchange rather than a locking-solution or thrombolytic intervention, since neither of those approaches addresses a mechanical positioning problem; recognizing which of these three distinct mechanisms — thrombus, fibrin sheath, or malposition — underlies a given episode of catheter dysfunction, rather than applying a single default intervention regardless of the underlying cause, is what allows the most efficient and effective corrective approach to be selected on the first attempt rather than through sequential trial of each possible intervention.

CLINICAL PEARL: A catheter that infuses easily but aspirates poorly suggests a fibrin sheath rather than intraluminal thrombus; this pattern, combined with a gradual rather than abrupt onset, helps direct the appropriate corrective intervention toward guidewire exchange or sheath disruption rather than thrombolytic instillation alone.

DIALYSIS RECOGNITION & RESPONSE SYSTEM — Catheter Care Arcs

The Pattern: A tunneled catheter shows a gradual decline in aspiration capability while infusion remains relatively preserved.

Stem Signature: Progressive difficulty achieving adequate blood flow for treatment, developing gradually over days to weeks, with the catheter still able to infuse fluid relatively easily but unable to aspirate blood adequately to support the prescribed blood flow rate.

The Decision: Recognize this asymmetric infuse-versus-aspirate pattern as characteristic of a fibrin sheath rather than acute intraluminal thrombus, and proceed toward guidewire exchange or fluoroscopic sheath disruption rather than relying on thrombolytic instillation alone, which is less effective against an external fibrin sheath than against intraluminal clot.

Trap Logic: Any catheter dysfunction can be treated reflexively with a first-line thrombolytic instillation regardless of the underlying mechanism, but a fibrin sheath's characteristic asymmetric pattern and gradual onset distinguish it from acute thrombus and predict a more limited response to thrombolytic therapy alone.

Response Anchor: An asymmetric infuse-easy, aspirate-poor pattern with gradual onset points to a fibrin sheath — proceed toward guidewire exchange or sheath disruption rather than relying on thrombolytic instillation alone.

Diagnosis and Management of Catheter-Related Bloodstream Infection

Recognizing Catheter-Related Bloodstream Infection

Catheter-related bloodstream infection presents with fever, rigors, or hemodynamic instability temporally associated with catheter use, most classically occurring during or shortly after a dialysis treatment as bacteria colonizing the catheter are flushed into the systemic circulation by the blood flow treatment requires, though presentation can also occur independent of treatment timing in a more indolent, chronically colonized catheter. Exit-site or tunnel-tract erythema, tenderness, or purulent drainage, when present, strongly supports a catheter source for a febrile episode, but their absence does not exclude catheter-related bloodstream infection, since infection can originate from the catheter's intraluminal surface without any visible external exit-site or tunnel involvement at all.

Distinguishing a simple exit-site infection, confined to the immediate skin surrounding the catheter's exit point without extending along the subcutaneous tunnel, from a true tunnel-tract infection extending along the cuff's subcutaneous course, matters considerably for management: a simple exit-site infection often responds to local wound care and oral or topical antibiotics without necessarily requiring catheter removal, while tunnel-tract infection, discussed further below, generally does require removal given the difficulty of clearing infection from tissue surrounding an embedded foreign cuff. Careful palpation along the full subcutaneous tunnel course, not merely inspection of the visible exit site itself, is necessary to make this distinction reliably, since tunnel involvement may not always be visually apparent from the skin surface alone.

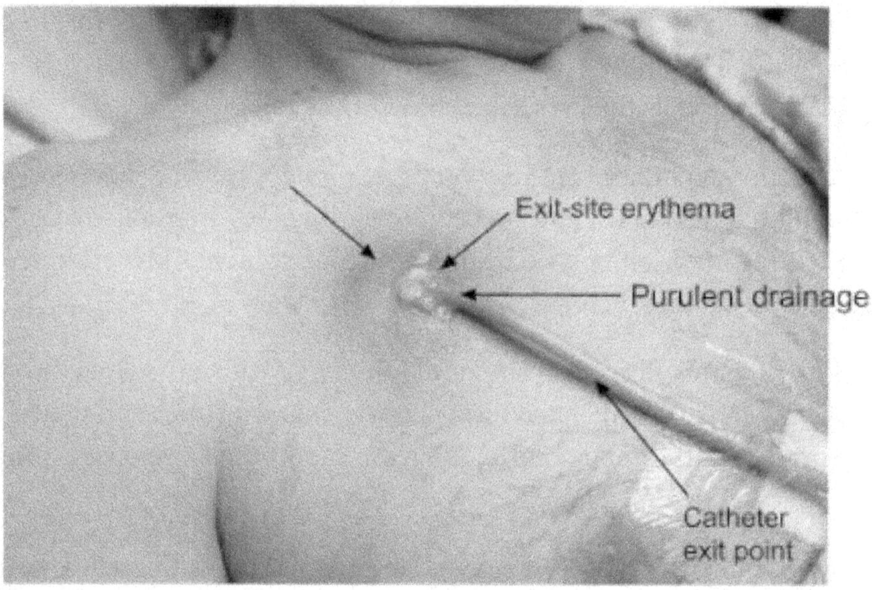

Paired blood cultures, one drawn through the catheter itself and one from a peripheral venipuncture site, support the diagnosis when the catheter-drawn culture becomes positive substantially earlier than the peripheral culture, a differential time to positivity reflecting the higher bacterial concentration typically present at the catheter's colonized surface relative to the patient's peripheral bloodstream; this paired culture technique, while not always practically obtained in every clinical circumstance, provides considerably more diagnostic specificity for a catheter source than a single culture drawn through the catheter alone, which cannot by itself distinguish catheter colonization from a bloodstream infection originating elsewhere and simply detected via the catheter-drawn sample.

Quantitative blood culture techniques, comparing the actual colony count from catheter-drawn versus peripheral samples rather than only the time to positivity, offer a further diagnostic refinement in centers with the laboratory capability to perform them, though differential time to positivity remains the more widely available and practically applied technique across most clinical settings; regardless of which specific comparative technique is used, the underlying diagnostic principle is the same: demonstrating that the catheter-associated sample carries a meaningfully higher bacterial burden than the peripheral sample supports attributing the bacteremia to the catheter rather than to some other, unrelated source.

Antibiotic Lock Therapy and Catheter Salvage

For a patient with confirmed catheter-related bloodstream infection who is hemodynamically stable, without evidence of severe sepsis, tunnel-tract infection, or a particularly virulent or difficult-to-treat organism, catheter salvage using systemic antibiotics combined with antibiotic lock therapy — instilling a high-concentration antibiotic solution within the catheter lumen between treatments, in addition to systemic therapy — offers a reasonable alternative to immediate catheter removal, particularly valuable for a patient with limited remaining vascular access options for whom catheter loss would be especially costly.

Salvage success depends considerably on the infecting organism: coagulase-negative staphylococci and many gram-negative organisms respond reasonably well to salvage attempts in appropriately selected patients, while Staphylococcus aureus bacteremia, fungal infection, and infections complicated by septic thrombosis or endocarditis generally warrant prompt catheter removal rather than a salvage attempt, given these organisms' and complications' associated risk of severe, difficult-to-clear infection and the more serious downstream consequences a failed salvage attempt would risk in these specific circumstances.

A defined trial period, typically several days of combined systemic and antibiotic lock therapy with close clinical monitoring and repeat blood cultures to confirm clearance, should be established at the outset of any salvage attempt, with a clear plan for proceeding to catheter removal if repeat cultures remain positive or clinical improvement does not occur within this defined window, rather than allowing a salvage attempt to continue indefinitely without a predetermined point at which it is deemed unsuccessful and removal is pursued instead.

When Catheter Removal Is Necessary

Catheter removal, with a new catheter placed at a different site once the infection has adequately cleared, is necessary when salvage is contraindicated by organism or clinical severity as discussed above, when a salvage attempt has already failed to clear the infection despite appropriate antibiotic lock and systemic therapy, or when tunnel-tract infection, evidenced by erythema and tenderness extending along the subcutaneous tunnel rather than confined to the immediate exit site, is present, since an infected tunnel tract cannot be adequately treated with antibiotics alone while the catheter and its incorporated cuff remain in place within the infected tissue.

A seventy-four-year-old man with a tunneled catheter as his only remaining access option, having exhausted surgical access possibilities per the extended evaluation described in Chapter 9, develops fever and rigors during a dialysis treatment. Paired blood cultures confirm catheter-related bloodstream infection with coagulase-negative staphylococci, without exit-site or tunnel-tract involvement on examination and without hemodynamic instability. Given his organism's generally favorable salvage prognosis and his lack of any remaining alternative access site, his nephrology team elects a salvage attempt with systemic antibiotics and antibiotic lock therapy rather than immediate catheter removal. His fevers resolve within forty-eight hours, repeat blood cultures clear, and his catheter remains in place and functional through a complete antibiotic course, avoiding the loss of his only remaining vascular access. This case illustrates why the salvage-versus-removal decision weighs both the specific infecting organism's salvage prognosis and the patient's remaining access options together, rather than defaulting reflexively to catheter removal for every confirmed infection regardless of these individualizing factors.

His team also documents the specific criteria that would have prompted a switch from salvage to removal had his clinical course diverged from the favorable trajectory actually observed — persistent fever or positive cultures beyond forty-eight to seventy-two hours of appropriate therapy, hemodynamic instability, or development of tunnel-tract involvement — ensuring that the salvage attempt proceeded with a defined endpoint for reassessment rather than as an open-ended trial without a clear point at which the team would have reconsidered the initial decision.

CAUTION: Tunnel-tract infection, Staphylococcus aureus bacteremia, fungal infection, and infection complicated by septic thrombosis or endocarditis generally warrant prompt catheter removal rather than a salvage attempt, given the substantially higher risk of a failed salvage attempt in these specific circumstances.

DIALYSIS RECOGNITION & RESPONSE SYSTEM — Catheter Care Arcs

The Pattern: A patient with a tunneled catheter and no remaining alternative vascular access develops confirmed catheter-related bloodstream infection.

Stem Signature: Fever and positive paired blood cultures confirming a catheter source, in a patient whose infecting organism is not Staphylococcus aureus or a fungal species, without tunnel-tract involvement, septic thrombosis, or endocarditis, and who has previously been assessed as having no remaining surgical access option.

The Decision: Attempt catheter salvage with systemic antibiotics and antibiotic lock therapy given the organism's favorable salvage prognosis and the patient's lack of alternative access, monitoring closely for treatment response rather than proceeding directly to catheter removal.

Trap Logic: Confirmed catheter infection can prompt reflexive catheter removal as the presumed safest default response, without weighing that removal itself carries real cost for a patient with no remaining access option, and that a favorable-prognosis organism without high-risk features genuinely supports a reasonable salvage attempt first.

Response Anchor: A favorable-prognosis organism without tunnel-tract involvement or other high-risk features, in a patient with no remaining access alternative, supports a salvage attempt — not reflexive catheter removal as the default first response.

Asymmetric Infuse-Easy, Aspirate-Poor Dysfunction: Recognize the fibrin sheath pattern and proceed toward guidewire exchange or sheath disruption rather than thrombolytic instillation alone.

Confirmed Infection With No Remaining Access Alternative: Weigh the organism's salvage prognosis and the patient's access options together, attempting salvage where both favor it rather than defaulting to reflexive removal.

Summary and Key Concepts

Tunneled catheters, anchored by an incorporated Dacron cuff within a subcutaneous tunnel, are suitable for weeks to months of use; non-tunneled catheters are intended for short-term bridging only, given their higher infection and dislodgement risk.

The right internal jugular vein is the preferred insertion site for essentially all patients; the subclavian vein is reserved for circumstances in which both internal jugular sites are unavailable, given its disproportionate central stenosis risk.

Ultrasound guidance and maximal sterile barrier precautions during insertion, combined with confirmed cavoatrial junction tip position, reduce both mechanical and infectious insertion complications.

Catheter dysfunction arises from intraluminal thrombus, an external fibrin sheath, or tip malposition, each requiring a distinct corrective approach; an asymmetric infuse-easy, aspirate-poor pattern points specifically toward a fibrin sheath.

Catheter-related bloodstream infection salvage with antibiotic lock therapy is reasonable for favorable-prognosis organisms in a hemodynamically stable patient without tunnel-tract involvement, particularly when the patient has no remaining access alternative; Staphylococcus aureus, fungal infection, and tunnel-tract or endovascular complications generally warrant prompt removal instead.

CHAPTER 13: INTRADIALYTIC HYPOTENSION AND HEMODYNAMIC INSTABILITY

Learning Objectives

Explain the physiologic mechanisms underlying intradialytic hypotension, including plasma refilling, autonomic compensation, and cardiac contribution.

Identify patient-level and prescription-level risk factors that predispose to intradialytic hypotension.

Recognize evolving intradialytic hypotension at the bedside and apply an immediate, staged response.

Apply sodium and ultrafiltration profiling, alongside other preventive strategies, to reduce the frequency of intradialytic hypotension in a susceptible patient.

Chapter Overview

Intradialytic hypotension is the most common complication encountered during hemodialysis treatment, occurring in a substantial proportion of sessions across the dialysis population as a whole and considerably more often in specific high-risk patients this chapter will characterize in detail. It is also among the most consequential: recurrent intradialytic hypotension is associated with reduced residual kidney function, myocardial and cerebral hypoperfusion with cumulative organ injury over repeated episodes, and a documented association with higher mortality in patients who experience it frequently. This chapter builds directly on the physiology established in Chapter 4, particularly the relationship between ultrafiltration rate and plasma refilling capacity, and extends that physiology into the practical bedside skills of recognition, immediate response, and prevention that every clinician and dialysis staff member managing hemodialysis patients must master. The chapter that follows addresses the narrower complications of cramps and dialyzer reactions, and the chapter after that addresses the rarer but more acutely dangerous emergencies of air embolism and arrhythmia; this chapter's subject, by contrast, is common enough that every experienced dialysis clinician will encounter it repeatedly across a career, making fluency with its recognition and management foundational rather than optional.

Pathogenesis of Intradialytic Hypotension

Plasma Refilling and Ultrafiltration Rate

As established in Chapter 4, ultrafiltration removes fluid directly from the plasma compartment, and maintaining adequate plasma volume during this removal depends on fluid moving from the interstitial and, to a lesser extent, intracellular compartments back into the vascular space at a rate that keeps pace with the ultrafiltration rate itself. This plasma refilling process is not instantaneous; it proceeds at a finite rate governed by the permeability of the capillary membrane, the hydrostatic and oncotic pressure gradients across it, and the total volume of interstitial fluid available to be mobilized, and when the prescribed ultrafiltration rate exceeds the rate at which refilling can occur, plasma volume falls progressively over the course of the treatment even though total body water is being removed at exactly the prescribed rate.

This mismatch between ultrafiltration rate and refilling capacity is the proximate mechanism underlying the majority of intradialytic hypotension episodes, and it explains several clinically familiar patterns: hypotension tends to cluster in the latter portion of a treatment, once a substantial fraction of readily mobilizable interstitial fluid has already been drawn down; it tends to occur more readily in patients with a large interdialytic weight gain, since a larger total ultrafiltration volume compressed into a fixed treatment time necessarily demands a higher average ultrafiltration rate; and it responds, at least partially, to the treatment-time extension strategy detailed in Chapter 6, since extending time for a fixed total fluid removal volume directly reduces the ultrafiltration rate the refilling process must keep pace with.

Refilling capacity itself is not a fixed, patient-independent constant; it varies with a patient's overall volume status, nutritional and albumin status, since oncotic pressure depends substantially on plasma protein concentration, and with any condition affecting capillary permeability or interstitial fluid volume, such as longstanding poor nutritional status producing a depleted interstitial reservoir with less fluid available to mobilize in the first place. This variability is part of why two patients undergoing what appears to be an identical ultrafiltration prescription can experience dramatically different hemodynamic tolerance, and why the risk factors detailed in the next section of this chapter must be assessed individually rather than assumed uniform across the general dialysis population.

The relationship between refilling capacity and ultrafiltration tolerance is not static across a single treatment either; as fluid is progressively removed and the interstitial reservoir depletes, the refilling rate itself tends to slow even at a constant ultrafiltration rate, meaning the same ultrafiltration rate that was well tolerated in the first hour of treatment may become poorly tolerated in the third hour simply because the physiologic reserve available to support refilling has been progressively consumed. This time-dependent decline in refilling capacity is the physiologic basis for the ultrafiltration profiling strategy discussed later in this chapter, which front-loads fluid removal specifically to take advantage of the greater refilling capacity available early in treatment.

Autonomic and Vascular Compensatory Mechanisms

As plasma volume falls during ultrafiltration, the body's normal compensatory response involves baroreceptor-mediated sympathetic activation, producing peripheral vasoconstriction to maintain central blood pressure despite the falling circulating volume, along with a compensatory increase in heart rate intended to preserve cardiac output as stroke volume declines with reduced venous return. In a patient with intact autonomic function, this compensatory sequence maintains blood pressure across a considerable range of volume depletion before hypotension actually manifests clinically, meaning symptomatic hypotension often represents the point at which compensatory capacity has been genuinely exhausted rather than the earliest possible sign of volume depletion.

Autonomic neuropathy, common in patients with longstanding diabetes and present to a lesser degree in the general dialysis population as a consequence of the uremic milieu itself, blunts this compensatory sequence considerably: a diabetic patient with significant autonomic neuropathy may show minimal heart rate response and inadequate vasoconstriction despite substantial volume depletion, producing a more abrupt, less gradually warned transition from apparently stable hemodynamics to frank hypotension than a patient with intact autonomic function would experience under the same ultrafiltration conditions. Recognizing which patients carry this blunted compensatory capacity, primarily through a known diabetes history and, where available, formal autonomic function testing, informs both risk stratification and bedside vigilance, since these patients may not display the gradual heart rate rise that would otherwise serve as an early warning sign in a patient with intact autonomic reflexes.

Vascular compliance and vasoconstrictive capacity also decline with age and with vascular calcification, a common finding in the long-term dialysis population given the mineral and bone disorder discussed in Chapter 23, further limiting the vasoconstrictive compensation available to older or more vascularly diseased patients relative to younger patients with more compliant, more reactive vasculature. This combination of factors — autonomic impairment and vascular stiffening — helps explain why intradialytic hypotension clusters so heavily among older patients with diabetes and established cardiovascular disease, a population in whom the compensatory mechanisms that would otherwise buffer against ultrafiltration-related volume depletion are most likely to be already compromised.

Cardiac Contributions to Hypotension

Beyond the peripheral vascular and autonomic mechanisms discussed above, cardiac factors contribute independently to intradialytic hypotension risk: diastolic dysfunction, extremely common in the long-term dialysis population given the combination of hypertension, left ventricular hypertrophy, and the chronic volume and pressure loading dialysis-dependent kidney failure imposes, produces a heart that is unusually sensitive to reductions in preload, since a stiff, poorly compliant left ventricle depends on adequate filling pressure to maintain stroke volume in a way a normally compliant ventricle does not.

Myocardial stunning, a transient, reversible impairment of regional myocardial contractility induced by the repeated ischemic stress of intradialytic hemodynamic instability itself, has been demonstrated in serial imaging studies of hemodialysis patients undergoing routine treatment, and represents a particularly concerning finding because it suggests a self-perpetuating cycle: episodes of intradialytic hypotension may themselves induce myocardial stunning that impairs cardiac reserve for subsequent treatments, increasing vulnerability to further hypotensive episodes in a pattern that, left unaddressed, compounds over repeated treatments rather than remaining a stable, one-time risk.

Arrhythmia, whether a preexisting condition or one precipitated acutely by the metabolic shifts discussed in Chapter 4's treatment of potassium and acid-base changes during treatment, can independently produce or worsen hypotension by disrupting the coordinated atrial and ventricular contraction sequence needed to maintain adequate cardiac output, and a patient whose hypotension does not respond to the standard interventions detailed later in this chapter should be assessed for a new or worsening arrhythmia as a potential contributing or primary cause rather than assuming straightforward volume-related hypotension in every case regardless of response to standard measures.

Pericardial effusion, whether from the uremic pericarditis discussed in Chapter 1 or another cause, represents a further, less common but important cardiac contributor to intradialytic hypotension, since even a modest effusion can produce enough pericardial constraint to limit ventricular filling further during the volume shifts of dialysis treatment, and a patient with known or suspected pericardial effusion warrants particular caution with ultrafiltration rate and closer hemodynamic monitoring than a patient without this additional cardiac constraint on filling.

KEY POINT: Intradialytic hypotension results from the interaction of ultrafiltration rate exceeding plasma refilling capacity, impaired autonomic and vascular compensation, and cardiac factors including diastolic dysfunction and myocardial stunning — not from any single mechanism operating in isolation.

Figure 13.1: Plasma Refilling and Ultrafiltration Rate Mismatch

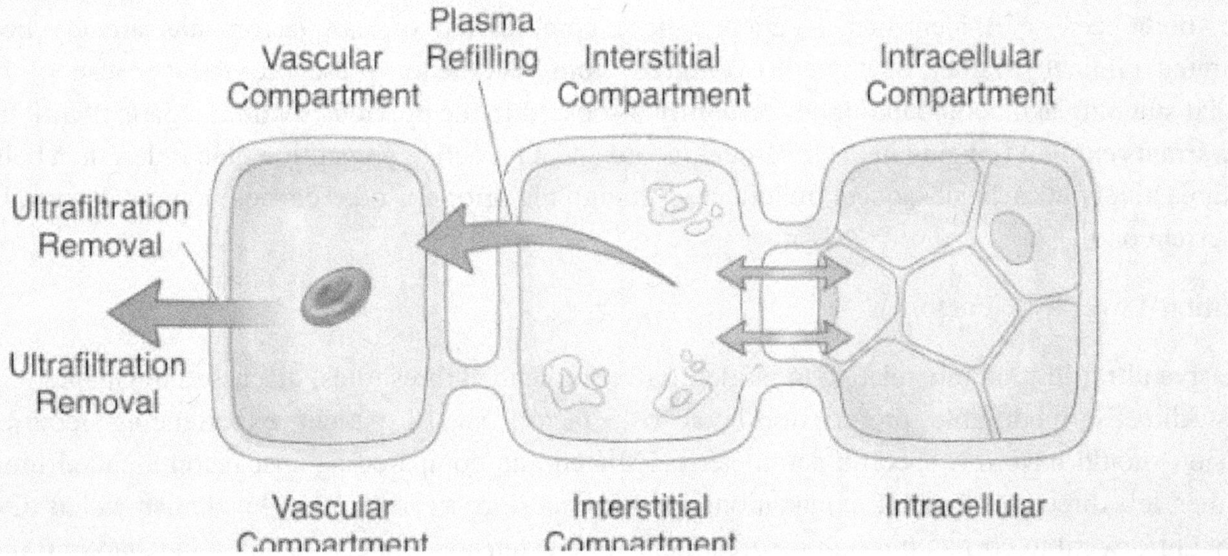

Predisposing Patient and Prescription Factors

Patient-Level Risk Factors

Advanced age, diabetes with autonomic neuropathy, established cardiovascular disease including diastolic dysfunction and prior myocardial infarction, and poor nutritional status with low serum albumin each independently increase intradialytic hypotension risk through the mechanisms detailed in the previous section, and a patient carrying several of these risk factors simultaneously experiences a compounding rather than simply additive increase in overall risk, since each factor tends to impair a different compensatory mechanism, leaving progressively fewer intact backup systems as risk factors accumulate.

Female sex and lower body weight have also been associated with somewhat higher intradialytic hypotension risk in some observational studies, plausibly reflecting the same body-size-dependent considerations discussed in Chapter 7's treatment of Kt/V interpretation: a smaller total blood volume relative to a given absolute ultrafiltration rate produces a proportionally larger fractional volume depletion than the same absolute rate would produce in a larger-bodied patient, underscoring again why absolute prescription parameters should be interpreted relative to the specific patient's body size and physiology rather than applied identically across a diverse patient population.

A low pre-dialysis blood pressure, whether from antihypertensive medication timing, autonomic dysfunction, or simply a patient's own baseline hemodynamic tendency, leaves less hemodynamic reserve to draw on before hypotension becomes clinically apparent, and identifying this pattern before treatment begins, through routine pre-dialysis vital sign assessment, allows anticipatory planning — a more conservative ultrafiltration rate, closer intradialytic monitoring, or a discussion with the patient's prescribing physician about antihypertensive medication timing relative to dialysis days — rather than discovering the elevated risk only once hypotension has already developed during treatment.

A history of recent or recurrent intradialytic hypotension is itself among the strongest predictors of future episodes, both because it identifies a patient whose combination of risk factors has already been demonstrated clinically rather than merely inferred from risk factor presence, and because of the myocardial stunning and compounding vulnerability discussed in the previous section; a patient with this history warrants explicit flagging in the treatment record and a proactive prevention plan rather than being managed reactively at each subsequent treatment as though the prior episodes carried no predictive value for the current one.

Prescription-Level Risk Factors

An excessive ultrafiltration rate relative to guideline-recommended thresholds, discussed in Chapter 6, is the most directly modifiable prescription-level risk factor, and a patient experiencing recurrent hypotension should have this specific parameter calculated and compared against recommended limits before other, less directly actionable explanations are pursued, since a prescription-level mismatch is often more straightforward to correct through the treatment-time extension strategy detailed in Chapter 6 than a patient-level risk factor such as diastolic dysfunction, which cannot be directly modified through prescription adjustment alone.

A dialysate sodium concentration set too low relative to the patient's own plasma sodium, discussed in Chapter 4, removes sodium from the blood by diffusion faster than is hemodynamically comfortable for some patients, compounding the volume-related hypotension risk with an additional osmotic and vascular refilling burden; similarly, a dialysate temperature set at standard body temperature rather than the modestly cooler setting discussed in Chapter 6 forgoes the mild vasoconstrictive benefit cooler dialysate provides, an easily overlooked prescription lever in a patient whose hypotension risk might benefit from this additional, low-cost adjustment.

Antihypertensive medication timing relative to the dialysis treatment itself is a further prescription-adjacent factor, though one residing partly outside the dialysis prescription proper and requiring coordination with the patient's broader medical care: a patient taking a short-acting antihypertensive shortly before a scheduled treatment may experience compounded hypotension from the medication's peak effect coinciding with the treatment's own hemodynamic stress, and holding or adjusting the timing of such medications on dialysis days, coordinated with the prescribing clinician, is a frequently underutilized but often effective prevention strategy for a patient whose hypotension pattern suggests this specific contributing factor.

Cumulative Risk Assessment

Because intradialytic hypotension risk arises from the interaction of multiple patient-level and prescription-level factors rather than any single dominant cause in most patients, a structured cumulative risk assessment, reviewing each factor discussed in this section systematically rather than addressing only the most recently identified or most obvious contributor, produces a more complete prevention plan than addressing factors piecemeal as they happen to be noticed. This structured approach mirrors the whole-patient adequacy assessment framework developed in Chapter 7 and the multidimensional prescription review recommended in Chapter 6: a single dominant explanation is convenient but often incomplete, and a patient's actual hypotension risk usually reflects the additive or compounding effect of several factors acting together.

Documenting this cumulative risk assessment explicitly in the patient's chart, rather than allowing it to exist only as an informal, undocumented impression among staff familiar with the patient, ensures that a covering clinician or a staff member less familiar with the patient's specific history has access to the same risk picture that has already been established, supporting consistent anticipatory management across every treatment rather than only when a staff member who happens to remember the patient's history is present.

Shift handoff communication specifically should include an explicit review of any patient flagged as high-risk for intradialytic hypotension under this cumulative assessment, since a staff member beginning a shift without this information has no way of knowing which patients warrant the heightened vigilance and increased monitoring frequency this chapter recommends, and a structured handoff checklist that explicitly prompts this review, rather than relying on incoming staff to independently notice a chart flag amid the many other handoff details competing for attention, better ensures this risk information actually transfers reliably from one shift to the next.

Risk Category	Specific Factor	Modifiability
Patient-Level	Diabetes with autonomic neuropathy	Not directly modifiable; informs vigilance

Patient-Level	Diastolic dysfunction and prior cardiac disease	Not directly modifiable; informs vigilance
Patient-Level	Low nutritional status and albumin	Modifiable over time through nutritional intervention
Prescription-Level	Excessive ultrafiltration rate	Directly modifiable through treatment time extension
Prescription-Level	Dialysate sodium and temperature settings	Directly modifiable through prescription adjustment
Prescription-Adjacent	Antihypertensive medication timing	Modifiable through coordination with prescribing clinician

Bedside Recognition and Immediate Response

Recognizing Evolving Intradialytic Hypotension

Early symptoms of evolving hypotension are frequently nonspecific and easily attributed to other causes: yawning, restlessness, nausea, and a vague sense of unease or discomfort often precede overt hypotension by several minutes, and staff trained to recognize this early symptom cluster as a potential harbinger of hypotension, rather than dismissing it as unrelated patient discomfort, can intervene before blood pressure has fallen to a level producing more dramatic symptoms such as dizziness, visual disturbance, or frank syncope.

Scheduled, frequent blood pressure monitoring throughout treatment, rather than only at the start and end, provides the objective data needed to catch a declining trend before it becomes symptomatic, and monitoring frequency should be increased specifically for patients identified as high-risk through the cumulative assessment described in the previous section, since a standard monitoring interval adequate for a low-risk patient may not catch a rapidly evolving episode in a high-risk patient with limited compensatory reserve and correspondingly less warning time between the onset of decline and the point of clinically significant hypotension.

Because ultrafiltration rate is typically highest, and therefore hypotension risk correspondingly greatest, during the middle-to-later portion of a standard treatment once a substantial fraction of the prescribed fluid removal has already occurred, this period warrants heightened attentiveness even in a patient without other specific risk factors, and staff scheduling and workflow within a busy dialysis unit should account for this pattern, ensuring that staff attention is not disproportionately concentrated at treatment initiation, when hypotension risk is typically lower, at the expense of the later treatment period when risk is often highest.

Continuous, automated blood pressure monitoring, available on many contemporary dialysis machines and capable of measuring at intervals considerably more frequent than the traditional fifteen-to-thirty-minute manual check, offers a further layer of surveillance particularly valuable for high-risk patients, providing a denser data stream from which a declining trend can be identified earlier than a sparser manual monitoring schedule would allow; where available, this automated capability should be preferentially applied to the highest-risk patients identified through the cumulative assessment process described earlier in this chapter, reserving the additional monitoring resource for the population most likely to benefit from the earlier warning it provides.

Immediate Bedside Response

Once hypotension is recognized, whether through symptoms, a measured blood pressure decline, or both, the immediate response follows a staged sequence: reducing or temporarily suspending the ultrafiltration rate to halt further volume removal, placing the patient in the Trendelenburg or a modified reverse-Trendelenburg position depending on unit protocol and patient tolerance to promote venous return, and administering a bolus of isotonic saline or, in some protocols, a hypertonic saline or dextrose solution to rapidly restore intravascular volume.

Reassessing blood pressure and symptoms within several minutes of these initial measures confirms whether the response has been adequate before deciding whether treatment can safely continue, whether ultrafiltration should resume at a reduced rate, or whether the treatment should be terminated early for that session; a patient whose hypotension resolves promptly with initial measures can often continue treatment, ideally at a lower ultrafiltration rate for the remainder of the session, while a patient whose hypotension persists or recurs despite these measures warrants a broader reassessment for one of the alternative or contributing causes discussed in the next subsection rather than simply repeating the same fluid bolus without further evaluation.

The specific volume and tonicity of fluid bolus used varies by unit protocol and patient circumstance: isotonic saline remains the most widely used first-line option given its simplicity and broad applicability, while hypertonic saline or dextrose solutions, used in some protocols specifically for their additional osmotic effect drawing fluid from the intracellular compartment into the vascular space, may be considered for a patient whose hypotension has proven resistant to isotonic saline alone, though these hypertonic options carry their own considerations, including the sodium load discussed in Chapter 4 for hypertonic saline and the glycemic effect discussed in Chapter 6 for dextrose-containing solutions, that should factor into the choice for a given patient.

Every episode of intradialytic hypotension, regardless of how promptly and successfully it was managed, should be documented with sufficient detail to inform the cumulative risk assessment discussed earlier in this chapter, including the ultrafiltration rate and volume at the time of the episode, the interventions used, and the response to those interventions; this documentation, reviewed at the patient's next prescription review as described in Chapter 6, is what allows a pattern across multiple episodes to be recognized and addressed proactively rather than each episode being managed in isolation without informing the patient's ongoing prevention plan.

CAUTION: Persistent or recurrent hypotension despite standard positional and fluid bolus measures warrants evaluation for an alternative or contributing cause — arrhythmia, occult bleeding, sepsis, or a dialyzer reaction — rather than repeated fluid administration alone.

Distinguishing Hypotension From Other Intradialytic Emergencies

Because several other intradialytic emergencies discussed in the next chapter, including air embolism, hemolysis, and severe allergic dialyzer reactions, can present with hypotension as a component of a broader symptom picture, a structured evaluation considering these alternative or contributing diagnoses is warranted whenever hypotension fails to respond promptly to standard measures, presents with an atypical accompanying symptom pattern such as chest pain, severe dyspnea, or a rash, or occurs in a context that raises specific suspicion for one of these alternative causes, such as a newly opened dialyzer or a recent line disconnection.

Occult bleeding, whether from a gastrointestinal source, a vascular access complication such as the rupture risk discussed in Chapter 11, or another site entirely, should also be considered in a patient whose hypotension is disproportionate to the ultrafiltration volume removed or accompanied by a falling hematocrit inconsistent with hemodilution alone, since volume-related hypotension from ultrafiltration and hypovolemic hypotension from bleeding require different immediate priorities, the latter demanding source identification and control rather than the standard positional and fluid bolus measures alone, however similar the two presentations may initially appear at the bedside.

Patient education regarding their own individual hypotension risk and warning signs, paralleling the vascular access self-monitoring education detailed in Chapter 10, empowers a patient to communicate proactively with staff at the earliest sign of the nonspecific symptoms discussed earlier in this chapter, rather than staff needing to detect every early warning sign entirely on their own through observation alone; a patient who understands that yawning or a vague sense of unease during their usual high-risk portion of treatment is worth mentioning immediately, rather than waiting to see if it resolves on its own, adds a valuable second layer of detection alongside staff vigilance and scheduled monitoring.

A sixty-nine-year-old man with diabetes, known diastolic dysfunction, and a history of recurrent intradialytic hypotension over the preceding two months is found on chart review to have a prescribed ultrafiltration rate consistently exceeding guideline-recommended thresholds on the two treatments following his longer interdialytic interval. His nephrology team implements a cumulative prevention bundle: extending treatment time by thirty minutes on those two specific treatments, adjusting his dialysate sodium to a modest upward profile early in treatment, reducing dialysate temperature by half a degree, and coordinating with his primary care physician to shift his morning antihypertensive dose to the evening on dialysis days. Over the following month, his hypotension episodes decline from an average of twice weekly to a single episode over four weeks, illustrating how a multimodal approach addressing several risk factors simultaneously, rather than a single isolated intervention, produced a meaningfully better outcome than any single measure would likely have achieved alone.

His team documents this bundle explicitly in his chart as his standing hypotension prevention protocol, ensuring any covering clinician or staff member treating him at a future session, including at another unit should he travel, has access to the specific combination of measures that proved effective for him individually, rather than each treating clinician needing to rediscover an effective approach independently through their own trial and error.

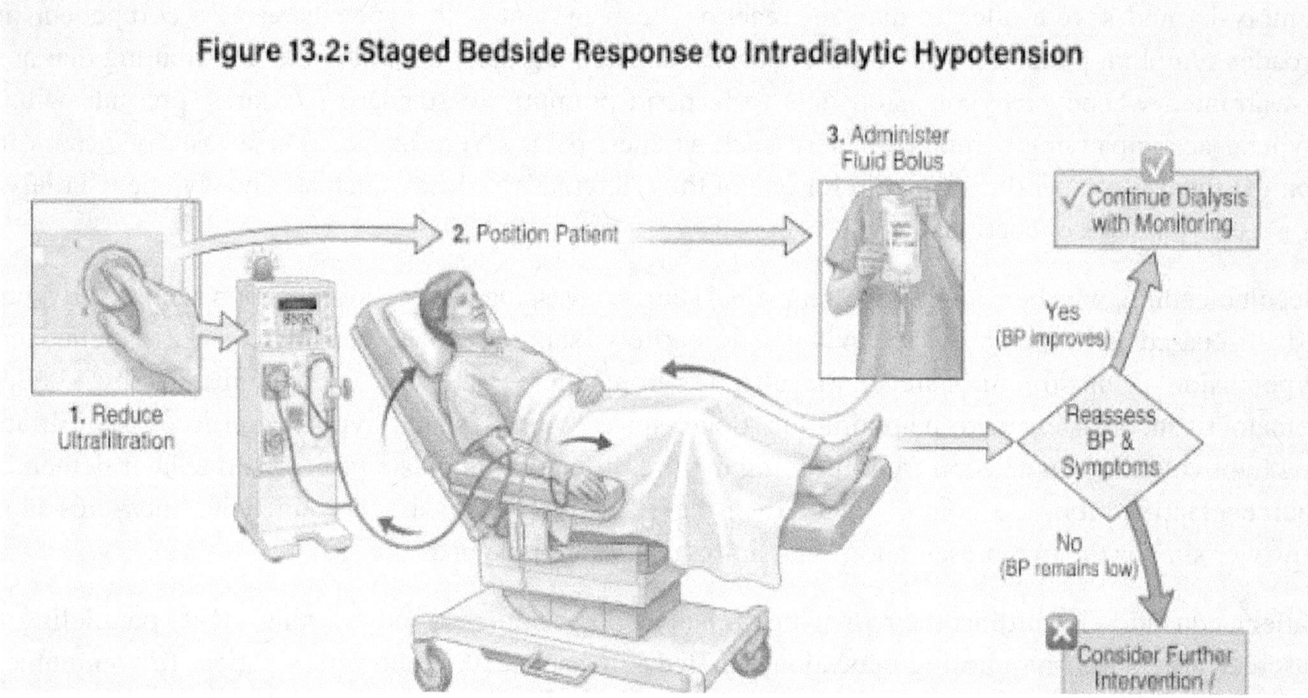

DIALYSIS RECOGNITION & RESPONSE SYSTEM — Hemodynamic Instability Arcs

The Pattern: A patient develops nonspecific symptoms such as yawning, restlessness, or mild nausea during the middle-to-later portion of treatment.

Stem Signature: Vague, nonspecific discomfort, yawning, or restlessness developing during the period of treatment when ultrafiltration rate is typically highest, without yet meeting a formal threshold for measured hypotension on the most recent blood pressure check.

The Decision: Treat these nonspecific symptoms as a potential early warning sign of evolving hypotension, obtain an immediate blood pressure check regardless of the scheduled monitoring interval, and consider reducing ultrafiltration rate proactively rather than waiting for the next scheduled check or for more dramatic symptoms to develop.

Trap Logic: Nonspecific symptoms like yawning or mild restlessness are easily dismissed as unrelated patient discomfort or simple boredom during a long treatment, when in fact they frequently precede overt, measurable hypotension by several minutes in susceptible patients.

Response Anchor: Nonspecific symptoms during the high-ultrafiltration-rate portion of treatment warrant an immediate, unscheduled blood pressure check — not dismissal as unrelated discomfort.

Preventive Strategies: Sodium and Ultrafiltration Profiling

Sodium Profiling Revisited

Sodium profiling, introduced in Chapter 4 as a technique for supporting plasma refilling during the higher-ultrafiltration-rate early portion of treatment while limiting net sodium load by treatment's end, is one of the most directly actionable prevention tools available for a patient with recurrent hypotension, and its implementation should be individualized to the specific patient's hypotension pattern rather than applied as a single generic profile uniformly: a patient whose hypotension clusters early in treatment may benefit from a more pronounced early sodium elevation than a patient whose hypotension clusters later, whose profile might instead extend a moderate sodium elevation further into the treatment before tapering.

The interdialytic weight gain and thirst consequences of sodium profiling, also discussed in Chapter 4, should be monitored explicitly when this technique is used preventively for hypotension, since a profile effective at reducing intradialytic hypotension but producing a substantial increase in interdialytic weight gain has simply shifted the clinical problem from intradialytic hemodynamic instability to a larger fluid burden the next treatment must remove, potentially perpetuating rather than resolving the underlying hypotension risk if the larger subsequent ultrafiltration volume itself produces further hypotension.

Individualizing a sodium profile requires reviewing several treatments' worth of blood pressure trend data alongside the specific profile used, rather than adjusting the profile based on a single treatment's outcome, since day-to-day variability in interdialytic weight gain and other factors can make a single treatment's response an unreliable guide to whether a given profile is genuinely effective for a specific patient; this trend-based approach to profile adjustment mirrors the same trend-over-single-value principle this book has applied to Kt/V interpretation in Chapter 7 and to vascular access surveillance in Chapter 11.

Ultrafiltration Profiling and Rate Limits

Ultrafiltration profiling, varying the ultrafiltration rate across the treatment rather than maintaining a constant rate throughout, typically front-loads a higher rate early in treatment when plasma refilling capacity is greatest, given the larger reservoir of readily mobilizable interstitial fluid available at that point, and tapers the rate toward the end of treatment as this reservoir becomes progressively depleted and refilling capacity correspondingly declines; this profiling approach can reduce hypotension frequency in some patients relative to a constant ultrafiltration rate, though, as with sodium profiling, its benefit is not universal across all patients and should be assessed individually against the specific patient's response.

Adherence to guideline-recommended maximum ultrafiltration rate thresholds, discussed in Chapter 6, remains foundational regardless of whether profiling is additionally employed, since profiling redistributes the ultrafiltration burden across the treatment but does not, by itself, reduce the total ultrafiltration volume that must be removed; a patient whose total ultrafiltration requirement genuinely exceeds what any redistribution of a fixed treatment time can safely accommodate still requires the treatment-time extension strategy discussed in Chapter 6 as the more fundamental intervention, with profiling serving as a complementary rather than a substitute measure.

Multimodal Prevention Bundles

As the case presented earlier in this chapter illustrated, the most effective prevention strategy for a patient with recurrent intradialytic hypotension typically combines several of the interventions discussed throughout this chapter — treatment time extension, sodium and ultrafiltration profiling, dialysate temperature reduction, and antihypertensive medication timing coordination — rather than relying on any single measure in isolation, reflecting the same multidimensional, cumulative-risk-based approach to prevention that this chapter's earlier discussion of risk assessment recommends for diagnosis.

Structuring this multimodal approach into a standardized, reusable prevention bundle that a dialysis unit can apply consistently whenever a patient is identified as high-risk, rather than reinventing an individualized plan from scratch for each newly identified high-risk patient, supports more consistent and more rapid implementation of effective prevention measures across a unit's full patient population, extending the same systemic, workflow-embedded principle this book has applied repeatedly to Life-Plan revision, prescription review, and vascular access surveillance to the specific domain of intradialytic hypotension prevention.

DIALYSIS RECOGNITION & RESPONSE SYSTEM — Hemodynamic Instability Arcs

The Pattern: A patient experiences recurrent intradialytic hypotension despite a single, isolated preventive measure already in place.

Stem Signature: Continued frequent hypotension episodes in a patient already receiving one preventive intervention, such as sodium profiling alone or dialysate temperature reduction alone, without the other complementary measures this chapter describes.

The Decision: Implement a multimodal prevention bundle combining several complementary measures — treatment time, sodium and ultrafiltration profiling, temperature, and medication timing — rather than escalating the single measure already in place or concluding that prevention has been fully attempted.

Trap Logic: A single preventive measure already in place can create a false sense that prevention has been adequately addressed, when in fact most patients with genuinely recurrent hypotension require several complementary interventions addressing different contributing mechanisms simultaneously.

Response Anchor: Recurrent hypotension despite a single preventive measure warrants a multimodal bundle addressing several mechanisms together — not escalation of the single measure already in place alone.

Nonspecific Symptoms During High-Ultrafiltration-Rate Periods: Obtain an immediate, unscheduled blood pressure check and consider proactive ultrafiltration reduction rather than dismissing the symptoms as unrelated discomfort.

Recurrent Hypotension Despite a Single Preventive Measure: Implement a multimodal prevention bundle addressing several contributing mechanisms together rather than escalating a single isolated measure.

Summary and Key Concepts

Intradialytic hypotension arises from the interaction of ultrafiltration rate exceeding plasma refilling capacity, impaired autonomic and vascular compensation, and cardiac factors including diastolic dysfunction and myocardial stunning.

Patient-level risk factors such as diabetes, cardiovascular disease, and poor nutrition compound with prescription-level factors such as excessive ultrafiltration rate, and a structured cumulative risk assessment identifies more complete prevention opportunities than addressing any single factor in isolation.

Nonspecific symptoms such as yawning or restlessness often precede measurable hypotension, and staff trained to recognize this early pattern can intervene before more dramatic symptoms develop.

The immediate bedside response follows a staged sequence of ultrafiltration reduction, positioning, and fluid administration, and persistent hypotension despite these measures warrants evaluation for an alternative or contributing cause.

Sodium profiling, ultrafiltration profiling, and other preventive measures are most effective combined into a multimodal, individualized prevention bundle rather than applied as a single isolated intervention.

CHAPTER 14: CRAMPS, DIALYZER REACTIONS, AND OTHER COMMON INTRADIALYTIC SYMPTOMS

Learning Objectives

Explain the pathophysiology of intradialytic muscle cramps and apply preventive and acute management strategies.

Distinguish the mechanisms of intradialytic nausea, vomiting, and headache and manage each appropriately.

Differentiate Type A and Type B dialyzer reactions by timing, presentation, and mechanism.

Recognize pyrogenic reactions and distinguish them from true catheter- or bloodstream-related bacteremia.

Chapter Overview

Chapter 13 addressed intradialytic hypotension, the single most common and most consequential intradialytic complication. This chapter addresses the remaining common symptom complexes that, while individually less dangerous than hypotension in the great majority of cases, occur frequently enough across a dialysis population that every clinician and dialysis staff member needs fluency in recognizing and managing each of them: muscle cramps, nausea and vomiting, headache, the dialyzer reactions introduced in Chapter 5, and pyrogenic reactions related to the water treatment and endotoxin exposure discussed in that same chapter. Several of these symptoms overlap in presentation with hypotension itself, and part of this chapter's purpose is to help the reader distinguish among them at the bedside, since the appropriate management for a cramp differs meaningfully from the appropriate management for early hypotension or an evolving dialyzer reaction, even though a patient experiencing any of these may present with a similar initial complaint of feeling unwell. A unifying theme across every symptom this chapter addresses is that an accurate first-response assessment, rather than an assumption based on which symptom complex happens to be most familiar or most recently encountered by the treating staff, determines whether the subsequent management proceeds efficiently toward the actual underlying cause or instead cycles through a series of interventions targeting the wrong mechanism before eventually arriving at an effective one.

Muscle Cramps: Mechanism and Management

Pathophysiology of Intradialytic Cramps

Intradialytic muscle cramps, most commonly affecting the calves, feet, and hands, are closely linked mechanistically to the intradialytic hypotension discussed in Chapter 13, sharing several of the same predisposing factors: rapid ultrafiltration reducing plasma volume and, correspondingly, muscle perfusion; a low dialysate sodium concentration relative to the patient's plasma sodium, producing an osmotic shift that affects muscle cell volume and excitability; and a low or rapidly falling calcium concentration during treatment, affecting neuromuscular excitability directly. Because cramps frequently precede or accompany intradialytic hypotension rather than occurring as an entirely separate phenomenon, evaluating for and addressing volume status is an appropriate first step even when cramps are the presenting complaint rather than measured hypotension itself, since the two frequently share the same underlying driver of excessive or rapid ultrafiltration relative to the patient's individual tolerance.

The precise cellular mechanism underlying the muscle cramp itself, beyond the volume and electrolyte contributors already described, likely involves altered muscle fiber membrane excitability and impaired neuromuscular junction function under conditions of relative hypoperfusion and electrolyte shift, producing the involuntary, painful, sustained muscle contraction characteristic of a cramp; this mechanism, while incompletely understood at the molecular level, is sufficiently well characterized at the clinical level to support the prevention and management strategies detailed in the remainder of this section, which target the upstream volume and electrolyte drivers rather than attempting to intervene directly at the muscle fiber level itself.

Carnitine deficiency, common in the long-term dialysis population given carnitine's partial dependence on kidney-mediated reabsorption and its removal during dialysis treatment itself, has been proposed as a contributing factor to cramp susceptibility in some patients, and carnitine supplementation has been studied as a targeted intervention for patients with frequent cramps refractory to the volume and electrolyte-focused measures detailed throughout this section, though the evidence supporting this approach remains less robust than the evidence supporting the primary prevention strategies this chapter emphasizes, and carnitine supplementation is generally reserved as a secondary consideration for refractory cases rather than a first-line intervention.

Risk Factors and Prevention

Patients experiencing frequent cramps share considerable overlap with the intradialytic hypotension risk factors detailed in Chapter 13: excessive interdialytic weight gain necessitating a high ultrafiltration rate, a dry weight set too low relative to the patient's true euvolemic weight, and a low dialysate sodium concentration each independently increase cramp frequency, and the same prevention strategies detailed in Chapter 13 for hypotension — treatment time extension, sodium and ultrafiltration profiling, and dry weight reassessment — correspondingly reduce cramp frequency in most affected patients, reflecting the shared underlying physiology between the two complications.

For patients whose cramps persist despite these standard measures, or whose cramps appear disproportionate to their apparent volume status, a dry weight reassessment specifically targeted at the possibility that the current dry weight is set below the patient's true euvolemic weight, discussed in Chapter

4, deserves particular consideration, since a dry weight set too aggressively low produces a state of chronic relative volume depletion that predisposes to cramps even on treatments without an unusually large ultrafiltration requirement, a pattern distinct from the more typical cramp pattern tied to an unusually large single-treatment ultrafiltration volume.

Patients using the ultrafiltration profiling technique discussed in Chapter 13, which front-loads fluid removal earlier in treatment when plasma refilling capacity is greatest, sometimes report a shift in when their cramps tend to occur, from the traditional late-treatment pattern toward a somewhat earlier onset corresponding to the profile's own front-loaded removal pattern; recognizing that a prevention strategy targeting one complication can shift the timing, though not necessarily eliminate the occurrence, of a mechanistically related complication is a useful general principle when evaluating whether a given intervention has been fully effective or has simply redistributed a symptom's timing without resolving its underlying cause.

Patients on hemodiafiltration, discussed in Chapter 4, have in some studies reported lower cramp frequency than patients on conventional hemodialysis at comparable ultrafiltration rates, plausibly reflecting the more favorable hemodynamic tolerance the greater convective clearance and associated technique refinements sometimes provide, though this association has not been demonstrated consistently across all comparative studies and should not be interpreted as suggesting hemodiafiltration should be selected primarily for cramp prevention rather than for the middle-molecule clearance benefits discussed in Chapter 4 that remain its primary clinical rationale.

Acute Management of Cramps

Once a cramp has developed, immediate measures include reducing or temporarily suspending the ultrafiltration rate, similar to the initial response to hypotension detailed in Chapter 13, and administering a small bolus of hypertonic saline or, in some protocols, hypertonic dextrose, both of which draw fluid osmotically into the vascular space and have demonstrated benefit in resolving an acute cramp episode; passive stretching of the affected muscle, applied gently rather than forcefully given the risk of exacerbating discomfort in an already painfully contracted muscle, provides additional symptomatic relief in many patients alongside these pharmacologic measures.

Quinine, historically used for cramp prophylaxis and treatment in the general population, carries a boxed warning regarding serious hematologic and cardiac adverse effects and is generally avoided in contemporary dialysis practice given these safety concerns relative to its modest efficacy, illustrating that a historically common intervention is not necessarily still an appropriate first-line choice once its full risk profile has become better characterized through subsequent pharmacovigilance experience.

Management of intradialytic cramps should rely on the physiologic interventions described above rather than on generic comfort measures applied without attention to the underlying volume and electrolyte mechanism, since a cramp that recurs repeatedly despite symptomatic treatment alone, without the underlying ultrafiltration rate or dry weight being reassessed, will simply recur at the next treatment and the one after that, reflecting an unaddressed prescription-level problem rather than a series of unrelated, isolated episodes.

CLINICAL PEARL: Recurrent intradialytic cramps share their underlying physiology with intradialytic hypotension; persistent cramps despite symptomatic treatment warrant dry weight and ultrafiltration rate reassessment rather than repeated symptomatic treatment alone.

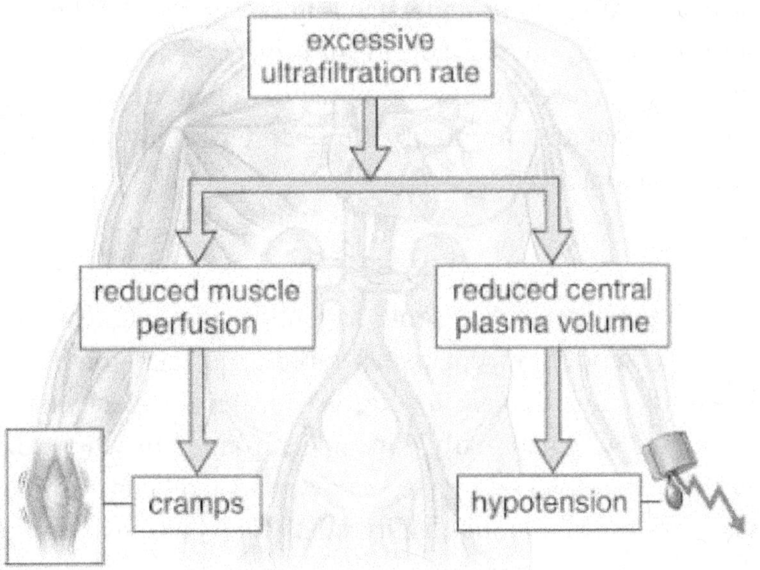

Figure 14.1 Shared Physiologic Pathway of Cramps and Hypotension

Nausea, Vomiting, and Headache During Treatment

Mechanisms of Intradialytic Nausea and Vomiting

Intradialytic nausea and vomiting most commonly reflect early or evolving hypotension, since reduced cerebral and splanchnic perfusion produces these symptoms through mechanisms similar to those underlying other forms of hypotension-related nausea, and any patient developing new intradialytic nausea should have blood pressure checked immediately as a first step, treating the nausea as a potential hypotension symptom until proven otherwise rather than assuming a benign, unrelated gastrointestinal cause without first excluding the more common and more directly actionable hypotension-related explanation.

Beyond hypotension, dialysis disequilibrium syndrome, discussed in Chapter 4 as a risk particularly relevant to new patients with severe azotemia, can also present with prominent nausea alongside its more classically emphasized headache and confusion, and a new patient developing nausea during an early treatment, particularly one with the severe starting azotemia discussed in that chapter, should be evaluated with disequilibrium syndrome specifically in mind rather than attributing the nausea to a nonspecific or unrelated cause. Rapid correction of acidosis, discussed in Chapter 4's treatment of bicarbonate dynamics, and rapid electrolyte shifts more broadly can also independently contribute to intradialytic nausea, providing a further mechanistic pathway distinct from hypotension or disequilibrium syndrome specifically.

Acetate, historically used as a dialysate buffer before bicarbonate-based dialysate became standard, was strongly associated with intradialytic nausea and vomiting and its replacement by bicarbonate buffering, discussed in Chapter 4, substantially reduced the overall prevalence of these symptoms across the dialysis population; this historical context is worth understanding because it illustrates how a symptom complex once considered a nearly universal, unavoidable feature of dialysis treatment was in fact substantially attributable to a specific, since-corrected prescription factor, a pattern worth keeping in mind whenever a symptom is assumed to be an inherent, unmodifiable feature of dialysis rather than a consequence of a specific, potentially correctable practice.

Intradialytic Headache

Intradialytic headache, common enough that some patients experience it with near every treatment, has been attributed to several overlapping mechanisms: rapid fluid and solute shifts producing changes in cerebral fluid dynamics similar in principle to the disequilibrium mechanism discussed in Chapter 4, caffeine withdrawal in patients who habitually consume caffeine but whose dialysis schedule interrupts their usual intake pattern, and, in some patients, a component related to blood pressure change itself, whether from hypotension or, less commonly, an intradialytic hypertensive response discussed further in Chapter 24.

Distinguishing a patient's typical, recurrent, mild-to-moderate intradialytic headache from a new, severe, or qualitatively different headache matters clinically, since the latter presentation should prompt evaluation for a more serious cause, including a hypertensive emergency or, rarely, an intracranial process, rather than being managed as though it were simply the patient's usual dialysis-related headache pattern; a patient's own report that a current headache feels different from their typical pattern deserves the same weight this book has assigned to other patient-reported subjective changes throughout Part III's discussion of vascular access surveillance.

An intradialytic hypertensive response, distinct from the intradialytic hypotension that dominates this book's treatment of blood pressure instability but discussed further in Chapter 24, occurs in a subset of patients whose blood pressure paradoxically rises rather than falls during ultrafiltration, and headache in this specific context may reflect the hypertensive process itself rather than the more commonly discussed hypotension-related or disequilibrium-related mechanisms; checking blood pressure as part of the initial headache assessment, rather than assuming a low or falling blood pressure by default, ensures this less common but clinically important alternative is not overlooked.

A structured approach to intradialytic headache assessment, checking blood pressure first given both hypotension and the less common hypertensive pattern as potential explanations, reviewing the timing relative to the patient's usual caffeine intake pattern, and considering the patient's specific dialysis history including whether they are a new patient at risk for disequilibrium syndrome, provides a more systematic evaluation than treating every headache as presumptively the patient's typical, benign pattern without this brief differential consideration each time a headache is reported, however routine that report may seem given a patient's prior history of similar episodes.

Management Approach

Management of intradialytic nausea, vomiting, and headache begins with excluding or addressing hypotension as the most common underlying driver, following the assessment and response framework detailed in Chapter 13, before pursuing symptomatic treatment of the specific complaint itself; antiemetics selected with attention to reduced renal clearance, as discussed in Chapter 3's treatment of symptom management pharmacology more broadly, and simple analgesics for headache, similarly selected with renal dosing considerations in mind, provide symptomatic relief once a more serious underlying cause has been reasonably excluded.

For a patient with recurrent, predictable intradialytic headache attributable substantially to caffeine withdrawal, a modest, consistent caffeine intake maintained on dialysis days, coordinated with the patient's usual routine, can reduce headache frequency more effectively than treating each episode symptomatically after it has already developed, illustrating that prevention, once the specific contributing mechanism is identified for an individual patient, is often more effective than repeated reactive symptomatic treatment.

Documenting each patient's individual symptom pattern — which of these common intradialytic symptoms they experience, their typical timing and severity, and which interventions have proven effective for them specifically — in the same structured, accessible format this book has recommended for other recurring clinical patterns throughout its earlier chapters allows any covering clinician to apply an already-established, individually effective management approach rather than starting from a generic protocol with each new episode.

DIALYSIS RECOGNITION & RESPONSE SYSTEM — Common Symptom Recognition Arcs

The Pattern: A patient develops new intradialytic nausea.

Stem Signature: New onset of nausea during treatment, without yet having a blood pressure check to correlate the symptom against, in a patient whose nausea could reflect evolving hypotension, disequilibrium syndrome, rapid electrolyte shift, or an unrelated cause.

The Decision: Check blood pressure immediately as the first response to any new intradialytic nausea, treating hypotension as the presumptive cause until excluded, before pursuing symptomatic antiemetic treatment or considering the less common alternative causes.

Trap Logic: New nausea can be treated symptomatically with an antiemetic as a reflexive first response, delaying recognition of evolving hypotension as the underlying and more urgently actionable cause in many cases.

Response Anchor: New intradialytic nausea warrants an immediate blood pressure check as the first response — not symptomatic antiemetic treatment before hypotension has been assessed.

First-Use and Anaphylactoid Dialyzer Reactions

Type A Reactions Revisited and Expanded

Type A dialyzer reactions, introduced in Chapter 5, present within the first several minutes of a treatment using a new dialyzer, with dyspnea, urticaria, and, in severe cases, frank anaphylaxis with hypotension and angioedema; this chapter revisits the topic specifically to integrate it into the broader intradialytic symptom framework this chapter is building, since a Type A reaction's early, minutes-into-treatment timing and its distinctive urticarial and respiratory presentation are the key features distinguishing it from the hypotension, cramps, and other symptom complexes discussed elsewhere in this chapter, which typically present later in treatment and lack the urticaria and acute respiratory component a Type A reaction produces.

Concurrent ACE inhibitor use combined with a negatively charged membrane surface, activating the bradykinin pathway through a mechanism distinct from classic IgE-mediated anaphylaxis, represents a specific, recognized risk factor for Type A reactions that deserves explicit medication reconciliation before a new dialyzer type is introduced for a given patient, and a patient with a prior Type A reaction history should have their specific reaction circumstances, including concurrent medications and the specific membrane and sterilization method involved, documented explicitly to guide future dialyzer selection and avoid re-exposure to the same precipitating combination.

Emergency management of a severe Type A reaction follows standard anaphylaxis protocol: immediate cessation of blood flow through the circuit, clamping the lines without returning the blood currently within the extracorporeal circuit to the patient given the ongoing exposure that blood represents, and administration of epinephrine, antihistamines, and corticosteroids according to the severity of the presentation and standard anaphylaxis management protocols applicable across any clinical setting. Staff training in recognizing and responding to a severe Type A reaction should be maintained with the same rigor as training for the other genuine emergencies discussed in the next chapter, since although Type A reactions are considerably less common than the milder symptoms detailed elsewhere in this chapter, a severe presentation requires the same rapid, practiced response any anaphylactic emergency demands.

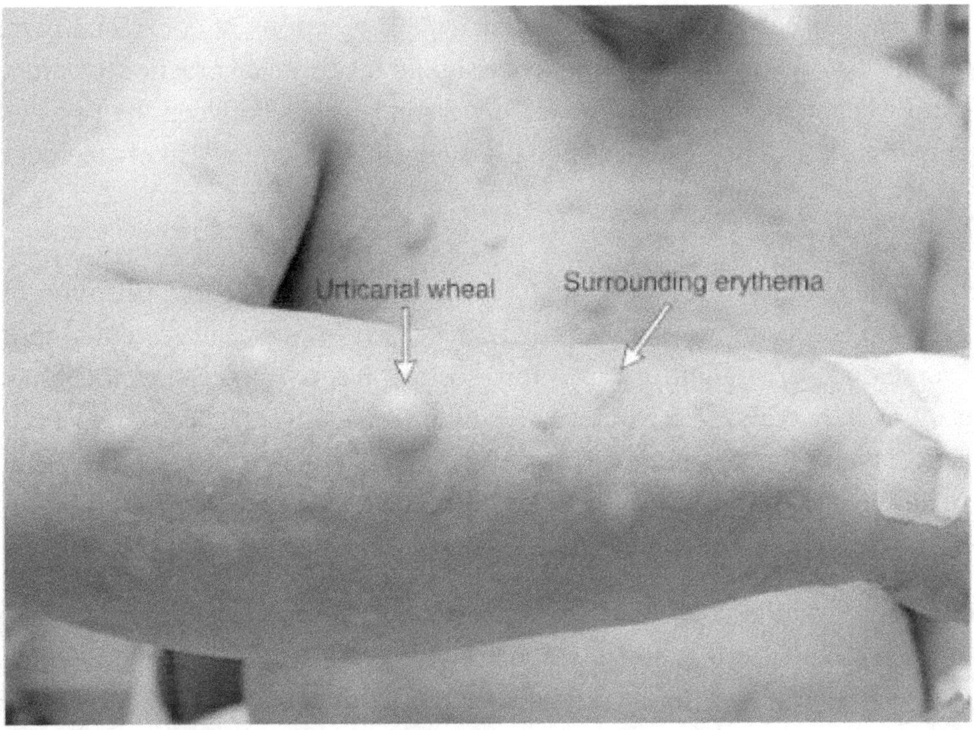

Type B Reactions

Type B reactions, also introduced in Chapter 5, present somewhat later than Type A, typically within the first half hour of treatment, with chest and back discomfort rather than the urticaria and severe hypotension characteristic of Type A, and are thought to relate to complement activation on contact with a less biocompatible membrane surface rather than the IgE- or bradykinin-mediated mechanisms underlying Type A reactions. Because Type B reactions are generally milder and more self-limited than Type A, management typically involves symptomatic support and continued observation rather than the immediate treatment discontinuation a severe Type A reaction requires, though a Type B reaction that fails to improve or that shows any accompanying hemodynamic instability should prompt the same treatment discontinuation and reassessment a Type A reaction would warrant.

Distinguishing Type B reactions from cardiac chest pain, particularly relevant given the elevated cardiovascular disease burden in the dialysis population discussed throughout Part VII of this book, deserves explicit attention: a Type B reaction's specific temporal association with treatment initiation on a new or infrequently used dialyzer, its typical resolution with symptomatic management and continued observation, and the absence of the electrocardiographic changes or other objective cardiac findings that would accompany a true cardiac event, together support a Type B reaction diagnosis, but a clinician should maintain a low threshold for cardiac evaluation, including electrocardiogram, in any patient with chest discomfort during dialysis given the population's elevated baseline cardiac risk, rather than assuming a Type B reaction reflexively without this basic cardiac screening.

Because the dialysis population carries a substantially elevated baseline prevalence of coronary artery disease relative to the general population, as discussed throughout Part VII of this book, the consequences of misattributing a true cardiac event to a presumed Type B reaction are considerably more serious than the reverse error, and this asymmetry in consequence should bias clinical practice toward a lower threshold for cardiac workup whenever genuine diagnostic uncertainty exists between the two possibilities, rather than treating the two misattribution errors as equally acceptable or equally likely to occur in practice.

Prevention and Reporting

Adequate dialyzer rinsing before use, following the manufacturer's specified rinsing protocol rather than an abbreviated version adopted informally to save time, removes sterilant residue implicated in Type A reactions and represents a straightforward, low-cost preventive measure that should be applied consistently for every new dialyzer regardless of how infrequently reactions are actually observed in a given unit's practice; a unit that has not experienced a Type A reaction in some time should not interpret this as license to abbreviate rinsing protocol, since consistent adherence to the full protocol is likely part of why reactions have remained infrequent in the first place.

Every dialyzer reaction, whether Type A or Type B, should be documented with sufficient detail — the specific dialyzer model and sterilization method, timing of onset relative to treatment start, and the patient's concurrent medications — to inform both that individual patient's future dialyzer selection and, aggregated across a unit's full patient population, to identify whether a particular dialyzer model, lot, or sterilization method is producing reactions at a higher-than-expected rate, a pattern that would warrant reporting to the manufacturer and potentially switching that specific product across the unit's broader formulary rather than treating each reaction as an isolated, patient-specific event unrelated to any broader pattern.

A structured symptom log, tracking every occurrence of the complications this chapter addresses across a unit's full patient population by date, patient, dialyzer lot where relevant, and specific presentation, supports exactly this kind of pattern detection at the institutional level, extending the same systemic, workflow-embedded surveillance principle this book has recommended repeatedly for vascular access complications in Part III and for the water treatment failures discussed in Chapter 5 to the broader category of common intradialytic symptoms this chapter addresses; a unit relying only on individual clinician memory to notice a developing pattern across multiple patients and multiple shifts is considerably less likely to detect that pattern promptly than one maintaining this kind of structured, centrally reviewed log.

KEY POINT: Type A reactions present within minutes with urticaria and respiratory symptoms; Type B reactions present somewhat later with chest and back discomfort and are generally milder; both should be documented in enough detail to inform future dialyzer selection and to detect any broader product-level pattern.

Pyrogenic and Febrile Reactions

Mechanism and Presentation

Pyrogenic reactions, presenting with fever, chills, and rigors developing during or shortly after a treatment, arise from bacterial endotoxin or other pyrogenic substances crossing the dialyzer membrane from contaminated dialysate into the blood, a mechanism directly connected to the water treatment quality standards discussed at length in Chapter 5, even when the dialyzer membrane itself remains fully intact and prevents whole bacteria from crossing; endotoxin fragments, considerably smaller than intact bacteria, can traverse an intact membrane under certain conditions, particularly with high-flux membranes and the backfiltration risk Chapter 5 describes, producing a pyrogenic reaction without requiring any breach in the membrane's basic bacterial barrier function.

The clinical presentation typically develops within the first hour of treatment, distinguishing it somewhat from catheter-related bloodstream infection, discussed in Chapter 12, which can present at variable points relative to treatment timing depending on the specific infection source and organism involved; this timing pattern, while not absolute, is a useful initial clue when a febrile episode's specific timing relative to treatment initiation is available to help distinguish among the several possible causes of intradialytic fever this chapter and Chapter 12 together describe.

Cytokine release, triggered by endotoxin or other pyrogenic substance contact with circulating monocytes and other immune cells as blood passes through the dialyzer, mediates the fever and rigors characteristic of a pyrogenic reaction through the same inflammatory cascade that produces fever in other, non-dialysis-related contexts, and the relatively rapid onset of symptoms once triggering exposure begins reflects the rapid kinetics of this cytokine-mediated inflammatory response once initiated. Repeated pyrogenic exposure over time, even at a level insufficient to produce an overt clinical reaction on any single treatment, has been proposed as a contributor to the chronic inflammatory state observed in some long-term dialysis patients, providing a further, longer-term rationale beyond acute reaction prevention for maintaining rigorous water treatment quality standards.

Figure 14.3: Temperature Trend During an Isolated Pyrogenic Reaction

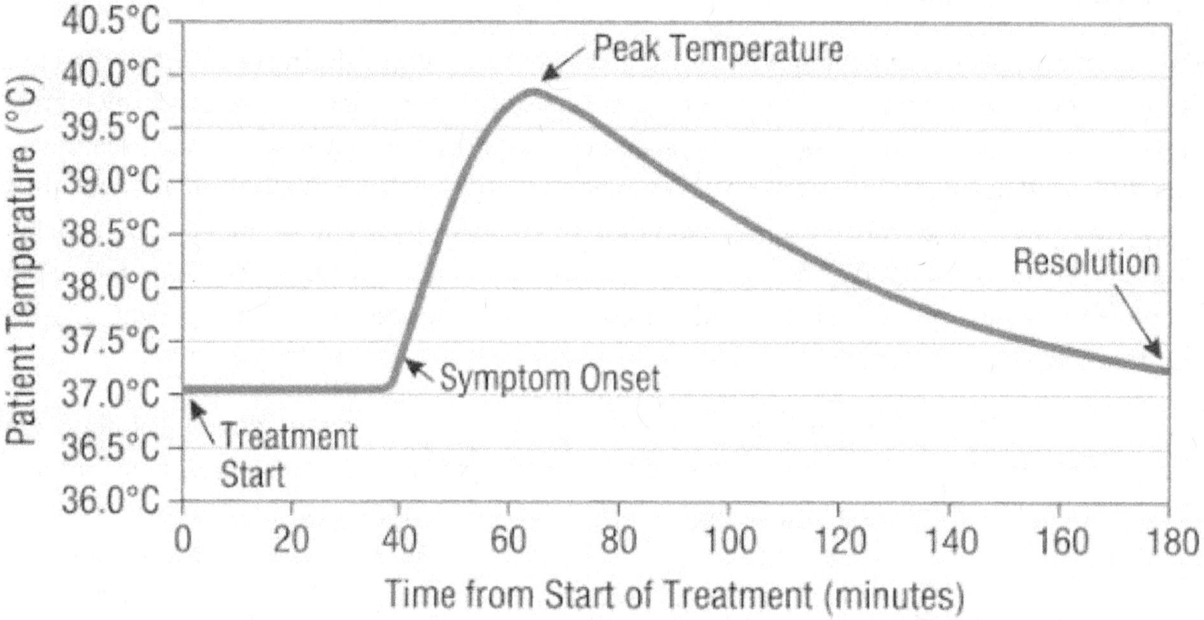

Distinguishing Pyrogenic Reactions From Bacteremia

Because pyrogenic reactions and true bacteremia, whether catheter-related as discussed in Chapter 12 or from another source entirely, can present with a similar febrile picture, blood cultures should be obtained for any significant febrile episode during dialysis rather than assuming a pyrogenic reaction reflexively, since a missed bacteremia carries considerably more serious consequences than the additional, relatively low-cost step of culturing blood in a patient who ultimately proves to have had a self-limited pyrogenic reaction rather than a true bloodstream infection.

The clustering pattern discussed in Chapter 5's water treatment failure case remains the single most useful distinguishing feature at the population level: multiple patients treated on the same water system within the same shift developing similar febrile symptoms strongly suggests a shared pyrogenic mechanism related to water or dialysate contamination, while an isolated febrile episode in a single patient, particularly one with a central venous catheter or other recognized bacteremia risk factor, more strongly suggests an individual bacteremic process requiring the catheter-specific evaluation detailed in Chapter 12 rather than a water-system-level investigation.

Investigation and Unit-Level Response

A confirmed or strongly suspected pyrogenic reaction should prompt water and dialysate quality testing at the affected treatment station and, if the pattern suggests a broader system-level issue, the water treatment system more generally, following the investigation approach detailed in Chapter 5; this testing should proceed even when the affected patient's symptoms resolve promptly with supportive care alone, since the goal of this investigation is preventing recurrence in this and other patients rather than solely managing the individual episode that prompted it.

A forty-seven-year-old man develops fever and rigors approximately forty minutes into a routine hemodialysis treatment, without any other patients on the same water system reporting similar symptoms that same shift and without any exit-site or catheter-related findings on his own examination. Blood cultures are obtained before symptomatic treatment with an antipyretic, and his symptoms resolve over the following two hours without antibiotic therapy. His blood cultures subsequently return negative at forty-eight hours, and given the absence of any clustering pattern among other patients and his negative cultures, his episode is classified as an isolated pyrogenic reaction rather than bacteremia, though his team notes that his negative cultures, while reassuring, do not entirely exclude a low-grade or partially treated bacterial process, and they document a plan for closer observation at his next several treatments to confirm his symptoms do not recur. This case illustrates the appropriate combined approach to an isolated febrile episode: obtaining cultures to rule out bacteremia despite a clinical picture suggestive of a self-limited pyrogenic reaction, rather than assuming the more benign diagnosis without this basic confirmatory step.

His unit's technical staff also perform a routine, precautionary water quality check at his treatment station despite the absence of any clustering pattern among other patients, reflecting a reasonably conservative practice of verifying water quality whenever a pyrogenic reaction is suspected in even a single patient, rather than reserving this verification only for confirmed multi-patient clusters; this precautionary check returns normal results, further supporting the isolated, rather than water-system-related, nature of his episode.

CAUTION: Any significant febrile episode during dialysis warrants blood cultures before attributing the presentation to a pyrogenic reaction, since missing a true bacteremia carries considerably more serious consequences than the added step of culturing.

DIALYSIS RECOGNITION & RESPONSE SYSTEM — Common Symptom Recognition Arcs

The Pattern: A patient develops fever and rigors during or shortly after a dialysis treatment.

Stem Signature: New fever, chills, or rigors developing during or within the hour following a treatment, without yet being characterized as either an isolated event or part of a cluster affecting other patients on the same water system.

The Decision: Obtain blood cultures before attributing the episode to a presumed pyrogenic reaction, and simultaneously check whether other patients on the same water system and shift are reporting similar symptoms, since this clustering assessment helps distinguish a water-system-level pyrogenic cause from an individual bacteremic process.

Trap Logic: A febrile episode with a clinical picture suggestive of a pyrogenic reaction can be assumed to be exactly that without confirmatory cultures, risking a missed true bacteremia that happened to present with a similar, non-specific febrile picture.

Response Anchor: Any significant intradialytic fever warrants blood cultures and a clustering check across other patients on the same water system — not an assumption of pyrogenic reaction without this confirmatory evaluation.

DIALYSIS RECOGNITION & RESPONSE SYSTEM — Common Symptom Recognition Arcs

New Intradialytic Nausea: Check blood pressure immediately as the first response, treating hypotension as the presumptive cause until excluded.

New Intradialytic Fever: Obtain blood cultures and check for clustering across other patients on the same water system before attributing the episode to a pyrogenic reaction alone.

Summary and Key Concepts

Intradialytic cramps share underlying physiology with hypotension, and persistent cramps despite symptomatic treatment warrant dry weight and ultrafiltration rate reassessment rather than repeated symptomatic management alone.

New intradialytic nausea should prompt an immediate blood pressure check as the first response, since hypotension is the most common underlying cause, alongside less common contributors including dialysis disequilibrium syndrome and rapid electrolyte shifts.

Type A dialyzer reactions present within minutes with urticaria and respiratory symptoms via an anaphylactoid or bradykinin-mediated mechanism; Type B reactions present somewhat later with milder chest and back discomfort via complement activation.

Every dialyzer reaction should be documented in enough detail to inform future dialyzer selection for that patient and to detect any broader product-level pattern across a unit's population.

Any significant intradialytic fever warrants blood cultures before attributing the episode to a pyrogenic reaction, and checking for symptom clustering across other patients on the same water system helps distinguish a water-related cause from an individual bacteremic process.

CHAPTER 15: LIFE-THREATENING INTRADIALYTIC EMERGENCIES: AIR EMBOLISM, ARRHYTHMIA, AND CARDIAC ARREST

Learning Objectives

Recognize air embolism and execute the immediate emergency response, including correct patient positioning.

Identify hyperkalemia-related and other causes of intradialytic arrhythmia and apply appropriate management.

Execute a modified resuscitation approach for cardiac arrest occurring during hemodialysis treatment.

Recognize acute hemolysis and line separation emergencies and respond immediately to limit patient harm.

Chapter Overview

The preceding two chapters addressed complications that, while sometimes serious, are common enough that most dialysis clinicians encounter them regularly and manage them as part of routine practice. This chapter addresses the rare but genuinely life-threatening emergencies that every dialysis unit must be prepared for even though any individual staff member may go months or years between actual occurrences: air embolism, life-threatening arrhythmia, cardiac arrest occurring during treatment, and the acute hemolysis and line separation emergencies that share a common feature of producing sudden, severe deterioration rather than the gradual, more readily anticipated decline characteristic of the complications discussed in Chapters 13 and 14. Because these events are rare, the skills needed to manage them well depend more heavily on structured protocol, drilled repetition, and equipment safeguards than on the kind of pattern-recognition experience that accumulates naturally through frequent exposure to common complications, and this chapter's emphasis reflects that reality throughout. This chapter closes Part IV of this book; Part V turns to the physiology and practice of peritoneal dialysis, a modality whose complications, while distinct in their specifics, follow the same recognition-decision-response logic this book has applied consistently across every chapter to this point.

Recognition and Immediate Management of Air Embolism

Mechanism and Presentation of Air Embolism

Air embolism occurs when air enters the extracorporeal circuit and passes into the patient's venous circulation, most commonly from a loose or disconnected line connection, an empty or improperly primed line, or, rarely, a failure of the air detector safety system discussed in Chapter 5 to catch air that has already entered the circuit before it reaches the patient. Once a sufficient volume of air enters the venous circulation, it travels to the right heart and pulmonary circulation, where it can obstruct pulmonary blood flow and, if the volume is substantial or the patient is positioned such that air migrates into the cerebral or coronary circulation through a patent foramen ovale or other right-to-left shunt, produce paradoxical embolization to the brain or heart with correspondingly severe neurologic or cardiac consequences.

Presentation depends heavily on the volume of air involved and the rate at which it enters the circulation: a small volume may produce only mild, transient dyspnea or coughing, while a larger or more rapid entry produces severe dyspnea, chest pain, hypotension, altered mental status, and, in the most severe cases, cardiac arrest, and the classic finding of a churning, machinery-like heart murmur reflects air mixing with blood within the cardiac chambers themselves, though this finding is neither universally present nor necessary to make the diagnosis in a patient with a compatible clinical presentation and circuit circumstance.

The volume of air required to produce clinically significant embolism in humans is not precisely established and likely varies by individual factors including body position and the rate of entry, but even a relatively modest volume, delivered rapidly, can produce severe symptoms, which is why the safety systems and staff vigilance discussed later in this chapter treat any suspected air entry as a potential emergency warranting the full response protocol rather than attempting to first estimate whether the volume involved was likely to be clinically significant before initiating a response.

A patient's underlying cardiopulmonary reserve also influences how a given volume of embolized air is tolerated: a patient with significant preexisting pulmonary hypertension or right heart dysfunction may decompensate with a volume of air that a patient with normal cardiopulmonary function would tolerate with only transient, self-limited symptoms, meaning the severity of a given air embolism event cannot be predicted from air volume alone without also considering the specific patient's baseline cardiopulmonary status, a consideration relevant to how aggressively the emergency response detailed below should be pursued and how closely the patient should be monitored following the acute event.

The specific circumstances under which air entrainment most commonly occurs are worth enumerating explicitly for staff training purposes: a central venous catheter accessed with the cap removed and left briefly open to air during connection or disconnection, a saline bag or priming solution allowed to run dry before the next bag is connected, a loose luer-lock connection anywhere along the arterial or venous line, and, less commonly, a defect in the tubing itself allowing air ingress under negative pressure conditions on the arterial side of the circuit. Recognizing these specific mechanical scenarios as the practical, everyday sources of this rare but dangerous emergency, rather than treating air embolism as an abstract risk disconnected from the concrete moments in a treatment where it actually arises, sharpens staff vigilance at precisely the junctures where vigilance matters most.

Catheter exchange procedures and any circumstance requiring temporary disconnection and reconnection of the extracorporeal circuit mid-treatment, whether for a dialyzer change following a suspected reaction discussed in Chapter 14 or for another reason, represent a period of elevated air entrainment risk distinct from routine, uninterrupted treatment, since each disconnection and reconnection introduces a fresh opportunity for air to enter the circuit at a connection point that would otherwise remain undisturbed for the full duration of a routine session; staff performing any mid-treatment circuit manipulation should apply the same rigor to confirming air-free reconnection as is applied during initial treatment setup, rather than treating a mid-treatment reconnection as a lower-risk, more routine event simply because the patient is already connected and treatment is already underway.

Immediate Emergency Response

The immediate response to suspected or confirmed air embolism follows a specific, protocol-driven sequence that every dialysis staff member should be able to execute without hesitation: clamp the venous line immediately to stop further air entry, stop the blood pump, and position the patient in the left lateral decubitus position with the head down, a position, sometimes termed the Durant position, intended to trap air within the right ventricle's apex away from the pulmonary outflow tract and to reduce the likelihood of air reaching the cerebral circulation through a right-to-left shunt should one be present.

High-flow oxygen administration by non-rebreather mask, immediate call for emergency medical support, and continuous monitoring for the arrhythmia and hemodynamic instability that can accompany significant air embolism should follow immediately alongside the positioning maneuver rather than in sequence after it, since these measures address different aspects of the emergency simultaneously and none should be delayed while another is completed; in facilities with rapid access to hyperbaric oxygen therapy, this treatment may be considered for a severe case, since hyperbaric oxygen reduces bubble size and improves oxygen delivery to compromised tissue, though its availability is limited in most community dialysis settings and transfer time to a hyperbaric facility must be weighed against the immediate supportive measures already described.

Prevention Through Equipment Safeguards

The air detector discussed in Chapter 5 is the primary engineered safeguard against air embolism, automatically clamping the venous line and stopping the blood pump upon detecting air within the returning blood line, and its proper function depends on correct line setup and priming at the start of every treatment, verified through the machine's automatic self-test sequence rather than assumed to be functioning correctly without this verification. Staff vigilance in checking every line connection for security at the start of treatment and periodically throughout, rather than relying on the air detector as the sole safeguard, provides a complementary layer of protection, since a connection that loosens gradually during treatment, allowing air to enter slowly rather than in a single detectable bolus, may present a more subtle detection challenge than the air detector's design primarily anticipates.

Regular equipment maintenance and calibration of the air detector, following the manufacturer's specified schedule, ensures this critical safety system continues to function as designed over the equipment's operational life, and any malfunction or bypass of the air detector, whether from equipment failure or, rarely, inappropriate manual override by staff attempting to work around a nuisance alarm, represents a serious safety lapse that should be addressed immediately through equipment service and, where relevant, staff retraining on the absolute prohibition against bypassing this specific safety system regardless of how frequently it may generate alarms judged to be false positives.

Proper priming technique at the start of every treatment, ensuring the entire extracorporeal circuit is fully purged of air before blood flow begins, represents a further foundational preventive measure that, while seemingly basic, remains a common source of air-related incidents when performed inconsistently or hurried under time pressure; standardized priming checklists, requiring explicit staff confirmation that priming has been completed and verified before treatment begins, reduce the risk of this foundational step being abbreviated or skipped entirely during a busy shift.

New staff orientation should include hands-on simulation of the air embolism response specifically, not merely didactic instruction describing the steps, since the psychomotor sequence of clamping, positioning, and calling for help under simulated time pressure builds the kind of rehearsed, automatic response this chapter's introduction identified as essential for an emergency too rare for most staff to develop fluency through real-world exposure alone; periodic refresher simulation, at an interval determined by unit policy, maintains this competency over time rather than allowing it to fade following initial training as staff move further from their orientation period without an actual event to reinforce the skill.

CAUTION: Suspected air embolism requires immediate venous line clamping, blood pump cessation, and left lateral decubitus head-down positioning — executed simultaneously with oxygen administration and an emergency call, not in sequence after any single measure is completed.

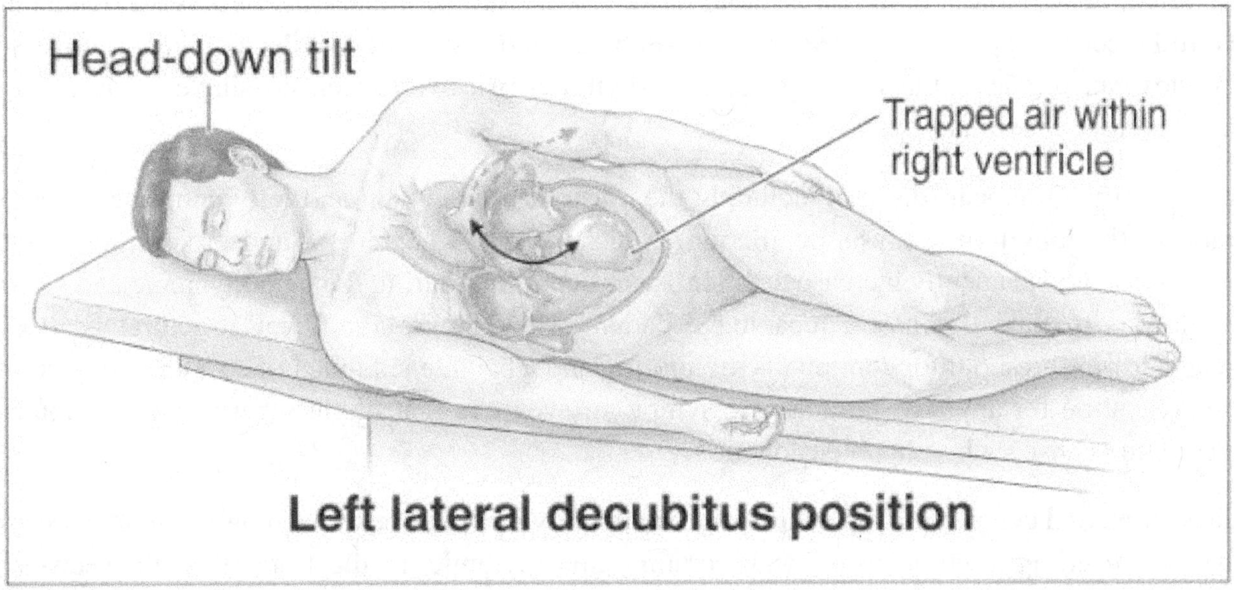

Figure 15.1: Durant Position for Suspected Air Embolism

Hyperkalemia-Related and Other Intradialytic Arrhythmias

Recognizing Hyperkalemia-Related Arrhythmia

Severe predialysis hyperkalemia, particularly when combined with a rapid diffusive potassium shift from an aggressively low dialysate potassium concentration as discussed in Chapter 6, can precipitate significant arrhythmia during the early portion of treatment, ranging from peaked T waves and QRS widening on continuous cardiac monitoring through more severe ventricular arrhythmia and, in the most extreme cases, cardiac arrest; recognizing this risk in advance, through the individualized dialysate potassium selection discussed in Chapter 6 for patients with severe hyperkalemia and cardiac disease, is the primary preventive strategy, but staff must remain prepared to recognize and respond to arrhythmia that develops despite this preventive individualization.

Continuous cardiac monitoring during the early portion of treatment for any patient with severe predialysis hyperkalemia, rather than relying solely on intermittent vital sign checks, provides the earliest possible detection of a developing arrhythmia, and staff should be trained to recognize the electrocardiographic progression from peaked T waves through PR interval prolongation and QRS widening to the sine-wave pattern that precedes frank ventricular arrhythmia, since intervention initiated at an earlier point in this progression carries a more favorable prognosis than intervention delayed until a more advanced, immediately life-threatening rhythm has already developed.

Other Causes of Intradialytic Arrhythmia

Beyond hyperkalemia, rapid shifts in other electrolytes, particularly calcium and magnesium, and the acid-base changes discussed in Chapter 4, can independently contribute to arrhythmia risk during treatment, and a patient developing arrhythmia without an obviously severe predialysis hyperkalemia should still have a full electrolyte panel reviewed, since a combination of more modest derangements across several electrolytes can produce clinically significant arrhythmia risk even when no single value in isolation appears severely abnormal.

Underlying structural heart disease, including the diastolic dysfunction and left ventricular hypertrophy common in the long-term dialysis population as discussed in Chapter 13, and preexisting conduction system disease independently increase arrhythmia susceptibility during the hemodynamic and electrolyte stress dialysis treatment imposes, meaning a patient with known significant structural heart disease warrants a lower threshold for continuous monitoring and a heightened index of suspicion for arrhythmia as an explanation for any new intradialytic symptom, even one that might otherwise be attributed to a more common cause such as hypotension alone.

Medication-related contributors, including digoxin toxicity in a patient whose renal clearance impairment predisposes to drug accumulation, and certain antiarrhythmic medications that themselves carry proarrhythmic potential under conditions of electrolyte shift, deserve specific consideration in a dialysis patient presenting with new arrhythmia, since these medication-related mechanisms may require a distinct management approach, including medication-specific reversal agents or dose adjustment, beyond the electrolyte and structural considerations already discussed in this section.

A comprehensive medication reconciliation, reviewing every medication a patient is taking specifically for arrhythmogenic potential in the context of the electrolyte shifts dialysis produces, is best performed proactively as part of routine care rather than reactively only after an arrhythmia has already occurred, and this reconciliation should be revisited whenever a new medication is added to a patient's regimen, since a medication with no prior arrhythmia history in that patient may nonetheless interact adversely with the specific electrolyte shift pattern a subsequent dialysis treatment produces, particularly in a patient whose dialysate potassium or other prescription parameters have also recently changed.

Management Approach

Management of intradialytic arrhythmia begins with immediate assessment of hemodynamic stability, since an unstable arrhythmia, producing hypotension, altered mental status, or cardiac arrest, requires immediate advanced cardiac life support intervention following standard resuscitation protocols, while a stable arrhythmia allows time for more deliberate evaluation of the underlying cause, particularly electrolyte and acid-base status, before determining whether antiarrhythmic intervention beyond correcting the underlying metabolic derangement is actually necessary.

Documentation of the specific arrhythmia, its temporal relationship to the treatment and to any electrolyte trend available from that session's labs, and the response to whatever intervention was applied, provides valuable information for the patient's subsequent prescription review, discussed in Chapter 6, allowing the treating team to determine whether a modified dialysate composition, an adjusted treatment schedule, or closer monitoring on future treatments is warranted to reduce recurrence risk, rather than treating each arrhythmia episode as an isolated event disconnected from the patient's ongoing prescription and monitoring plan.

A fifty-six-year-old man with a predialysis potassium of 7.2 mEq/L and known coronary artery disease is noted on continuous cardiac monitoring, initiated specifically given his severe hyperkalemia, to develop peaked T waves and mild QRS widening approximately fifteen minutes into treatment. His treating team, having anticipated this risk, had already individualized his dialysate potassium to a more gradual correction profile as described in Chapter 6, and continues close monitoring while administering calcium gluconate to stabilize the cardiac membrane pending further potassium correction through the ongoing dialysis treatment itself. His electrocardiographic changes resolve gradually over the following thirty minutes as his potassium falls, without progression to a more severe arrhythmia, and he completes his treatment without further incident. This case illustrates the value of anticipatory monitoring and prescription individualization discussed in Chapter 6 working in concert with prompt bedside recognition and pharmacologic membrane stabilization when early electrocardiographic changes do develop despite that anticipatory planning.

DIALYSIS RECOGNITION & RESPONSE SYSTEM — Critical Emergency Arcs

The Pattern: A patient with severe predialysis hyperkalemia shows early electrocardiographic changes during treatment.

Stem Signature: Peaked T waves or QRS widening on continuous monitoring in a patient with severe predialysis hyperkalemia, developing within the first portion of treatment, without yet progressing to a hemodynamically unstable rhythm.

The Decision: Administer calcium gluconate for cardiac membrane stabilization, continue close monitoring, and allow the ongoing dialysis treatment to continue correcting the underlying potassium, escalating to advanced cardiac life support only if progression to an unstable rhythm occurs.

Trap Logic: Early electrocardiographic changes in a stable patient can be under-recognized as merely an expected feature of severe hyperkalemia not yet requiring specific intervention, when membrane-stabilizing treatment at this early stage can prevent progression to a more dangerous, unstable arrhythmia.

Response Anchor: Early peaked T waves or QRS widening in a hyperkalemic patient warrant calcium gluconate administration for membrane stabilization — not simply continued observation while awaiting further potassium correction alone.

Cardiac Arrest on the Dialysis Unit

Immediate Response and Circuit Disconnection

Cardiac arrest occurring during hemodialysis treatment requires immediate disconnection from the extracorporeal circuit as the first step, returning the patient's blood if this can be accomplished within seconds without meaningfully delaying resuscitation, or clamping the lines and disconnecting without returning the blood if immediate return would delay chest compressions and other resuscitation measures;

this disconnection is a modification to standard resuscitation protocol specific to the dialysis setting, since continued connection to the extracorporeal circuit during chest compressions and defibrillation both interferes with resuscitation efforts physically and risks equipment damage or further patient harm from a circuit not designed to remain connected during active resuscitation.

Modified Resuscitation Considerations

Beyond circuit disconnection, resuscitation of a dialysis patient follows standard advanced cardiac life support protocols, but with specific attention to the electrolyte and metabolic factors that may have precipitated the arrest, particularly hyperkalemia, discussed earlier in this chapter, which should be treated empirically with calcium, insulin and glucose, and bicarbonate as part of the resuscitation effort in a dialysis patient with cardiac arrest of uncertain immediate cause, given the disproportionately high prevalence of hyperkalemia as a contributing or precipitating factor in this specific patient population relative to the general population experiencing cardiac arrest.

Vascular access considerations also factor into resuscitation planning: a patient's existing fistula, graft, or catheter, while not the primary route for resuscitation medications during active arrest given the more standard peripheral or central venous access typically used, should be protected from inadvertent damage during the physical activity of resuscitation, and staff performing chest compressions or other resuscitation maneuvers should be mindful of the access location to avoid unnecessary additional trauma to it during an already critical situation.

Volume status also factors into resuscitation medication dosing and fluid administration decisions in a way distinct from resuscitating a patient without kidney failure: a dialysis patient in cardiac arrest is often already volume overloaded relative to a non-dialysis patient, given the interdialytic fluid accumulation discussed throughout this book, meaning aggressive fluid resuscitation as part of standard shock management should be approached with more caution than in a patient with normal fluid-handling capacity, weighing the potential benefit of volume expansion against the risk of exacerbating an already volume-overloaded state in a patient whose kidneys cannot independently correct any resulting excess.

Defibrillation and cardioversion, where indicated by the specific rhythm identified during resuscitation, proceed according to standard advanced cardiac life support protocols without modification specific to the dialysis setting beyond the circuit disconnection already emphasized, and staff should not delay indicated defibrillation while completing circuit disconnection if the two cannot be accomplished simultaneously, since a shockable rhythm requiring immediate defibrillation takes priority over the circuit disconnection, however important that disconnection remains for the reasons already discussed.

Post-Arrest Care and Debrief

Following successful resuscitation, transfer to an appropriate higher level of care for post-arrest management, including targeted temperature management where indicated and ongoing evaluation of the arrest's underlying cause, proceeds according to standard post-arrest care protocols, with dialysis-specific considerations, particularly ongoing electrolyte and volume management, coordinated between the receiving team and the patient's nephrology team going forward.

A structured debrief following any cardiac arrest occurring on the dialysis unit, involving all staff present during the event, reviews the timeline of recognition and response, identifies any specific process or equipment issues that either supported or hindered an effective response, and provides an opportunity for staff to process the emotional impact of a genuinely rare and inherently distressing event; this debrief practice, similar in spirit to the withdrawal-decision debrief discussed in Chapter 3, serves both a quality-improvement function and a staff-support function, and units that conduct this debrief consistently after every such event report better staff confidence and preparedness for subsequent emergencies than units that do not.

Family communication following a cardiac arrest, whether the resuscitation is ultimately successful or not, deserves the same deliberate, compassionate approach this book has recommended for other difficult conversations throughout its earlier chapters, particularly Chapter 3's treatment of goals-of-care and withdrawal discussions; a designated staff member, ideally one with specific training in delivering difficult news, should communicate with the patient's family promptly and honestly, and this communication responsibility should be assigned explicitly as part of the unit's arrest response protocol rather than left unassigned amid the other urgent demands the event itself has placed on the treating team.

Because dialysis units typically care for the same patient population over months and years, staff frequently develop genuine relationships with their patients that make a cardiac arrest, whatever its outcome, an emotionally significant event for the treating team in a way distinct from an arrest occurring in a less continuous care relationship such as an emergency department encountering a patient for the first time; acknowledging this dimension explicitly within the debrief process, rather than treating the event as a purely clinical or procedural matter to be reviewed only for technical performance, supports the staff wellbeing this book has emphasized is relevant not only to patients but to the clinicians and staff caring for them throughout a long-term treatment relationship.

KEY POINT: Cardiac arrest during hemodialysis requires immediate circuit disconnection before or alongside standard resuscitation, with empiric treatment for hyperkalemia given its disproportionately high prevalence as a contributing cause in this population.

Figure 15.2: Circuit Disconnection Sequence at Cardiac Arrest

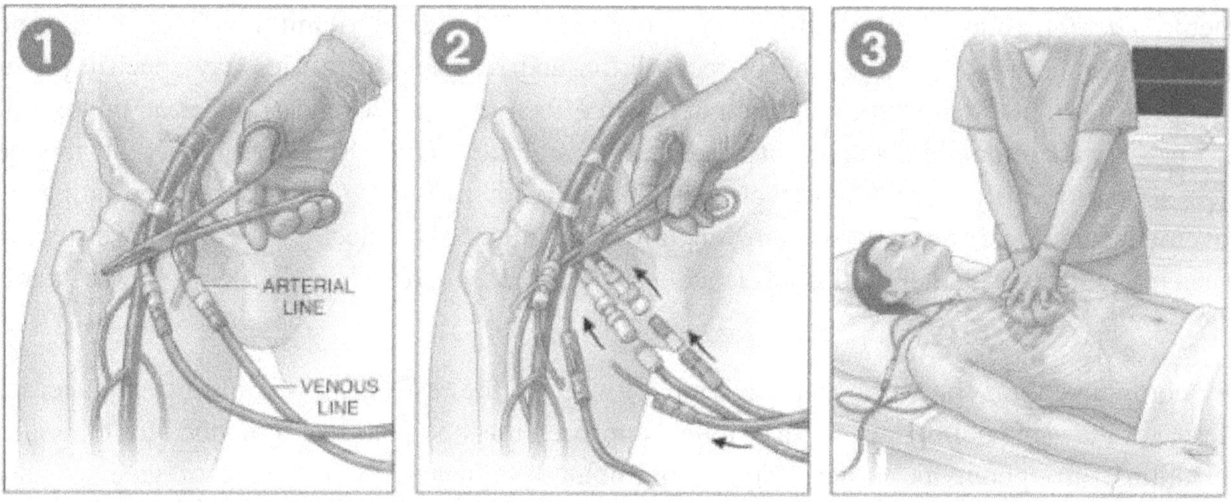

1. CLAMP LINES 2. DISCONNECT PATIENT 3. BEGIN COMPRESSIONS

Staff drilling for this specific sequence, using simulation exercises that combine standard advanced cardiac life support training with the dialysis-specific circuit disconnection step, ensures the disconnection becomes an automatic, practiced reflex rather than an additional cognitive step staff must consciously remember to perform amid the stress of an actual arrest; units that incorporate this combined drilling report faster and more consistent circuit disconnection during real events than units relying on standard resuscitation training alone without the dialysis-specific addition.

Hemolysis and Line Separation Emergencies

Recognizing Acute Hemolysis

Acute intradialytic hemolysis, whether from the chloramine exposure discussed in Chapter 5, a kinked or malfunctioning blood pump segment causing mechanical red cell trauma, or an overheated dialysate, presents with back or chest pain, a distinctive pink or red discoloration of plasma visible in the blood lines themselves, and, in severe cases, hyperkalemia from the released intracellular potassium content of lysed red cells compounding whatever baseline potassium status the patient had before the hemolytic event began.

Recognizing this visible plasma discoloration, sometimes described as a cherry or burgundy color distinct from normal blood appearance, is a critical bedside skill, and any staff member noticing this finding should stop the blood pump immediately and avoid returning the hemolyzed blood to the patient given the severe hyperkalemia risk this returned blood would pose, clamping the lines and disconnecting the patient from the circuit while the underlying cause, most urgently a water treatment or machine malfunction potentially affecting other patients simultaneously, is investigated following the clustering-assessment principle developed in Chapter 5.

Laboratory confirmation of hemolysis, including a markedly elevated lactate dehydrogenase, low haptoglobin, and an elevated free hemoglobin level, supports the bedside visual diagnosis and helps quantify severity, though laboratory confirmation should never delay the immediate bedside response already described, since the visible plasma discoloration itself is sufficiently specific to warrant immediate action without awaiting laboratory confirmation that would introduce a delay measured in tens of minutes to hours depending on the receiving laboratory's turnaround time, a delay entirely incompatible with the urgency this presentation demands.

Because hemolysis from a water treatment or machine-level cause can affect multiple patients simultaneously, exactly as the chloramine exposure case in Chapter 5 illustrated, any confirmed or strongly suspected hemolysis event should prompt immediate notification of technical staff to check whether other patients on the same water system or machine are showing similar findings, proceeding in parallel with the individual patient's clinical management rather than only after that individual management has been fully addressed, since a delay in this parallel notification risks additional patients being exposed to the same causative process while the first affected patient is being managed.

Clearly defined staff roles during any of the emergencies this chapter describes, established in advance through unit protocol and reinforced through the drilling discussed elsewhere in this chapter, prevent the confusion and duplicated or omitted actions that can otherwise occur when multiple staff members respond to a sudden emergency without a predetermined division of responsibility: one designated staff member managing the circuit and immediate mechanical response, another managing patient assessment and any indicated resuscitation measures, and a third managing communication, including calling for additional help and, once the immediate crisis has stabilized, notifying the patient's family and the broader care team; assigning these roles explicitly as part of routine unit training, rather than leaving role assignment to be worked out spontaneously in the moment an actual emergency unfolds, is what allows a well-drilled team to respond with the coordinated efficiency this chapter's rare, high-stakes emergencies demand.

Line Separation and Blood Loss Emergencies

Venous line separation, in which the venous needle or line disconnects from the patient's access during treatment, allows blood to be pumped out of the patient's body at the full prescribed blood flow rate, and given hemodialysis blood flow rates commonly ranging from two to four hundred milliliters per minute or more, this represents a genuine, rapidly developing hemorrhagic emergency capable of producing life-threatening blood loss within minutes if not recognized and addressed immediately; blood loss detection systems on modern dialysis machines, monitoring for the pressure and volume changes a line separation produces, provide an important safeguard, but should not be relied upon as a sole protection against a complication that direct visual and physical monitoring of line connections throughout treatment can often catch even more rapidly.

Immediate response to a recognized or suspected line separation includes stopping the blood pump immediately, clamping the affected line, applying direct pressure to the access site to control ongoing bleeding, and assessing the patient for signs of significant blood loss, including hypotension and tachycardia, with volume resuscitation initiated promptly if these signs are present; because the visible blood loss at the treatment station itself may not fully convey the actual volume lost, especially if separation occurred gradually before being fully recognized, clinical assessment of the patient's hemodynamic status, not merely the visible blood volume at the bedside, should guide the urgency and intensity of the resuscitative response that follows.

Arterial line disconnection, though somewhat less commonly discussed than venous line separation given the venous side's more direct connection to ongoing blood loss from the patient, carries its own risk profile, including air entrainment into the arterial line that can then be pumped toward the patient, connecting this specific complication back to the air embolism risk discussed at the start of this chapter; both arterial and venous line security therefore warrant the same rigorous, periodic verification throughout treatment rather than treating venous line security as the sole priority given its more immediately obvious blood-loss consequence.

A dialysis unit's overnight or lower-staffed shifts deserve particular attention to line separation risk, since a patient dialyzing with reduced direct staff observation, whether during a home treatment or an in-center nocturnal shift with a lower staff-to-patient ratio, has less opportunity for a separation to be caught through direct visual observation alone before the blood loss detection system, if present, triggers its own alarm; units and home programs operating under these lower-observation conditions should ensure blood loss detection technology is functioning and appropriately configured, and that patients trained for home or self-monitored treatment understand the line security checks and immediate response actions this section describes.

Regular inspection and secure taping or fastening of both arterial and venous needle connections at the start of treatment, combined with keeping the access site visible rather than covered by bedding or clothing throughout treatment wherever clinically feasible, allows both staff and, in a home setting, the patient's care partner to notice a developing separation visually before it progresses to the point of triggering a machine-based blood loss alarm, providing an additional, low-cost layer of protection alongside the engineered safeguards this section has already described.

CAUTION: Venous line separation can produce life-threatening blood loss within minutes at standard blood flow rates; immediate blood pump cessation, line clamping, and direct pressure are required the moment separation is recognized or suspected, with hemodynamic assessment guiding subsequent resuscitation.

DIALYSIS RECOGNITION & RESPONSE SYSTEM — Critical Emergency Arcs

The Pattern: Blood lines show a distinctive pink or red discoloration of the plasma component during treatment.

Stem Signature: Visible cherry or burgundy discoloration of the plasma within the blood lines, with or without the patient reporting back or chest pain, raising concern for acute hemolysis.

The Decision: Stop the blood pump immediately, do not return the hemolyzed blood to the patient given the severe hyperkalemia risk it carries, and investigate the underlying cause following the water-treatment and machine-malfunction clustering assessment described in Chapter 5.

Trap Logic: Subtle plasma discoloration can be missed or dismissed if staff are not specifically trained to look for it, and blood already hemolyzed can be reflexively returned to the patient before its severe hyperkalemia risk is recognized.

Response Anchor: Visible plasma discoloration is acute hemolysis until proven otherwise — stop the pump immediately and do not return the affected blood to the patient.

DIALYSIS RECOGNITION & RESPONSE SYSTEM — Critical Emergency Arcs

Early Hyperkalemic Electrocardiographic Changes: Administer calcium gluconate for membrane stabilization rather than continued observation while awaiting further potassium correction.

Visible Plasma Discoloration Suggesting Hemolysis: Stop the blood pump immediately, do not return the affected blood, and investigate for a shared water-treatment or machine cause.

Summary and Key Concepts

Air embolism requires immediate venous line clamping, blood pump cessation, and left lateral decubitus head-down positioning, executed simultaneously with oxygen administration and an emergency call.

Severe hyperkalemia can precipitate a recognizable electrocardiographic progression toward dangerous arrhythmia, and early calcium gluconate administration for membrane stabilization can prevent progression to a more unstable rhythm.

Cardiac arrest during hemodialysis requires immediate circuit disconnection before or alongside standard resuscitation, with empiric hyperkalemia treatment given its disproportionate prevalence as a contributing cause in this population.

Visible plasma discoloration signals acute hemolysis and requires immediate blood pump cessation without returning the affected blood, given the severe hyperkalemia risk hemolyzed blood carries.

Venous line separation can produce life-threatening blood loss within minutes at standard blood flow rates, and immediate cessation, clamping, and direct pressure are required the moment separation is recognized or suspected.

CHAPTER 16: PERITONEAL PHYSIOLOGY AND MEMBRANE TRANSPORT CHARACTERISTICS

Learning Objectives

Describe peritoneal membrane structure and the three-pore model of solute and water transport.

Perform and interpret a peritoneal equilibration test.

Classify a patient's transport category and match prescription strategy to that category.

Compare dextrose and alternative osmotic agents and explain the mechanisms underlying peritoneal ultrafiltration failure.

Chapter Overview

Part V of this book turns from hemodialysis, the subject of every chapter to this point, to peritoneal dialysis, a modality that uses the patient's own peritoneal membrane as the dialyzing surface rather than an extracorporeal circuit and synthetic membrane. This chapter establishes the physiologic foundation the remainder of Part V builds on: how the peritoneal membrane itself is structured, how solutes and water actually cross it, how a peritoneal equilibration test characterizes an individual patient's specific membrane behavior, and how osmotic agents drive the ultrafiltration that a diffusion-based clearance mechanism alone cannot achieve. Readers arriving from Part II's treatment of hemodialysis physiology will recognize a familiar structure to this chapter, since diffusion, convection, and osmotically driven fluid movement all appear here as they did in Chapter 4, but the peritoneal membrane's biology, its patient-to-patient variability, and the clinical consequences of that variability are distinct enough from a synthetic dialyzer membrane to warrant this chapter's dedicated, thorough treatment before Chapter 17 turns to how this physiology translates into an actual prescription. The chapters that follow this one work through that prescription in detail, through the adequacy assessment framework distinct from but conceptually related to the Kt/V approach developed in Chapter 7, and through the peritonitis and access complications that parallel, in a different anatomic and physiologic context, the vascular access complications addressed in Part III.

Peritoneal Membrane Anatomy and Transport Physiology

Peritoneal Membrane Structure and the Three-Pore Model

The peritoneal membrane, a continuous serosal layer lining the abdominal cavity and covering the abdominal viscera, consists of a single layer of mesothelial cells overlying an interstitial matrix rich in capillaries, and it is these capillaries, not the mesothelial layer itself, that constitute the actual functional barrier across which solutes and water move during peritoneal dialysis; the mesothelium is highly permeable and offers little resistance to transport, meaning the capillary endothelium and its associated basement membrane are where the meaningful selectivity of peritoneal transport actually resides.

The peritoneal membrane's total surface area, considerably larger than the body surface area it overlies given the extensive folding of the mesentery and visceral peritoneum, provides substantially more anatomic surface than is ever fully recruited during a typical dwell, since dialysate distributes unevenly within the peritoneal cavity and does not contact the membrane's full anatomic extent uniformly; this distinction between total anatomic surface area and the effectively perfused, dialysate-contacted surface area actually available for transport at any given moment is a recurring theme in understanding why interventions such as increased fill volume, discussed later in this chapter, can meaningfully increase effective transport capacity without requiring any change to the membrane's underlying anatomic properties.

The three-pore model, the framework most widely used to explain peritoneal membrane transport behavior, proposes three functionally distinct pathways across this capillary barrier: large pores, relatively few in number but permitting passage of large molecules including proteins; small pores, the most numerous pathway and the primary route for small solute diffusion such as urea and creatinine; and ultrasmall pores, corresponding to aquaporin channels that permit water passage without accompanying solute, accounting for a purely osmotic, solute-free component of ultrafiltration distinct from the solute-coupled fluid movement occurring through the small-pore pathway.

This three-pore framework explains several clinically important observations that a single-pore model could not: the disproportionate free-water removal seen with a rapid osmotic gradient early in a dwell, reflecting the ultrasmall aquaporin pathway's rapid but self-limited contribution; the more gradual sodium removal that lags behind free-water removal for this same reason, since sodium is largely excluded from the aquaporin pathway and depends instead on the small-pore route; and the small but clinically relevant protein loss that occurs through the large-pore pathway, a loss factored into the nutritional considerations discussed in Chapter 25.

Protein loss through the large-pore pathway varies meaningfully by transport category, with faster transporters generally losing more protein per exchange than slower transporters, given the faster transporter's generally more permeable membrane across all three pore pathways simultaneously rather than a selective increase confined to the small-pore pathway alone; this pattern means a high transporter's nutritional management, discussed in Chapter 25, must account for a correspondingly greater protein replacement need than a low transporter would require, layering an additional individualization consideration on top of the prescription-matching principles this chapter develops for clearance and ultrafiltration specifically.

Solute Transport Across the Peritoneal Membrane

Diffusive solute transport across the peritoneal membrane follows the same fundamental concentration-gradient principle established in Chapter 4 for hemodialysis, with solute moving from the higher concentration in peritoneal capillary blood to the lower concentration in the instilled dialysate, and, as in hemodialysis, this diffusive process favors small solutes such as urea over larger molecules, since molecular size determines how readily a given solute can traverse the small-pore pathway that carries the majority of diffusive transport.

Unlike hemodialysis, where blood and dialysate flow continuously past a fixed membrane at controlled, prescribed rates, peritoneal dialysis diffusion occurs across a membrane bathed in a static pool of dialysate that remains in the peritoneal cavity for the duration of a dwell, meaning the concentration gradient driving diffusion is not continuously replenished as it is in hemodialysis but instead narrows progressively over the course of the dwell as solute equilibrates between blood and dialysate; this progressive narrowing is precisely what the peritoneal equilibration test, detailed in the next section, is designed to characterize for an individual patient.

Peritoneal surface area actually in contact with dialysate, rather than the membrane's total anatomic surface area, determines the effective area available for diffusive transport at any given moment, and this contact area itself varies with instilled dialysate volume, meaning a larger fill volume, up to the point of patient tolerance, generally increases effective diffusive surface area and correspondingly increases solute clearance per dwell, a consideration directly relevant to the prescription decisions detailed in Chapter 17.

Solute size dependence in peritoneal diffusion parallels, but is not identical to, the same size dependence discussed in Chapter 4 for hemodialysis: larger middle molecules cross the peritoneal membrane more slowly than urea, similarly to the pattern seen across a hemodialysis dialyzer membrane, but the peritoneal membrane's continuous, extended dwell exposure, in contrast to a hemodialysis treatment's finite few-hour session, allows even comparatively slow-diffusing middle molecules considerably more cumulative time to cross the membrane over a full day's dwells than a hemodialysis session provides, which is part of the physiologic basis for the somewhat different middle-molecule clearance profile peritoneal dialysis achieves relative to conventional hemodialysis, a comparison relevant to the modality selection discussion in Chapter 2.

Peritoneal Membrane Blood Flow and Its Regulation

Peritoneal capillary blood flow, rather than membrane permeability alone, is a further determinant of achievable diffusive clearance, since even a maximally permeable membrane cannot support diffusion faster than blood flow can deliver and remove solute at the capillary level; under normal physiologic conditions peritoneal blood flow substantially exceeds what is needed to support achievable diffusive clearance rates, meaning blood flow is not typically the rate-limiting factor for most patients, but conditions that reduce peritoneal perfusion, including peritonitis with its associated inflammatory vasodilation paradoxically increasing early clearance before later fibrotic changes reduce it, or severe systemic hypotension, can shift blood flow into a genuinely rate-limiting role.

Vasoactive substances and inflammatory mediators, released locally within the peritoneal cavity during an episode of peritonitis discussed in Chapter 19, transiently increase peritoneal blood flow and effective vascular surface area, producing the paradoxical finding of increased small-solute clearance during acute peritonitis despite the membrane being under active inflammatory insult; this transient increase is not a sign of improved membrane health but rather a marker of acute inflammation, and it typically reverses, sometimes overshooting into reduced transport capacity, as the peritonitis resolves and the membrane's more chronic inflammatory and fibrotic response, discussed further in Chapter 19, potentially develops.

Systemic conditions beyond peritonitis itself can also influence peritoneal blood flow and, correspondingly, transport characteristics measured on a given day's testing: an intercurrent febrile illness, significant systemic inflammation from an unrelated cause, or even substantial physical exertion shortly before testing can transiently alter peritoneal blood flow and produce a PET result that does not reflect the patient's true, stable baseline transport category. For this reason, PET testing is ideally scheduled during a period of the patient's usual clinical stability, deferred if the patient is acutely unwell from an intercurrent illness at the time testing would otherwise be performed, and a transport category result obtained during any such acute intercurrent process should be interpreted cautiously and, where the clinical picture allows, repeated once the patient has returned to their usual baseline state.

KEY POINT: The three-pore model explains peritoneal transport through small pores carrying most diffusive solute clearance, ultrasmall aquaporin channels carrying solute-free water removal, and large pores accounting for protein loss; peritoneal blood flow, while not typically rate-limiting, can become so during peritonitis or severe hypotension.

Figure 16.1: The Three-Pore Model of Peritoneal Membrane Transport

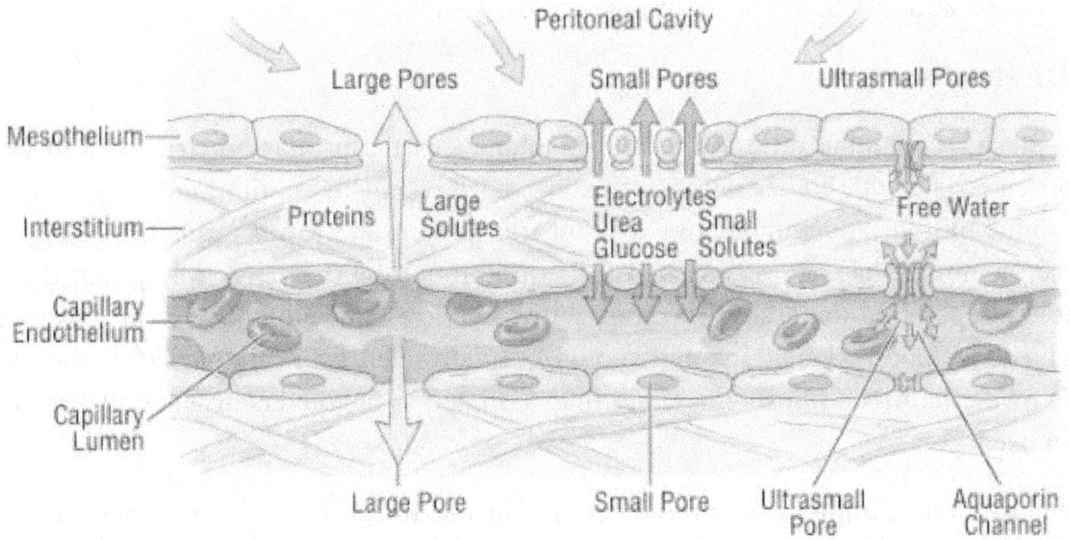

The Peritoneal Equilibration Test

Performing the Standard PET

The peritoneal equilibration test characterizes an individual patient's specific membrane transport behavior by measuring the ratio of dialysate-to-plasma creatinine and the ratio of dialysate glucose concentration at a given time point to its initial instilled concentration, across a standardized dwell using a defined dextrose concentration, typically performed with samples drawn at dwell initiation and at defined intervals, most commonly at the four-hour mark, with drainage volume also measured to characterize ultrafiltration capacity alongside the diffusive transport characteristics the creatinine and glucose ratios capture.

Standardization of the test conditions, including the specific dextrose concentration used, the dwell duration, and the timing of sample collection, is essential to obtaining results comparable across different patients and across serial testing of the same patient over time, since a patient's apparent transport category can shift artifactually if the test itself is performed under inconsistent conditions from one occasion to the next rather than reflecting a genuine change in the patient's underlying membrane physiology.

Timing the initial PET appropriately relative to peritoneal dialysis catheter placement and initiation, generally performed after an initial period of several weeks once the peritoneum has recovered from the catheter insertion procedure itself, avoids the confounding effect of postoperative peritoneal inflammation, which can transiently alter transport characteristics in a manner similar to, though generally milder than, the acute peritonitis-related changes discussed earlier in this chapter, potentially producing a misleading initial transport classification if the test is performed too early in the postoperative course.

Interpreting PET Results

The dialysate-to-plasma creatinine ratio at the four-hour mark is the primary metric used to classify a patient's transport category, with higher ratios, reflecting more complete equilibration between dialysate and plasma creatinine by four hours, indicating a faster transporter, and lower ratios indicating a slower transporter whose membrane has not yet reached full equilibration by the same time point; the specific numeric thresholds separating high, high-average, low-average, and low transport categories are standardized against reference populations and should be interpreted using the specific laboratory and testing protocol's own established thresholds rather than assumed to be universally identical across every testing method in use.

The dialysate glucose ratio, declining over the dwell as glucose diffuses from the higher-concentration dialysate into blood, moves in the opposite direction from the creatinine ratio and provides a complementary, cross-validating measure of the same underlying transport characteristic: a fast transporter shows both a high creatinine ratio and a low glucose ratio at four hours, since rapid diffusion in both directions has already progressed further toward equilibration by that time point, while a slow transporter shows the opposite pattern of both ratios remaining further from their eventual equilibration value.

Drain volume at the end of the standard test dwell, reflecting net ultrafiltration achieved under the standardized test conditions, provides a further data point beyond the creatinine and glucose ratios themselves, and a patient whose drain volume is unexpectedly low relative to what their creatinine-and-glucose-based transport classification would predict may be showing early signs of the ultrafiltration failure discussed later in this chapter, even before a formal transport category shift becomes apparent on the diffusive solute measures alone, underscoring why all three data points from a single PET — creatinine ratio, glucose ratio, and drain volume — are interpreted together rather than any single measure in isolation.

Because the reference population and specific testing protocol used to establish the standard transport-category thresholds can vary somewhat between different published classification systems, a patient transferring care between centers or having testing performed through a different laboratory should ideally have their transport category reassessed under the receiving center's own protocol rather than assuming a classification obtained elsewhere under a different protocol necessarily translates precisely into the receiving center's own categorical framework; this consideration parallels the standardized-sampling-technique caution this book raised in Chapter 7 regarding hemodialysis adequacy measurement, where consistent methodology, not merely a numeric result taken in isolation, is what makes a given measurement clinically meaningful and comparable over time.

Limitations and Modified Testing

The standard PET's fixed dextrose concentration and dwell duration, while providing the standardization needed for reliable classification and comparison across patients, do not fully capture how a given patient's membrane behaves under the specific dwell durations and dextrose concentrations their actual individualized prescription may use, and a modified PET, using a shorter dwell duration or an alternative dextrose concentration matched more closely to a patient's anticipated actual prescription, can provide more directly applicable information for prescription design in select circumstances, discussed further in Chapter 17.

A mini-PET or other abbreviated testing protocol, sampling at fewer time points or over a shorter total duration than the standard four-hour test, offers a lower-burden alternative for routine reassessment once a patient's baseline transport category has already been established through a full standard PET, trading some precision for reduced patient burden in a testing modality intended for periodic monitoring rather than initial, definitive classification.

Transport Category	4-Hour D/P Creatinine	Diffusive Clearance	Ultrafiltration Capacity
High	Highest ratio	Most rapid and complete	Lowest, given rapid glucose absorption dissipating osmotic gradient
High-Average	Above average	Rapid	Moderate

Low-Average	Below average	Slower	Better sustained
Low	Lowest ratio	Slowest	Best sustained, given slow glucose absorption

Fast, Average, and Slow Transporter Categories

Clinical Implications of Transport Category

A high transporter achieves rapid, extensive diffusive solute clearance but, because glucose also diffuses rapidly from dialysate into blood, loses the osmotic gradient driving ultrafiltration correspondingly quickly, meaning a high transporter tends to achieve excellent small-solute clearance but comparatively poor sustained ultrafiltration, particularly over a longer dwell where the osmotic gradient has already substantially dissipated well before the dwell concludes; this pattern is the physiologic basis for high transporters generally being better suited to a prescription using shorter, more frequent dwells rather than the longer dwells that work well for a slower transporter, a matching principle developed fully in the next subsection.

A low transporter shows the inverse pattern: slower diffusive clearance but better-sustained ultrafiltration over a longer dwell, since the osmotic gradient dissipates more gradually as glucose diffuses across the membrane more slowly; this pattern makes low transporters generally well suited to longer dwells, including the extended overnight dwell characteristic of continuous ambulatory peritoneal dialysis discussed in Chapter 17, since the longer time available allows adequate diffusive clearance to accumulate despite the slower rate, without sacrificing ultrafiltration to the same degree a high transporter would experience over an equally long dwell.

CLINICAL PEARL: High transporters achieve excellent diffusive clearance but poor sustained ultrafiltration over long dwells; low transporters show the inverse pattern, making transport category a direct determinant of which dwell duration and frequency strategy will actually work for a given patient.

Matching Prescription to Transport Category

A high transporter's prescription generally favors shorter, more frequent exchanges, most readily accommodated through automated peritoneal dialysis using a cycler to deliver multiple short dwells overnight, discussed fully in Chapter 17, rather than the extended dwells of continuous ambulatory peritoneal dialysis that would leave a high transporter's osmotic gradient dissipated for a large fraction of each dwell, wasting much of the dwell's duration without contributing meaningfully to either clearance or ultrafiltration once equilibration has already been substantially reached well before the dwell concludes.

A low transporter, conversely, benefits from longer dwells that allow adequate time for the slower diffusive process to achieve sufficient clearance, and this patient's prescription can reasonably incorporate the extended overnight dwell of continuous ambulatory peritoneal dialysis, or a cycler prescription with longer individual dwell times than would suit a high transporter, without the wasted-duration problem a high transporter would experience under the same extended-dwell approach; a low transporter placed on a rapid-cycling, short-dwell prescription designed for a high transporter would likely show inadequate clearance, since the shorter dwells would not allow sufficient time for this patient's slower diffusive process to reach an adequate degree of equilibration.

Transport Category Change Over Time

A patient's transport category is not necessarily fixed for the duration of their peritoneal dialysis course; a gradual shift toward a faster transport category over months to years of peritoneal dialysis use has been documented in some patients, plausibly reflecting cumulative membrane changes from repeated exposure to dextrose-based dialysate and, in some cases, episodes of peritonitis, discussed in Chapter 19, each of which can leave lasting membrane changes even after the acute episode itself has resolved.

Periodic PET reassessment, rather than relying indefinitely on a single baseline classification obtained near the start of a patient's peritoneal dialysis course, allows this kind of transport category drift to be identified and the prescription adjusted accordingly, following the same trigger-based reassessment principle this book has applied throughout to the Life-Plan, dialysis prescriptions, and vascular access surveillance; a patient whose clearance or ultrafiltration has begun to decline despite an apparently unchanged prescription, discussed further in the peritoneal dialysis adequacy treatment of Chapter 18, is a specific circumstance that should prompt repeat PET testing to determine whether a transport category shift, rather than a fixed prescription inadequacy, explains the change.

Osmotic Agents and Ultrafiltration Physiology

Dextrose as the Standard Osmotic Agent

Dextrose, available in several standardized concentrations, remains the most widely used osmotic agent in peritoneal dialysate, creating the osmotic gradient that drives ultrafiltration through the mechanism described earlier in this chapter; higher dextrose concentrations produce a steeper initial osmotic gradient and correspondingly greater initial ultrafiltration, though this benefit comes at the cost of greater glucose absorption into the patient's systemic circulation, with implications for glycemic control, particularly relevant in the diabetic peritoneal dialysis population, and for long-term metabolic and membrane health given the cumulative glucose exposure repeated use of higher-concentration dextrose solutions imposes over time.

Because the osmotic gradient dextrose provides dissipates progressively over a dwell as glucose diffuses from dialysate into blood, the choice of dextrose concentration for a given dwell should be matched to that dwell's anticipated duration and the patient's transport category, following the prescription-matching principles detailed earlier in this chapter, rather than using a single dextrose concentration uniformly across every dwell regardless of its specific duration and the patient's specific transport characteristics.

Long-term dextrose exposure, particularly at higher concentrations used repeatedly over years of peritoneal dialysis treatment, has been implicated in the gradual peritoneal membrane fibrosis and vasculopathy some long-term peritoneal dialysis patients develop, a process related to but distinct from the acute peritonitis-related membrane changes discussed in Chapter 19, and this cumulative concern is part of the rationale for minimizing dextrose concentration and total glucose exposure where clinically feasible, using the lowest dextrose concentration that achieves adequate ultrafiltration for a given dwell rather than defaulting to a higher concentration for a larger initial safety margin that may not be necessary for that specific patient and dwell.

Icodextrin and Alternative Osmotic Agents

Icodextrin, a glucose polymer too large to be readily absorbed across the small-pore pathway, provides sustained ultrafiltration through a colloid osmotic mechanism distinct from dextrose's crystalloid osmotic mechanism, maintaining an effective osmotic gradient over a considerably longer dwell duration than any dextrose concentration can sustain, making it particularly well suited to the single long dwell, whether the extended daytime dwell in automated peritoneal dialysis or the overnight dwell in continuous ambulatory peritoneal dialysis, where dextrose's osmotic effect would have already substantially dissipated well before the dwell concludes.

Icodextrin's benefit is most pronounced specifically in high transporters, whose rapid glucose absorption otherwise limits dextrose-based ultrafiltration most severely over an extended dwell, making icodextrin a particularly valuable prescription tool for exactly the patient population whose transport category creates the greatest sustained-ultrafiltration challenge; icodextrin is not, however, a universal substitute for dextrose across every dwell in a prescription, since its slower initial osmotic onset makes it less suited to a short dwell where dextrose's more rapid initial gradient better serves that dwell's specific clearance and ultrafiltration goals.

Glucose polymer absorption from icodextrin, while considerably slower than dextrose absorption given the polymer's larger molecular size, does occur to some degree over an extended dwell, and the maltose and other glucose-polymer metabolites this absorption produces can interfere with certain point-of-care glucose monitoring technologies, producing falsely elevated glucose readings in a patient using icodextrin; awareness of this specific interaction, and use of a glucose monitoring method verified compatible with icodextrin use, prevents a patient or clinician from misinterpreting a falsely elevated glucose reading as evidence of poor glycemic control requiring insulin or other diabetes medication adjustment when the elevated reading in fact reflects this assay interference rather than a genuine glycemic change.

Ultrafiltration Failure Mechanisms

Ultrafiltration failure, defined as inadequate fluid removal despite an appropriately prescribed osmotic agent and dwell duration, arises from several distinct mechanisms requiring different management approaches: a transport category shift toward faster transport, discussed earlier in this chapter, dissipating the osmotic gradient more rapidly than the prescription accounts for; a reduced effective peritoneal surface area from adhesions or membrane fibrosis, often related to prior peritonitis episodes; or, less commonly, a genuine loss of aquaporin-mediated free-water transport specifically, producing a pattern of preserved small-solute clearance but disproportionately impaired ultrafiltration relative to what the patient's overall transport category would otherwise predict.

Distinguishing among these mechanisms in a patient presenting with ultrafiltration failure requires more than a standard PET alone in some cases: a modified PET using pure glucose polymer or other specialized testing protocols can help isolate an aquaporin-specific defect from the more common transport category shift or membrane fibrosis explanations, and referral to a center with experience in this more specialized testing is reasonable for a patient whose ultrafiltration failure remains unexplained after standard PET testing and the more common explanations have been reasonably excluded through the evaluation this chapter and Chapter 18 together describe.

A fifty-eight-year-old woman on continuous ambulatory peritoneal dialysis for four years reports increasing difficulty achieving adequate fluid removal over the preceding two months, with progressive lower extremity edema despite maintaining her established prescription unchanged. A repeat PET reveals a shift from her baseline low-average transport category toward high-average transport, consistent with the membrane transport drift discussed earlier in this chapter. Recognizing that her current prescription, built around longer dwells appropriate for her original slower transport category, is now poorly matched to her new, faster transport status, her nephrology team transitions her to automated peritoneal dialysis with shorter, more frequent cycler dwells better suited to her new transport category, incorporating icodextrin for her single long daytime dwell to sustain ultrafiltration despite her faster transport. Her volume status improves over the following weeks on this revised prescription. This case illustrates why declining ultrafiltration despite an unchanged prescription should prompt repeat PET testing to assess for a transport category shift, rather than assuming the original prescription remains correctly matched to a membrane that itself may have changed.

CAUTION: Declining ultrafiltration despite an unchanged peritoneal dialysis prescription warrants repeat PET testing to assess for a transport category shift, rather than assuming the prescription itself has simply become inadequate without reassessing the membrane's current transport characteristics.

Figure 16.2
Dextrose Versus Icodextrin Osmotic Gradient Over a Dwell

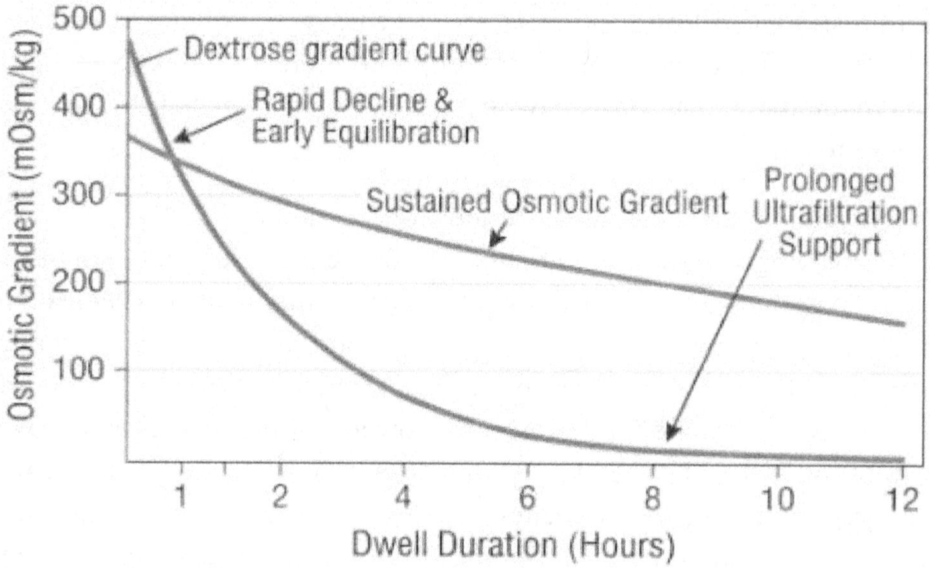

DIALYSIS RECOGNITION & RESPONSE SYSTEM — Peritoneal Physiology Arcs

The Pattern: A peritoneal dialysis patient develops declining ultrafiltration despite an unchanged prescription.

Stem Signature: Progressive difficulty achieving adequate fluid removal, with new or worsening volume overload symptoms, in a patient whose peritoneal dialysis prescription has not been recently modified and who has not had transport category reassessed in some time.

The Decision: Obtain a repeat PET to assess for a transport category shift, distinguishing this specific, correctable mechanism from other causes of ultrafiltration failure such as membrane fibrosis or aquaporin dysfunction, and revise the prescription to match whatever transport category the repeat test reveals.

Trap Logic: Declining ultrafiltration on an unchanged prescription can be attributed reflexively to a generic, unspecified membrane failure without distinguishing which of several specific mechanisms is actually responsible, delaying the transport-category-specific prescription correction that a repeat PET would directly inform.

Response Anchor: Declining ultrafiltration on an unchanged prescription warrants a repeat PET to assess for a transport category shift specifically — not an assumption of generic, unspecified membrane failure.

Declining Ultrafiltration on an Unchanged Prescription: Obtain a repeat PET to assess for a transport category shift and revise the prescription to match the current transport category, rather than assuming generic membrane failure.

Summary and Key Concepts

The three-pore model explains peritoneal transport through small pores carrying diffusive solute clearance, ultrasmall aquaporin channels carrying solute-free water removal, and large pores accounting for protein loss.

The peritoneal equilibration test, using standardized dialysate-to-plasma creatinine and dialysate glucose ratios at four hours, classifies a patient into a transport category ranging from high to low.

High transporters achieve rapid diffusive clearance but poor sustained ultrafiltration over long dwells; low transporters show the inverse pattern, directly determining which dwell duration and frequency strategy suits a given patient.

Dextrose provides rapid but self-limited osmotic ultrafiltration; icodextrin sustains ultrafiltration over considerably longer dwells through a colloid osmotic mechanism, particularly valuable for high transporters and extended dwells.

Declining ultrafiltration despite an unchanged prescription should prompt repeat PET testing to assess for a transport category shift, since a patient's transport category can drift over years of peritoneal dialysis use.

CHAPTER 17: PERITONEAL DIALYSIS CATHETERS AND PRESCRIPTION DESIGN

Learning Objectives

Describe peritoneal dialysis catheter design, insertion technique, and appropriate break-in care.

Design a continuous ambulatory peritoneal dialysis prescription and individualize it to a patient's transport category.

Design an automated peritoneal dialysis prescription using a cycler and match it to transport category and lifestyle.

Apply incremental peritoneal dialysis principles to a patient with meaningful residual kidney function.

Chapter Overview

Chapter 16 established the physiologic foundation of peritoneal transport: how the membrane is structured, how the peritoneal equilibration test characterizes an individual patient's transport category, and how osmotic agents drive ultrafiltration. This chapter translates that physiology into the two concrete building blocks every peritoneal dialysis patient depends on: the catheter that provides physical access to the peritoneal cavity, and the prescription, whether manually exchanged throughout the day under continuous ambulatory peritoneal dialysis or delivered by machine overnight under automated peritoneal dialysis, that determines how effectively that access is actually used. The chapter closes with incremental peritoneal dialysis, a prescription philosophy that treats residual kidney function as an active partner in a patient's overall clearance rather than an incidental bonus, extending the same individualized, trajectory-aware reasoning this book has applied to hemodialysis prescription in Chapter 6 to the peritoneal context specifically.

Catheter Types and Insertion Technique

Catheter Design and Configuration

The peritoneal dialysis catheter, most commonly a flexible silicone tube with one or two Dacron cuffs anchoring it within the subcutaneous tissue and rectus muscle, provides the physical conduit between the external dialysate connection and the peritoneal cavity itself, and its design shares a conceptual similarity with the tunneled hemodialysis catheter discussed in Chapter 12: a subcutaneous tunnel and incorporated cuff anchor the catheter securely and create a barrier against organism migration along the catheter's external surface, protecting against the peritonitis discussed in Chapter 19 in much the same way the hemodialysis catheter's tunnel protects against catheter-related bloodstream infection.

The intraperitoneal segment's specific configuration, whether a straight or coiled design, and the number of side holes along this segment, influence both drainage efficiency and the catheter's tendency toward the mechanical complications, including catheter tip migration and omental wrapping, discussed further in this chapter; a coiled intraperitoneal segment is generally thought to distribute mechanical stress more evenly and may reduce the risk of the catheter tip migrating out of the pelvis, its intended resting position, though comparative outcome data across different specific catheter designs remains less extensive than the comparative data available for hemodialysis vascular access options detailed in Part III of this book.

Catheter material selection has remained largely stable over decades of clinical use, with silicone favored over polyurethane in most contemporary practice given silicone's greater flexibility and reduced tendency toward the kinking that a stiffer material can produce, particularly at the point where the catheter transitions from its subcutaneous course into the peritoneal cavity itself; this material choice, while less frequently revisited than the configuration and cuff-number decisions discussed elsewhere in this section, reflects an accumulated clinical consensus favoring the material properties that best support long-term, trouble-free catheter function over years of daily use.

Two-cuff catheters, incorporating both a deep cuff within the rectus muscle and a superficial cuff within the subcutaneous tissue closer to the exit site, provide a more extensive barrier against organism migration than a single-cuff design, and the superficial cuff's position relative to the skin exit site, ideally positioned so the cuff itself does not extrude through the skin, deserves careful surgical planning, since an extruding cuff creates a chronic source of local irritation and infection risk that undermines the very protective function the cuff is intended to provide.

Insertion Techniques and Timing

Catheter insertion can be performed surgically through an open or laparoscopic approach, or percutaneously using a modified Seldinger technique under imaging guidance, with selection among these approaches depending substantially on local expertise and available resources; laparoscopic insertion offers the specific advantage of direct visualization allowing simultaneous adhesiolysis or other corrective procedures if unexpected intraperitoneal findings are encountered, while percutaneous insertion, where the necessary expertise and imaging support are available, offers a less invasive approach with a shorter procedure time for an appropriately selected, uncomplicated candidate.

Prophylactic antibiotic administration at the time of catheter insertion, following a defined protocol timed to peak antibiotic tissue concentration at the moment of the procedure itself, reduces early postoperative infection risk and represents a straightforward, well-supported perioperative measure that should be applied consistently regardless of which specific insertion technique is used, mirroring the maximal sterile barrier and perioperative infection-prevention principles this book has applied to hemodialysis catheter insertion in Chapter 12.

Catheter exit-site positioning deserves the same deliberate planning discussed in Chapter 12 for hemodialysis catheters: an exit site positioned to point downward or laterally rather than directly upward reduces the tendency for fluid and debris to pool at the exit site, and positioning that avoids the beltline, skin folds, and areas of friction from clothing supports easier patient self-care, a consideration that should be discussed with the patient before the procedure, including trialing the planned exit site position with the patient in both sitting and standing positions to confirm it does not conflict with typical clothing or belt placement.

Timing catheter insertion relative to anticipated dialysis initiation follows the same Life-Plan-driven principle established in Chapter 2 and applied to hemodialysis vascular access in Chapter 9: insertion timed to allow an adequate break-in period, discussed in the next subsection, before the catheter must actually be used, avoids the compressed, higher-complication-risk urgent insertion and immediate use that a late-referred patient, discussed in Chapter 2, may otherwise require.

Break-In Period and Early Catheter Care

A break-in period of at least two weeks, and ideally longer where the clinical trajectory permits it, following catheter insertion and before beginning regular dialysis exchanges, allows the exit site and subcutaneous tunnel to heal and the cuffs to become incorporated by surrounding fibrous tissue, similarly to the tunneled hemodialysis catheter incorporation process discussed in Chapter 12; using the catheter for dialysis before this incorporation is complete increases the risk of pericatheter leak, in which dialysate tracks along the still-unincorporated tunnel to the skin surface or into surrounding tissue, and of exit-site trauma that can predispose to earlier infection.

During the break-in period, exit-site care follows a defined protocol emphasizing minimal manipulation, gentle cleansing according to unit protocol, and avoiding any dressing change technique that applies tension or rotational stress to the catheter at the exit site, since the still-forming tissue tract is more vulnerable to disruption from mechanical stress during this period than it will be once healing is complete; immobilizing the external catheter segment securely against the skin, preventing it from dangling and pulling at the exit site with ordinary patient movement, is a further practical measure supporting undisturbed healing during this window.

Recognizing Early Mechanical Catheter Complications

Catheter tip migration, in which the intraperitoneal segment moves out of its intended pelvic position, most commonly upward toward the upper abdomen, is among the more common early mechanical complications and typically presents as slow or incomplete drainage rather than an inability to instill fluid, since inflow is generally less position-dependent than the gravity-assisted drainage phase of an exchange; a plain abdominal radiograph confirms tip position directly and should be obtained whenever migration is suspected on the basis of this characteristic drainage pattern, distinguishing migration from the fibrin obstruction and constipation-related drainage problems discussed below, each of which requires a different corrective approach.

Omental wrapping, in which the omentum, a fold of peritoneal tissue rich in immune and vascular elements, envelops the catheter's side holes and obstructs flow, produces a similar drainage pattern to tip migration but is not correctable by the positional or laxative measures that address migration or constipation respectively; omental wrapping often requires surgical or laparoscopic revision, in some cases combined with omentopexy, securing the omentum away from the catheter, to prevent recurrence following revision, and this specific complication, along with migration, together account for a substantial share of early mechanical catheter dysfunction requiring surgical rather than purely medical correction.

Constipation, a far more common and far more easily corrected cause of impaired drainage than either migration or omental wrapping, restricts catheter drainage simply through the mechanical effect of a loaded colon crowding the pelvis and displacing the catheter tip or compressing the drainage pathway, and a bowel regimen addressing constipation proactively, rather than reactively only once drainage problems have already developed, is a simple, low-cost preventive measure that should be part of routine peritoneal dialysis patient care from the outset rather than considered only after a drainage complaint has already arisen; distinguishing constipation-related drainage impairment from the more structural causes discussed above is most reliably accomplished by first addressing constipation directly and reassessing drainage before pursuing radiographic or surgical evaluation, given how frequently this simple, reversible cause explains an otherwise concerning drainage pattern.

A sixty-one-year-old man on continuous ambulatory peritoneal dialysis for three months reports progressively slower drainage over the preceding week, with each exchange now taking noticeably longer to complete than his usual routine. His nephrology team's first response, following the evaluation sequence this chapter recommends, is to review his bowel habit, which reveals he has had markedly reduced stool frequency over the same period coinciding with a recent reduction in his oral fluid intake during a period of hot weather. A bowel regimen is initiated, and his drainage returns to its prior baseline within several days without any further intervention required. This case illustrates why constipation, the most common and most easily reversible cause of impaired peritoneal drainage, is appropriately investigated and addressed first, before pursuing the radiographic evaluation for catheter migration or the surgical evaluation for omental wrapping that a persistent, unresponsive drainage problem would subsequently warrant.

CLINICAL PEARL: Impaired peritoneal drainage is most commonly caused by constipation; addressing bowel habit first, before pursuing radiographic evaluation for catheter migration or surgical evaluation for omental wrapping, resolves the majority of drainage complaints without further intervention.

DIALYSIS RECOGNITION & RESPONSE SYSTEM — Peritoneal Prescription Arcs

The Pattern: A peritoneal dialysis patient reports progressively slower or incomplete drainage during exchanges.

Stem Signature: Gradually worsening drainage time or incomplete drainage volume over days to weeks, without fever, abdominal pain, or cloudy effluent that would instead suggest the peritonitis discussed in Chapter 19.

The Decision: Evaluate and address bowel habit and constipation first, since this is the most common and most readily reversible cause, before pursuing an abdominal radiograph to assess for catheter tip migration or considering surgical evaluation for omental wrapping if the drainage problem persists despite an adequate bowel regimen.

Trap Logic: Impaired drainage can prompt immediate radiographic or surgical evaluation without first addressing the far more common and more easily corrected cause of constipation, leading to unnecessary imaging and specialist referral for a problem that a simple bowel regimen would have resolved.

Response Anchor: Impaired peritoneal drainage warrants addressing constipation first — not immediate radiographic or surgical evaluation before this simple, common, and reversible cause has been excluded.

Pericatheter leak, in which dialysate tracks along the catheter tunnel to the exit site or into surrounding subcutaneous tissue, presents as visible fluid drainage at the exit site distinct from normal exit-site secretions, or as localized subcutaneous swelling near the catheter tract, and is most common during the vulnerable break-in period discussed earlier in this chapter, before the cuffs have fully incorporated, though it can also occur later following a sudden increase in intra-abdominal pressure from heavy lifting, severe coughing, or another Valsalva-type maneuver in a catheter that had previously been functioning without leak. Management of an early leak typically involves temporarily reducing or suspending dialysate fill volume, allowing the tunnel tract additional time to heal, while a later leak occurring in a previously well-functioning catheter warrants investigation for the specific precipitating activity and, in some cases, temporary transition to lower-volume or supine-only exchanges while healing is supported.

KEY POINT: A break-in period of at least two weeks before beginning regular exchanges allows catheter cuff incorporation to complete, reducing the risk of pericatheter leak and early exit-site trauma that using the catheter too soon would otherwise risk.

Figure 17.1: Two-Cuff Peritoneal Dialysis Catheter Configuration

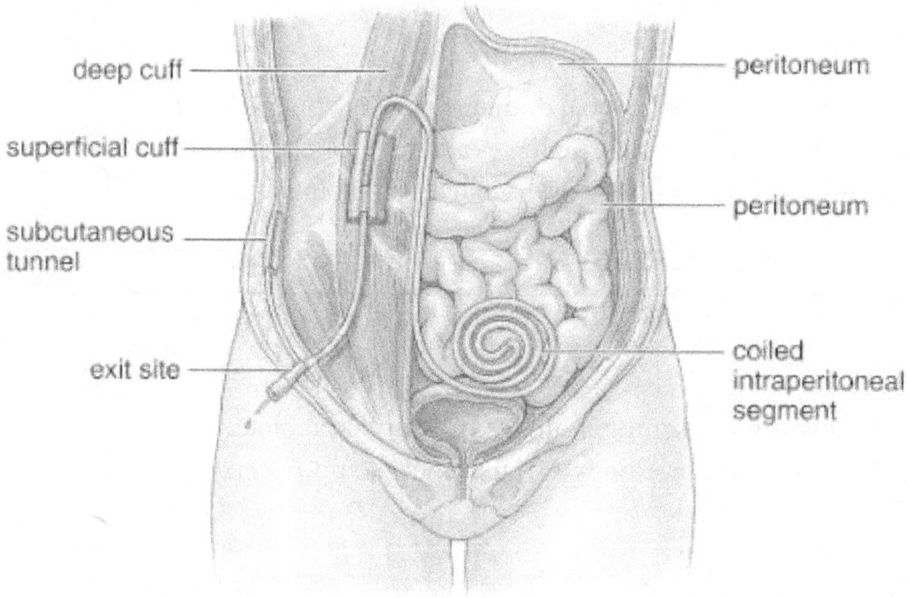

Continuous Ambulatory Peritoneal Dialysis Prescriptions

Standard CAPD Exchange Schedule

Continuous ambulatory peritoneal dialysis, the manual exchange approach performed by the patient without a machine, typically involves three to five exchanges daily, each consisting of draining the previous dwell, instilling fresh dialysate, and allowing that fresh fill to dwell for a period ranging from approximately four hours during the day to a longer, roughly eight-to-ten-hour dwell overnight; this schedule distributes exchanges across the patient's waking hours with a final exchange before sleep providing the long overnight dwell, a pattern that has remained the standard CAPD structure since the modality's earliest clinical use given its reasonable balance of adequate clearance against the practical burden of manual exchanges performed while awake.

Figure 17.2: CAPD Manual Exchange Sequence

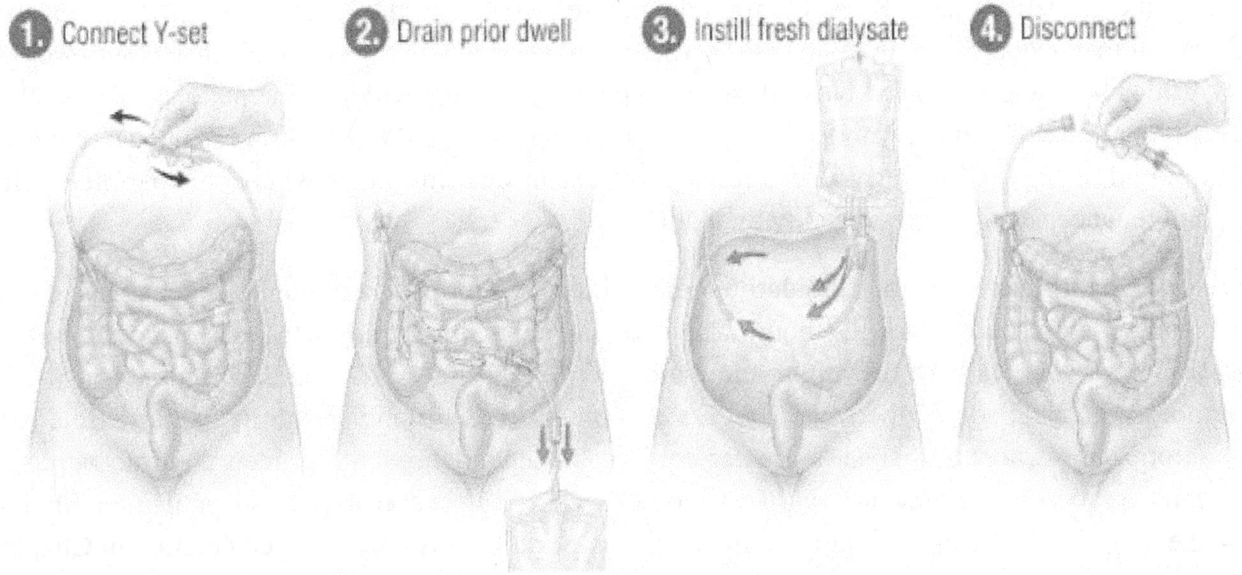

Each exchange requires the patient to perform a defined sequence of steps using sterile technique: connecting the fresh dialysate bag and drain bag to the catheter using a Y-set or twin-bag system designed to minimize touch contamination risk, draining the prior dwell by gravity, instilling the fresh fill, and disconnecting, with the entire process typically requiring twenty to thirty minutes per exchange once a patient is proficient; this hands-on, multiple-times-daily process is precisely the daily commitment discussed in Chapter 2's treatment of modality education, and a patient's actual tolerance for this specific daily routine, rather than an abstract preference for peritoneal dialysis in principle, should be confirmed through the hands-on training process before a patient commits fully to a CAPD-based prescription.

Individualizing the CAPD Prescription

Fill volume, typically starting in a range tolerable for a new patient and advanced gradually as the patient's abdominal capacity and comfort allow, directly affects both clearance and ultrafiltration per exchange, following the same surface-area-and-volume relationship discussed in Chapter 16, and a patient's individual tolerance for a given fill volume, reflecting their body size, abdominal wall compliance, and any intra-abdominal pathology, should guide this advancement rather than defaulting immediately to a standard adult fill volume regardless of individual tolerance.

Dwell duration and dextrose concentration for each of the day's exchanges should be individualized according to the patient's PET-determined transport category discussed in Chapter 16: a high transporter's CAPD prescription may benefit from a shorter daytime dwell duration than the standard four hours, given this patient's more rapid equilibration, potentially requiring an additional daytime exchange to maintain adequate total daily clearance despite the shorter individual dwell times, while a low transporter can tolerate the standard or even somewhat extended dwell durations without the diminishing marginal clearance return a high transporter would experience over an equally extended dwell.

Advantages and Limitations of CAPD

CAPD's principal advantage is its continuous nature, avoiding the peaks and troughs of solute concentration that accompany the more discrete treatment sessions of hemodialysis discussed throughout Part II of this book, and its lack of dependence on a cycler machine, which some patients find preferable specifically because it requires no equipment beyond dialysate bags and simple manual connection supplies, an advantage particularly relevant for a patient in circumstances where reliable electricity or cycler maintenance support is less readily available.

CAPD's principal limitation is the cumulative time burden of multiple daily manual exchanges, a burden that falls specifically during waking hours and can conflict with employment, travel, and other daily activities in a way the largely overnight automated peritoneal dialysis schedule discussed next in this chapter does not; this trade-off between CAPD's equipment-free simplicity and its daytime time burden versus automated peritoneal dialysis's greater equipment dependence but reduced daytime burden is a central consideration in the modality-within-a-modality choice a peritoneal dialysis patient and their care team make, paralleling the broader hemodialysis-versus-peritoneal-dialysis choice detailed in Chapter 2.

Automated Peritoneal Dialysis Prescriptions

Cycler-Based Prescription Design

Automated peritoneal dialysis uses a cycler machine to perform multiple exchanges automatically overnight while the patient sleeps, typically delivering three to six cycles over an eight-to-ten-hour period, with the specific number of cycles, fill volume per cycle, and total overnight dwell time all programmable and individualized to the patient's transport category and clearance needs following the same principles established in Chapter 16 and applied to CAPD earlier in this chapter.

A last-fill volume, instilled by the cycler at the end of the overnight session and left to dwell throughout the following day until the patient's next connection that evening, extends the prescription's clearance and ultrafiltration into the daytime hours without requiring a manual daytime exchange, and the dextrose concentration or, where appropriate, icodextrin selection for this last-fill dwell should be individualized to the patient's transport category exactly as discussed in Chapter 16, given this dwell's typically much longer duration than any individual overnight cycle.

Modern cyclers record detailed treatment data for every session, including actual fill and drain volumes achieved, cycle duration, and any alarms triggered during the night, and reviewing this downloaded data at routine follow-up visits provides an objective record of prescription adherence and technical performance considerably more detailed than what a patient can reliably recall and report from memory; a discrepancy between the prescribed and actually delivered treatment parameters, identified through this downloaded data, should prompt investigation into whether the discrepancy reflects a mechanical issue with the cycler or catheter, a patient-initiated adjustment made without informing the treating team, or a systematic pattern such as consistently incomplete drainage that itself warrants the mechanical complication evaluation detailed earlier in this chapter.

Alarm patterns recorded by the cycler over multiple nights, rather than any single night's alarm considered in isolation, can reveal a developing mechanical problem before it becomes severe enough to produce a clinically obvious drainage complaint the patient would otherwise report proactively; a cycler generating an increasing frequency of low-drain-volume alarms over consecutive nights, for example, may reflect an early, still-mild degree of the catheter migration or omental wrapping discussed earlier in this chapter, and reviewing this trend at scheduled follow-up, rather than waiting for the patient to notice and report a subjective drainage change, extends the same proactive, trend-based surveillance principle this book has applied throughout to vascular access monitoring and dialysis adequacy assessment.

Matching APD to Transport Category and Lifestyle

High transporters are particularly well suited to automated peritoneal dialysis, since the multiple short overnight cycles align closely with this patient's need for frequent, brief dwells to avoid the rapid osmotic gradient dissipation discussed in Chapter 16, while the extended last-fill daytime dwell, using icodextrin specifically to sustain ultrafiltration through the day despite this patient's rapid transport, addresses the daytime clearance and ultrafiltration need without requiring a manual daytime exchange this patient's rapid transport would otherwise make comparatively inefficient.

Beyond the physiologic matching considerations already discussed, lifestyle factors weigh heavily in the CAPD-versus-APD choice: a working patient or one with significant daytime obligations may strongly prefer automated peritoneal dialysis's overnight-concentrated schedule, freeing daytime hours from the manual exchange burden CAPD imposes, while a patient with a strong preference for avoiding equipment dependence, or one whose home environment poses practical challenges to cycler setup and maintenance, may reasonably prefer CAPD despite its greater daytime time burden; this choice, like the broader modality choices detailed in Chapter 2, is best made collaboratively, weighing physiologic fit against the patient's own priorities and circumstances rather than defaulting to either approach as a universal default.

Sleep quality and cycler noise deserve explicit discussion during modality education specifically for automated peritoneal dialysis, since the cycler's operating sounds, while generally modest, can disrupt sleep for some patients or their bed partners, and this consideration, while seemingly minor relative to the physiologic factors this chapter has emphasized, meaningfully affects a patient's actual long-term satisfaction and adherence with an automated prescription; addressing this concern proactively, including discussing cycler placement options that minimize noise disruption, supports better long-term tolerance than treating it as an incidental detail unworthy of explicit attention during the initial prescription discussion.

The Daytime Dwell in APD

Some automated peritoneal dialysis prescriptions incorporate an additional manual daytime exchange beyond the cycler-delivered overnight cycles and last-fill dwell, particularly for a patient whose combined overnight and last-fill clearance falls short of their adequacy target discussed in Chapter 18, extending the prescription's total clearance without requiring the patient to return to a full CAPD-equivalent daytime exchange burden; this hybrid approach illustrates that CAPD and APD are not always mutually exclusive categories but can be combined flexibly to meet an individual patient's specific clearance needs.

A patient's residual kidney function, discussed further in the incremental peritoneal dialysis treatment later in this chapter, factors directly into whether this additional daytime exchange is actually necessary, since a patient with meaningful residual function may achieve adequate total clearance from overnight cycling and last-fill dwell alone, without needing the additional daytime exchange a patient with negligible residual function might require to reach the same total adequacy target.

Incremental Peritoneal Dialysis Strategies

Rationale for Incremental PD

Incremental peritoneal dialysis begins a patient at a reduced dialysis dose, whether through fewer exchanges, shorter dwells, or lower fill volumes than a full-dose prescription would use, explicitly accounting for the patient's own residual kidney function as an active contributor to total clearance rather than an incidental bonus layered on top of a full-dose peritoneal prescription calculated as though residual function did not exist; this approach mirrors the individualized, whole-patient adequacy reasoning developed in Chapter 7 for hemodialysis, extended here to the peritoneal context where residual function often remains more substantial and more clinically consequential for a longer period than in the typical hemodialysis patient, given peritoneal dialysis's gentler hemodynamic profile discussed in Chapter 2.

Reducing the initial dialysis dose in a patient with substantial residual function offers several practical advantages beyond simply avoiding an unnecessarily intensive prescription: fewer exchanges or a shorter cycler session reduces the daily time burden and equipment cost during the period residual function remains substantial, and some evidence suggests incremental approaches may help preserve residual function longer than an immediately full-dose prescription, plausibly by avoiding the additional dextrose exposure and osmotic stress a full-dose prescription would impose on residual native kidney tissue that a reduced initial dose spares.

The evidence base supporting residual-function preservation specifically as a benefit of incremental peritoneal dialysis remains less robust and less consistent across studies than the more straightforward, well-established practical burden-reduction benefit, and clinicians should present the residual-preservation rationale to patients with appropriate epistemic humility, framing the reduced initial burden as the primary, well-supported advantage while noting the preservation benefit as a plausible additional consideration rather than a firmly established, guaranteed outcome of the incremental approach.

Implementing and Advancing an Incremental Prescription

Implementing an incremental prescription requires accurately measuring residual kidney function at initiation, typically through a timed urine collection assessing residual urea and creatinine clearance similarly to the residual function assessment discussed in Chapter 7 for hemodialysis, and calculating the peritoneal dialysis dose needed to supplement this residual contribution to reach an appropriate total clearance target, rather than prescribing a reduced peritoneal dose without this explicit calculation confirming the combined total is actually adequate.

Because residual kidney function typically declines over time, an incremental prescription requires scheduled reassessment, following the same trigger-based and periodic reassessment principle this book has applied throughout to prescriptions across every modality, with the peritoneal dose increased proportionally as residual function declines to maintain adequate total clearance; a patient started on an incremental prescription should have residual function reassessed at defined intervals, with an explicit, proactive plan for advancing the prescription as that function declines, rather than waiting for symptoms of inadequate total clearance to develop before recognizing that the incremental approach's initial calculation no longer reflects the patient's current physiologic reality.

A forty-four-year-old man beginning peritoneal dialysis is found to have a residual kidney function contributing meaningfully to his overall clearance, measured through a timed urine collection at initiation. Rather than starting him on a full-dose four-exchange CAPD prescription, his nephrology team calculates that three exchanges daily, combined with his residual function, achieve an adequate total clearance target, and he begins this reduced, incremental prescription, benefiting from a lower daily time burden during this initial period. His residual function is reassessed every three months, and eighteen months into treatment, a meaningful decline is identified; his prescription is advanced to four exchanges daily to compensate for this decline, maintaining adequate total clearance despite his residual function's continued decline. This case illustrates the incremental approach's full lifecycle: an individualized reduced starting prescription justified by measured residual function, followed by scheduled reassessment and proactive advancement as that function predictably declines over time, rather than either a one-time reduced prescription left unexamined indefinitely or an immediately full-dose prescription that would have imposed unnecessary burden during his initial period of substantial residual function.

CLINICAL PEARL: An incremental peritoneal dialysis prescription requires the same scheduled reassessment and proactive advancement this book has applied to every other prescription-and-residual-function relationship; a reduced starting dose justified by residual function today does not remain adequate once that function has meaningfully declined.

DIALYSIS RECOGNITION & RESPONSE SYSTEM — Peritoneal Prescription Arcs

The Pattern: A patient on an incremental peritoneal dialysis prescription has not had residual kidney function reassessed in an extended period.

Stem Signature: A patient started on a reduced, incremental peritoneal dialysis prescription based on residual function measured at initiation, now well beyond the interval at which reassessment was originally planned, with no repeat measurement yet obtained despite the predictable, expected decline in residual function over time.

The Decision: Obtain a repeat residual function measurement and advance the peritoneal prescription proportionally if a meaningful decline is confirmed, rather than allowing the original reduced prescription to continue by default simply because no symptom has yet prompted reconsideration.

Trap Logic: An incremental prescription that has functioned without apparent problems can create a false sense that the original reduced dose remains adequate indefinitely, when residual function's predictable decline means the original calculation's justification is itself eroding even before any symptom of inadequate clearance becomes apparent.

Response Anchor: An overdue residual function reassessment on an incremental prescription warrants proactive repeat measurement and prescription advancement — not continuation of the original reduced dose by default until symptoms eventually appear.

DIALYSIS RECOGNITION & RESPONSE SYSTEM — Peritoneal Prescription Arcs

Impaired Peritoneal Drainage: Address constipation first, since it is the most common and most readily reversible cause, before pursuing radiographic evaluation for catheter migration or surgical evaluation for omental wrapping.

Overdue Residual Function Reassessment on an Incremental Prescription: Obtain a repeat measurement and advance the prescription proportionally rather than allowing the original reduced dose to continue by default.

Summary and Key Concepts

The peritoneal dialysis catheter's tunnel and cuff design parallels the tunneled hemodialysis catheter, providing a barrier against organism migration, and requires an adequate break-in period before regular use to allow proper incorporation.

CAPD's manual exchange schedule should be individualized in fill volume, dwell duration, and dextrose concentration according to a patient's PET-determined transport category, trading equipment-free simplicity against a daytime time burden.

Automated peritoneal dialysis concentrates exchanges overnight via cycler, particularly well suited to high transporters, and can incorporate a last-fill dwell or additional daytime exchange to extend clearance into daytime hours.

Incremental peritoneal dialysis accounts explicitly for residual kidney function in calculating the initial prescription dose, reducing early treatment burden while residual function remains substantial.

An incremental prescription requires scheduled reassessment of residual function and proportional prescription advancement as that function predictably declines, rather than continuing an initial reduced dose indefinitely without reassessment.

CHAPTER 18: PERITONEAL DIALYSIS ADEQUACY AND INDIVIDUALIZED PRESCRIPTION

Learning Objectives

Calculate peritoneal Kt/V and weekly creatinine clearance, combining dialysate and residual contributions.

Explain why residual kidney function carries particular weight in peritoneal dialysis adequacy and apply strategies to preserve it.

Assess volume status in a peritoneal dialysis patient and integrate ultrafiltration failure into adequacy assessment.

Construct a whole-patient peritoneal dialysis adequacy framework extending beyond a single Kt/V target.

Chapter Overview

Chapter 7 established that hemodialysis adequacy is a necessary but insufficient concept when reduced to Kt/V alone, and that whole-patient assessment integrating residual function, nutrition, and symptom burden provides a more complete picture. This chapter develops the parallel argument for peritoneal dialysis, where the same underlying principle applies with even greater force: residual kidney function typically remains more substantial and more clinically consequential for longer in peritoneal dialysis patients than in hemodialysis patients, making its explicit incorporation into adequacy assessment not an optional refinement but a central requirement for accurate evaluation. This chapter works through the specific calculations peritoneal adequacy assessment uses, the particular reasons residual function preservation deserves active attention in this population, how ultrafiltration failure integrates into the adequacy picture, and how the field has evolved away from a single numeric target toward the whole-patient framework this chapter's final section develops. Readers will recognize throughout this chapter a close structural parallel to Chapter 7's hemodialysis adequacy treatment, and this parallel is deliberate: the underlying argument that a single small-solute clearance number cannot substitute for genuine whole-patient assessment applies with equal force across both modalities, even though the specific calculations, the relative weight residual function carries, and the specific complications requiring integration into that assessment differ meaningfully between them.

Peritoneal Kt/V and Creatinine Clearance

Calculating Peritoneal Kt/V

Peritoneal Kt/V, conceptually parallel to the hemodialysis Kt/V developed in Chapter 7, expresses total urea clearance relative to estimated total body water, but differs in calculation because peritoneal clearance is continuous rather than delivered in discrete treatment sessions: rather than measuring clearance across a single treatment as hemodialysis Kt/V does, peritoneal Kt/V is calculated from the total urea removed in dialysate drained over a full twenty-four-hour period, or more practically a representative collection period, extrapolated to a weekly total and expressed relative to the same estimated body water volume.

This continuous-clearance calculation means peritoneal Kt/V does not carry the single-pool-versus-equilibrated distinction that complicates hemodialysis Kt/V interpretation, since there is no discrete treatment-end moment at which urea disequilibrium between compartments would need to be corrected for; the continuous nature of peritoneal clearance means blood and dialysate urea concentrations remain in a more consistent, steady-state relationship throughout the day rather than showing the treatment-and-rebound pattern hemodialysis produces, simplifying peritoneal Kt/V calculation relative to its hemodialysis counterpart in this specific respect even as it introduces the residual-function-weighting considerations detailed later in this chapter.

Practical collection technique matters considerably to the accuracy of this calculation: a patient must drain and save every dialysate exchange over the full collection period, typically twenty-four hours, into designated collection containers rather than discarding any portion, since even a single missed or partially discarded exchange introduces a systematic underestimate of total clearance that a formula extrapolating from an incomplete collection cannot correct for. Structured patient education specifically addressing this collection technique, reinforced periodically rather than delivered only once at the time a patient is first trained on peritoneal dialysis generally, reduces the collection errors that would otherwise produce an artifactually low Kt/V result misread as evidence of inadequate clearance rather than a correctable collection technique problem.

Weekly Creatinine Clearance

Weekly creatinine clearance, calculated similarly from total creatinine removed in dialysate over a representative collection period and extrapolated to a weekly total, provides a complementary measure to peritoneal Kt/V, and, as with the urea reduction ratio discussed in Chapter 7 as a hemodialysis cross-check against Kt/V, creatinine clearance and Kt/V can occasionally diverge in a peritoneal dialysis patient, most commonly when a patient's muscle mass is unusually low or high relative to the population average the standard reference calculations assume, echoing the same body-composition-dependent interpretation caution Chapter 7 raised for hemodialysis Kt/V.

Because creatinine generation depends on muscle mass in a way total body water does not directly track, a patient with significant muscle wasting may show a creatinine clearance that appears more favorable relative to their actual clinical adequacy than their Kt/V would suggest, since a smaller creatinine generation rate is more easily cleared to a seemingly adequate degree even by a modest absolute clearance;

recognizing this potential distortion, particularly in a frail or malnourished patient, is part of why the whole-patient framework this chapter develops incorporates nutritional assessment as a complementary measure rather than relying on either clearance metric considered in isolation.

A thirty-six-year-old woman on automated peritoneal dialysis for eight months presents for routine adequacy testing with a Kt/V result substantially below her prior consistent readings, without any accompanying symptoms suggesting genuine clinical decline and without any recent prescription change. Rather than immediately escalating her prescription in response to this apparently low result, her nephrology team reviews her collection technique in detail and discovers she had inadvertently discarded one of her cycler's overnight drain bags rather than saving it for collection, having misunderstood a recent change in her cycler's bag configuration. A repeat, correctly performed collection the following week returns a result consistent with her prior stable baseline, confirming the initial low value reflected a collection error rather than a genuine adequacy problem. This case illustrates why an unexpected adequacy result, particularly one inconsistent with the patient's prior stable trend and unaccompanied by any corresponding clinical change, should prompt review of collection technique before triggering a prescription escalation that would not address a problem that does not, in fact, exist.

Combining Dialysate and Residual Contributions

Total peritoneal dialysis adequacy, whether expressed as Kt/V or creatinine clearance, is calculated as the sum of the dialysate-derived contribution and the residual native kidney contribution, a combination made explicit and routine in peritoneal dialysis adequacy reporting in a way that, as Chapter 7 noted, is less consistently incorporated into routine hemodialysis Kt/V reporting despite residual function's relevance there as well; this explicit combination reflects peritoneal dialysis's typically longer preservation of meaningful residual function and the correspondingly larger share of total clearance that residual function often represents, particularly in the early years of a patient's peritoneal dialysis course.

Because residual function's contribution to total clearance can be substantial, a patient's dialysate-only Kt/V may fall meaningfully below what would be considered adequate if considered as the sole clearance source, while their combined total, incorporating a still-meaningful residual contribution, remains fully adequate; interpreting a peritoneal Kt/V value therefore requires knowing both the dialysate and residual components separately, not merely the combined total, since a declining residual contribution masked by a stable combined total can herald an approaching adequacy problem that will become apparent only once residual function has declined further, a pattern this chapter's third section develops in more detail.

Adequacy Component	What It Measures	Key Interpretation Point
Dialysate Kt/V	Urea clearance from drained dialysate alone	Reflects prescription-delivered clearance specifically
Residual Kt/V	Urea clearance from native kidney function	Declines over time; requires separate tracking from the combined total

Total Kt/V	Sum of dialysate and residual contributions	The adequacy target is applied to this combined value
Weekly Creatinine Clearance	Creatinine removal, dialysate plus residual	Can diverge from Kt/V in patients with atypical muscle mass

KEY POINT: Peritoneal dialysis adequacy is calculated as the sum of dialysate and residual kidney contributions; tracking these components separately, not only the combined total, is essential to recognizing a declining residual contribution before it becomes clinically apparent.

Residual Kidney Function and Its Preservation

Why Residual Function Matters More in PD

Residual kidney function tends to decline more slowly in peritoneal dialysis patients than in hemodialysis patients, plausibly reflecting peritoneal dialysis's gentler, continuous physiologic profile relative to hemodialysis's intermittent, larger-volume hemodynamic shifts discussed in Chapter 13, meaning residual function's contribution to total clearance remains clinically significant for a meaningfully longer period in the typical peritoneal dialysis patient's course than in the typical hemodialysis patient's course.

This slower decline is part of the physiologic rationale underlying the incremental peritoneal dialysis approach discussed in Chapter 17, since a prescription strategy explicitly built around leveraging a substantial and durable residual contribution is more clinically justified in a population where that contribution genuinely persists for years rather than declining rapidly over months; residual function's outsized and prolonged importance in peritoneal dialysis is precisely why this chapter, unlike the hemodialysis adequacy treatment in Chapter 7, integrates residual function as a foundational rather than supplementary component of the adequacy calculation itself.

Strategies to Preserve Residual Function

Avoiding nephrotoxic medications and minimizing episodes of volume depletion or acute kidney injury, principles applicable across the entire chronic kidney disease trajectory discussed in Chapter 1, remain directly relevant once a patient has started peritoneal dialysis, since residual function, though already reduced, retains real value worth actively protecting rather than treating as a lost cause simply because the patient has already reached kidney failure and initiated replacement therapy.

Angiotensin-converting enzyme inhibitors and angiotensin receptor blockers, beyond their established role earlier in chronic kidney disease progression, have shown some evidence of residual-function-preserving benefit specifically in the peritoneal dialysis population, plausibly through the same intraglomerular hemodynamic mechanisms relevant to their use earlier in chronic kidney disease, and continuing or initiating these agents in a peritoneal dialysis patient, where not otherwise contraindicated by hyperkalemia or hypotension risk, represents a reasonable, evidence-informed component of a residual-function preservation strategy rather than a medication class to be reflexively discontinued once a patient has started dialysis simply because its original chronic-kidney-disease-progression indication has technically been superseded by dialysis initiation itself.

Diuretic therapy, often continued in peritoneal dialysis patients specifically to support residual urine output and volume management even after dialysis initiation, differs in this respect from typical hemodialysis practice, where diuretics are frequently discontinued once dialysis begins given the treatment's own capacity for fluid removal; in peritoneal dialysis, however, a loop diuretic at an appropriately titrated dose can meaningfully support residual urine output and thereby ease the volume-management burden the peritoneal prescription alone would otherwise need to carry entirely, making diuretic continuation a reasonable, evidence-informed component of the residual-function and volume-preservation strategy this section develops, rather than an automatically discontinued medication simply because the patient has technically become dialysis-dependent.

Avoiding or minimizing exposure to iodinated contrast media and other nephrotoxic diagnostic or therapeutic agents wherever a reasonable alternative exists remains relevant even after dialysis initiation, since residual function, though already substantially reduced, can still be acutely and sometimes permanently injured by an avoidable nephrotoxic exposure in the same way native kidney function earlier in the chronic kidney disease trajectory can be; this consideration deserves explicit communication to any non-nephrology clinician ordering a contrast-enhanced study or other potentially nephrotoxic intervention for a peritoneal dialysis patient, since a clinician unfamiliar with this patient's ongoing residual-function-preservation goals might not otherwise weigh this consideration into their own ordering decision.

Figure 18.2 Residual Kidney Function Decline Trajectory in Peritoneal Dialysis

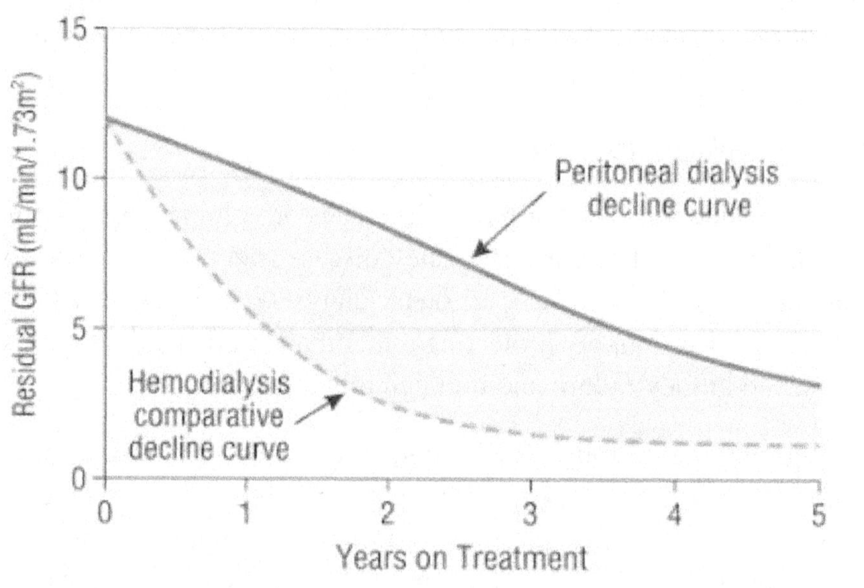

Measuring and Monitoring Residual Function

Residual function is measured through a timed urine collection, typically performed alongside the dialysate collection used for the total Kt/V and creatinine clearance calculations discussed earlier in this chapter, allowing both the dialysate and residual components to be captured from the same overall collection period rather than requiring separate, differently timed assessments; because residual function in a patient with even minimal remaining urine output can be measured this way, only a patient who has become fully anuric can be assumed to have no residual contribution requiring this separate measurement and tracking.

Scheduled reassessment of residual function, at an interval determined by the patient's individual trajectory and rate of prior decline, allows the gradual decline this chapter has emphasized to be tracked proactively, with the peritoneal prescription adjusted to compensate as that decline progresses, following the same trigger-based and periodic reassessment principle this book has applied to every other prescription-and-residual-function relationship throughout its treatment of both hemodialysis and peritoneal dialysis.

DIALYSIS RECOGNITION & RESPONSE SYSTEM — Peritoneal Adequacy Arcs

The Pattern: A peritoneal dialysis patient's combined total Kt/V remains stable while their residual function has not been separately reassessed recently.

Stem Signature: A stable, at-target combined total Kt/V on routine monitoring in a patient whose residual and dialysate components have not been separately reviewed, and whose residual function has not been formally reassessed within the interval this chapter recommends.

The Decision: Review the dialysate and residual components of the total Kt/V separately, and obtain a fresh residual function measurement if due, rather than accepting a stable combined total as confirmation that no meaningful change has occurred in either underlying component.

Trap Logic: A stable combined total can mask a declining residual contribution that has been offset, whether coincidentally or through an unremarked prescription change, by a rising dialysate contribution, delaying recognition of a residual decline that the total Kt/V alone does not reveal.

Response Anchor: A stable combined Kt/V does not confirm stable residual function — review the components separately and reassess residual function on schedule rather than inferring stability from the total alone.

Volume Status and Ultrafiltration Failure

Assessing Volume Status in PD Patients

Volume assessment in a peritoneal dialysis patient draws on the same clinical examination elements discussed in Chapter 4 for hemodialysis — jugular venous pressure, peripheral edema, lung auscultation, and blood pressure trends — supplemented, as in hemodialysis, by bioimpedance spectroscopy or point-of-care ultrasound assessment of inferior vena cava characteristics where available, but interpreted against a continuous rather than intermittent fluid removal pattern, since a peritoneal dialysis patient does not experience the same interdialytic accumulation-and-removal cycle a hemodialysis patient does.

This continuous pattern means volume status in a well-managed peritoneal dialysis patient should, in principle, remain more stable day to day than the sawtooth pattern characteristic of hemodialysis, and a peritoneal dialysis patient showing significant day-to-day volume fluctuation, rather than the expected greater stability, should prompt evaluation for an underlying cause such as inconsistent adherence to the prescribed exchange schedule, an evolving ultrafiltration problem discussed in the next subsection, or a dietary sodium and fluid intake pattern exceeding what the current prescription can accommodate.

Consequences of Chronic Volume Overload

Chronic volume overload in a peritoneal dialysis patient, similarly to the hemodialysis population discussed throughout Part VII of this book, contributes to hypertension, left ventricular hypertrophy, and cardiovascular morbidity over time, and because peritoneal dialysis's continuous fluid removal profile can make volume overload less immediately symptomatic on a day-to-day basis than the more acute hemodialysis-related fluid shifts a clinician might be more accustomed to recognizing, volume status deserves explicit, deliberate assessment at every peritoneal dialysis follow-up visit rather than being inferred only from the absence of overt symptoms a patient might not yet be reporting.

Because peritoneal dialysis patients often maintain better-preserved residual function and correspondingly better-preserved urine output than hemodialysis patients, at least in the earlier years of treatment, this residual urine output itself contributes to volume management and should be incorporated into the overall volume assessment rather than considered separately from the dialysate-derived ultrafiltration this chapter and Chapter 16 both address; a declining residual urine output, tracked alongside the residual clearance function discussed earlier in this chapter, is a further signal that the peritoneal prescription's ultrafiltration contribution may need to increase to compensate for this declining native contribution to overall fluid balance.

Structured volume assessment documentation at every follow-up visit, using a consistent format that captures examination findings, any objective bioimpedance or ultrasound data available, residual urine output, and the patient's own interval weight trend, supports the same kind of trend-based recognition this book has emphasized throughout for other gradually evolving clinical patterns, allowing a slowly developing volume overload to be recognized from the accumulated trend across several visits even when no single visit's findings alone would have prompted concern.

Integrating Ultrafiltration Failure Into Adequacy Assessment

Ultrafiltration failure, discussed mechanistically in Chapter 16, integrates directly into the adequacy framework this chapter develops: a patient with adequate solute clearance by Kt/V but declining ultrafiltration capacity is not adequately dialyzed in the whole-patient sense this chapter and Chapter 7 both emphasize, since inadequate fluid removal produces the volume-related morbidity discussed above regardless of how favorable the solute clearance numbers otherwise appear.

A peritoneal dialysis adequacy review that reports Kt/V and creatinine clearance without also explicitly reporting ultrafiltration capacity and trend, alongside the volume assessment findings detailed earlier in this section, provides an incomplete picture in the same way a hemodialysis adequacy review reporting Kt/V alone without volume status, discussed in Chapter 7, would be incomplete; this chapter's recommended adequacy framework therefore treats ultrafiltration capacity as a co-equal component alongside solute clearance rather than a secondary consideration addressed only once solute clearance targets have already been confirmed satisfactory.

Recognizing When Transition to Hemodialysis Becomes Appropriate

Refractory ultrafiltration failure or inadequate solute clearance despite prescription optimization, recurrent peritonitis discussed in Chapter 19, or a patient's own preference shift away from peritoneal dialysis are each reasonable grounds for transitioning to hemodialysis, and recognizing when this transition has become the more appropriate path, rather than continuing to escalate an already-optimized peritoneal prescription indefinitely, reflects the same individualized, trajectory-aware Life-Plan reasoning developed in Chapter 2, now applied to a modality change occurring later in a patient's course rather than only at initial modality selection.

This transition, when it becomes necessary, benefits from the same proactive, well-planned sequencing this book has emphasized throughout Part III's treatment of hemodialysis access: initiating vascular access evaluation and creation in advance of an anticipated transition, wherever the clinical trajectory allows this advance planning, rather than waiting until peritoneal dialysis has already failed outright and an urgent catheter-based hemodialysis bridge becomes the only immediately available option; a patient whose peritoneal adequacy or ultrafiltration trend is declining in a way that suggests transition may eventually become necessary is a reasonable candidate for early, parallel vascular access planning, mirroring the same proactive sequencing this book recommended for a patient transitioning from peritoneal dialysis toward an anticipated hemodialysis need in Chapter 9's treatment of access timing relative to the Life-Plan.

CAUTION: Adequate Kt/V does not confirm adequate peritoneal dialysis adequacy in the whole-patient sense; ultrafiltration capacity and volume status require explicit, co-equal assessment alongside solute clearance at every adequacy review.

Figure 18.1: Combined Dialysate and Residual Contributions to Total Peritoneal Clearance

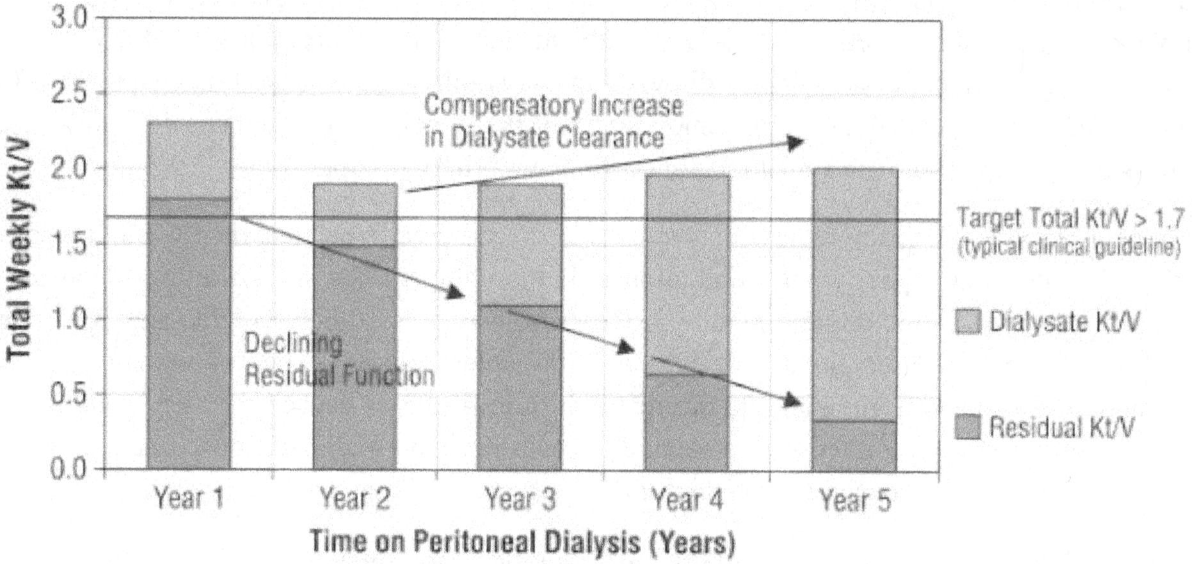

Beyond Kt/V: Patient-Centered Adequacy Measures

The Evolution Away From a Single Kt/V Target

Early peritoneal dialysis adequacy guidelines, similarly to the early hemodialysis dose-escalation history discussed in Chapter 7, emphasized progressively higher Kt/V targets based on observational associations between higher clearance and better outcomes, and subsequent randomized evidence testing whether prospectively raising peritoneal Kt/V above a more modest, already-adequate threshold produced additional benefit generally failed to confirm the anticipated further improvement, prompting the same shift away from escalating a single small-solute target that Chapter 7 described for hemodialysis.

This evolution has been particularly influential in the peritoneal dialysis context because achieving a very high Kt/V target through dialysate clearance alone, once residual function has been exhausted, typically requires an intensified prescription that meaningfully increases either exchange frequency or dwell volume, imposing a real burden on the patient without the confirmed corresponding benefit the earlier, more escalation-oriented targets assumed; recognizing this has shifted contemporary practice toward accepting a more modest total Kt/V target, particularly once residual function has substantially declined, rather than pursuing progressively higher dialysate-derived clearance as an end in itself.

This evidence-driven de-escalation of numeric targets should not be mistaken for a suggestion that adequacy monitoring itself has become less important; rather, it redirects clinical attention away from chasing an ever-higher single number and toward the broader, whole-patient assessment this chapter's final section develops, in the same way Chapter 7 redirected hemodialysis adequacy attention away from Kt/V escalation and toward residual function, nutrition, and symptom burden once dose-escalation trials in that modality similarly failed to show benefit from pushing small-solute clearance higher once an adequate threshold was reached.

Quality of Life and Symptom Burden

A patient's own reported quality of life, symptom burden, and functional status provide information about peritoneal dialysis adequacy that Kt/V and creatinine clearance cannot, mirroring exactly the whole-patient clinical markers Chapter 7 recommended incorporating into hemodialysis adequacy review; a peritoneal dialysis patient with numerically adequate Kt/V who nonetheless reports declining appetite, increasing fatigue, or reduced functional capacity warrants the same broader evaluation Chapter 7 recommended for an analogous hemodialysis presentation, rather than reassurance that a passing Kt/V excludes a dialysis-related explanation for these symptoms.

The burden peritoneal dialysis itself imposes, including the exchange schedule's daily time cost discussed in Chapter 17 and any accumulated frustration with recurrent mechanical or infectious complications discussed in Chapters 17 and 19, also factors into a genuinely patient-centered adequacy assessment, since a technically adequate prescription that a patient finds unsustainable in practice will not deliver its intended clinical benefit if the patient's actual adherence to it erodes under the weight of this burden; periodically and explicitly asking a patient how the prescription is actually working for them in daily life, not only what their laboratory-based adequacy metrics show, closes this gap between technical and lived adequacy.

Validated quality-of-life instruments specific to the dialysis population, incorporating domains such as physical functioning, symptom burden, and treatment satisfaction, offer a more structured and comparable way to capture this patient-centered dimension than an informal conversation alone, and incorporating periodic administration of such an instrument into routine peritoneal dialysis follow-up, alongside the laboratory-based adequacy metrics this chapter has detailed, operationalizes the whole-patient principle in a way that a purely informal, unstructured check-in risks applying inconsistently across different patients and different clinic visits.

A Practical Whole-Patient PD Adequacy Framework

A structured peritoneal dialysis adequacy review, integrating total Kt/V with its separately tracked dialysate and residual components, weekly creatinine clearance, ultrafiltration capacity and volume status trend, residual urine output, nutritional markers, and the patient's own reported symptom burden and prescription tolerance, provides a considerably more complete picture than any single metric considered in isolation, extending the whole-patient adequacy principle Chapter 7 developed for hemodialysis into its full, peritoneal-specific form.

A sixty-seven-year-old man on peritoneal dialysis for two years has maintained a combined total Kt/V consistently at target, but his most recent review, prompted by his report of increasing fatigue and reduced appetite over the preceding month, reveals on closer examination that his residual Kt/V component has declined substantially while his dialysate component has correspondingly increased to compensate, keeping the combined total stable despite this underlying shift. His residual urine output has also declined over the same period, and his team recognizes that his total clearance number, while numerically reassuring, obscures a genuine decline in his overall physiologic reserve that his reported symptoms are now reflecting. Rather than reassuring him that his adequate Kt/V excludes a dialysis-related cause for his symptoms, his team pursues nutritional assessment, finds early evidence of protein-energy wasting, and adjusts his dietary counseling and peritoneal prescription accordingly. His symptoms improve over the following weeks. This case illustrates precisely the pattern this chapter has developed throughout: a stable combined total can mask a meaningful underlying decline, and genuinely whole-patient adequacy assessment, not the total Kt/V number alone, is what catches it.

CLINICAL PEARL: A stable total Kt/V does not exclude declining residual function or emerging nutritional compromise; new symptoms in a numerically adequate patient warrant the same whole-patient review this book recommends throughout, not reassurance based on the total number alone.

DIALYSIS RECOGNITION & RESPONSE SYSTEM — Peritoneal Adequacy Arcs

The Pattern: A peritoneal dialysis patient with a stable, at-target total Kt/V develops new fatigue or declining appetite.

Stem Signature: New constitutional symptoms and a declining nutritional marker in a patient whose combined total Kt/V has remained at target throughout, without an obvious change in the prescription itself.

The Decision: Pursue a whole-patient adequacy review, including separate residual and dialysate component tracking, residual urine output trend, and nutritional assessment, rather than reassuring the patient that a numerically adequate total Kt/V excludes a dialysis-related explanation.

Trap Logic: A stable total Kt/V can be mistaken for confirmation that the peritoneal dialysis prescription is fully adequate in every respect, when the total may be masking a declining residual contribution that only component-level review and nutritional assessment would reveal.

Response Anchor: New symptoms despite a stable total Kt/V warrant a whole-patient adequacy review — not reassurance based on the combined total number alone.

Stable Total Kt/V Without Recent Component Review: Review the dialysate and residual components separately and reassess residual function on schedule rather than inferring stability from the total alone.

New Symptoms Despite At-Target Total Kt/V: Pursue a whole-patient adequacy review — components, residual urine output, nutrition — rather than reassurance based on the total number alone.

Summary and Key Concepts

Peritoneal Kt/V and weekly creatinine clearance are calculated from dialysate collected over a representative period, combined with the residual native kidney contribution, which should be tracked separately rather than only as part of the combined total.

Residual kidney function typically declines more slowly and remains clinically significant longer in peritoneal dialysis than in hemodialysis, making its preservation and monitoring a foundational rather than supplementary component of adequacy assessment.

Volume status and ultrafiltration capacity require explicit, co-equal assessment alongside solute clearance, since adequate Kt/V does not confirm adequate fluid management.

Dose-escalation evidence in peritoneal dialysis parallels the hemodialysis experience described in Chapter 7, showing no additional benefit from pursuing progressively higher Kt/V once an adequate threshold is reached.

A whole-patient adequacy framework integrating Kt/V components, ultrafiltration and volume status, residual urine output, nutrition, and patient-reported symptom burden and prescription tolerance provides a more complete picture than any single metric considered alone.

CHAPTER 19: PERITONITIS AND PERITONEAL ACCESS INFECTIONS

Learning Objectives

Apply the three diagnostic criteria for peritoneal dialysis peritonitis and interpret effluent cell count and culture results.

Select empiric antibiotic therapy, choose an appropriate route of administration, and tailor therapy once culture results return.

Distinguish exit-site infection from tunnel infection and apply prevention strategies to reduce both.

Recognize indications for catheter removal and technique failure, and manage recurrent peritonitis within defined catheter-salvage limits.

Chapter Overview

Peritonitis is the complication most feared by patients and clinicians alike in peritoneal dialysis, and for good reason: it is the leading cause of technique failure and catheter loss, a recognized contributor to the membrane fibrosis and transport changes discussed in Chapter 16, and, in its most severe or recurrent forms, a direct threat to a patient's continued ability to remain on the modality at all. This chapter closes Part V of this book by working through peritonitis from first recognition to final resolution or, where resolution proves impossible, to the catheter removal and modality transition that recurrent or refractory infection sometimes demands. Exit-site and tunnel infections, related but mechanistically and clinically distinct complications sharing the same anatomic access this chapter's subject depends on, receive their own dedicated treatment, since a clinician who conflates these related infections risks either overtreating a simple exit-site process or, more dangerously, undertreating a tunnel infection whose relationship to peritonitis carries different management implications entirely. Throughout, this chapter applies the same recognition-decision-response logic this book has used consistently since Chapter 1: early, structured recognition followed by decisive, protocol-driven action outperforms delayed or uncertain response, and nowhere in this book is that principle more consequential than in a peritonitis episode, where hours, not days, meaningfully affect the eventual outcome.

This chapter's four sections trace a single episode's natural progression: recognizing that peritonitis has occurred using the diagnostic criteria the first section develops, initiating and then tailoring appropriate antibiotic therapy as the second section describes, distinguishing this process from the related but distinct exit-site and tunnel infections the third section addresses, and, where an episode proves refractory or recurrent, recognizing the point at which catheter removal becomes the more appropriate path forward, developed in the chapter's final section. Readers should approach this chapter not as four independent topics but as a single connected clinical pathway, since a genuine understanding of peritonitis management requires holding all four stages in view simultaneously rather than treating diagnosis, treatment, related infections, and eventual catheter decisions as separable concerns addressed in isolation from one another.

Diagnostic Criteria for Peritoneal Dialysis Peritonitis

The Three Diagnostic Criteria

Peritoneal dialysis peritonitis is diagnosed when at least two of three criteria are present: clinical features consistent with peritonitis, most commonly abdominal pain and cloudy dialysate effluent; an effluent white cell count exceeding the standard diagnostic threshold with a predominance of polymorphonuclear cells, reflecting an acute bacterial inflammatory response rather than the more chronic or reactive cellular patterns other conditions can produce; and a positive effluent culture identifying a causative organism. Because any two of these three criteria are sufficient for diagnosis, a patient with compatible symptoms and an elevated effluent white cell count can and should be diagnosed and treated presumptively even before culture results return, since awaiting culture confirmation before initiating treatment would introduce a treatment delay this chapter's introduction has already identified as directly consequential to outcome.

The specific numeric threshold for effluent white cell count used to satisfy the second diagnostic criterion is well established in published guideline recommendations and should be interpreted alongside the differential, since a total cell count near this threshold with a genuinely polymorphonuclear predominance carries different diagnostic weight than the same total count with a lymphocyte or mixed-cell predominance more suggestive of a non-infectious or resolving process; laboratories reporting only a total cell count without a differential breakdown provide meaningfully less diagnostic information than one reporting both, and requesting a differential as a routine component of any effluent cell count ordered for suspected peritonitis ensures this additional diagnostic information is available at the time the initial treatment decision must be made.

Abdominal pain in peritonitis ranges from mild and diffuse to severe and localized, and its absence does not exclude the diagnosis in a patient whose effluent shows the cloudiness and elevated white cell count otherwise diagnostic of the condition; some patients, particularly those with a more indolent or early-presenting infection, report minimal or no pain despite an unambiguously abnormal effluent, and clinicians should not require pain as a mandatory diagnostic feature when the effluent findings themselves already satisfy two of the three criteria without it. Fever, present in only a minority of peritonitis episodes, is similarly not a required diagnostic feature, and its absence should not delay treatment in a patient whose effluent findings and clinical picture otherwise support the diagnosis.

Cloudy effluent, the finding most likely to be first noticed by the patient themselves during a routine exchange, deserves particular emphasis in patient education, discussed further in Chapter 17's treatment of peritoneal dialysis self-care: a patient trained to recognize cloudy effluent as an urgent finding requiring same-day contact with their dialysis unit, rather than a concerning but non-urgent observation to mention at their next scheduled visit, is functioning as the frontline detection system this diagnosis depends on in a modality where the patient, not clinical staff, is present at the moment the earliest sign typically first appears.

Effluent Cell Count and Culture Technique

Effluent white cell count, obtained from a sample of drained dialysate sent for cell count and differential, requires a dwell time of at least several hours to be interpretable, since a very short dwell may not allow sufficient time for white cells to accumulate in the effluent even in a patient with genuine peritonitis; a patient presenting with suspected peritonitis on a very short, recently instilled dwell should have that dwell allowed to continue for a more diagnostically adequate duration, or a fresh sample instilled and dwelled for an adequate period, rather than basing a diagnostic decision on a cell count obtained from an inadequately short dwell that could produce a falsely reassuring result.

Culture technique matters as much as the decision to culture at all: inoculating blood culture bottles directly with effluent, rather than sending effluent alone to the microbiology laboratory for standard culture plating, meaningfully improves organism recovery rates, since the blood culture bottle's enriched broth medium supports growth of organisms present in the comparatively low concentrations typical of peritoneal dialysis effluent more reliably than standard culture technique optimized for higher-concentration specimens. Centrifugation of a larger effluent volume before culture, concentrating any organisms present into a smaller processed volume, further improves yield in some laboratory protocols, and a unit's specific culture technique should be reviewed and, where feasible, upgraded to these higher-yield methods if culture-negative peritonitis rates, discussed further below, are running higher than would be expected.

Culture-negative peritonitis, in which clinical and cell-count criteria are met but no organism is ultimately identified despite adequate culture technique, occurs in a meaningful minority of episodes and should prompt review of culture technique specifically, including whether blood culture bottle inoculation and adequate incubation duration were both properly applied, before concluding that the episode is genuinely culture-negative; a persistently high culture-negative rate across a unit's overall peritonitis experience, rather than an occasional isolated culture-negative episode, is the more informative signal that technique improvement, rather than simple chance, explains the pattern.

Gram stain, performed on the effluent sample while awaiting full culture results, can provide preliminary organism-category information within hours rather than the one to several days full culture typically requires, and while gram stain sensitivity in peritoneal dialysis effluent is limited relative to culture given the comparatively low organism concentrations typical of this specimen type, a positive gram stain identifying gram-positive cocci in clusters, for example, can support an early, more targeted empiric adjustment ahead of full culture and sensitivity results, particularly valuable in a patient whose presentation raises specific concern that might warrant earlier-than-usual antibiotic tailoring rather than waiting the full standard interval for complete culture data.

Communicating a gram stain result to the patient and, where relevant, to covering staff who may see the patient before full culture results return, should be framed explicitly as preliminary and subject to revision once full culture and sensitivity data are available, since overconfidence in an early gram stain finding, particularly given its limited sensitivity in this specific specimen type discussed above, risks a premature and potentially incorrect narrowing of therapy before the more definitive full culture data has actually had the opportunity to confirm or revise that preliminary impression.

Differential Diagnosis of Cloudy Effluent

Not every instance of cloudy effluent reflects infectious peritonitis: a markedly eosinophilic effluent cell count, rather than the polymorphonuclear predominance characteristic of bacterial infection, suggests a sterile, hypersensitivity-type reaction, sometimes related to a new dialysate formulation, tubing material, or medication instilled intraperitoneally, and this eosinophilic pattern, once recognized, generally resolves with removal of the presumed offending agent rather than requiring the antibiotic course discussed later in this chapter. Chylous effluent, a milky rather than simply cloudy appearance related to lymphatic fluid leakage into the peritoneal cavity, is a distinct and considerably rarer finding with its own separate differential diagnosis, including intra-abdominal malignancy or lymphatic obstruction, and should not be conflated with the infectious cloudiness this chapter primarily addresses.

Intra-abdominal pathology unrelated to the peritoneal dialysis catheter itself, including appendicitis, diverticulitis, or cholecystitis, can occasionally produce a secondary peritonitis with cloudy effluent as a downstream consequence of the primary intra-abdominal process, and this possibility deserves consideration specifically when an episode's clinical picture includes localized findings atypical for straightforward catheter-related peritonitis, or when initial empiric therapy fails to produce the improvement typically expected, prompting broader imaging evaluation to exclude an underlying surgical abdominal process that catheter-directed antibiotic therapy alone would not address.

A recent invasive gynecologic or colonoscopic procedure, or a history of diverticular disease, inflammatory bowel disease, or prior abdominal surgery creating adhesions or altered bowel anatomy, each raise the prior probability that an apparent peritonitis episode may in fact represent a secondary process originating from an unrelated intra-abdominal source rather than a primary catheter-related infection, and eliciting this history explicitly as part of the initial peritonitis evaluation, rather than proceeding directly to standard empiric treatment without this brief additional history, helps identify the patients for whom broader evaluation should be considered proactively rather than only after an unexpectedly poor response to standard therapy has already occurred.

Effluent Finding	Likely Cause	Management Implication
Cloudy, PMN-predominant, culture-positive	Bacterial peritonitis	Initiate empiric antibiotic therapy immediately
Cloudy, PMN-predominant, culture-negative	Culture-negative peritonitis	Treat empirically; review culture technique

Cloudy, eosinophil-predominant	Sterile hypersensitivity reaction	Remove suspected offending agent; antibiotics generally unnecessary
Milky (chylous)	Lymphatic leak or intra-abdominal pathology	Separate evaluation distinct from infectious peritonitis workup

Figure 19.1

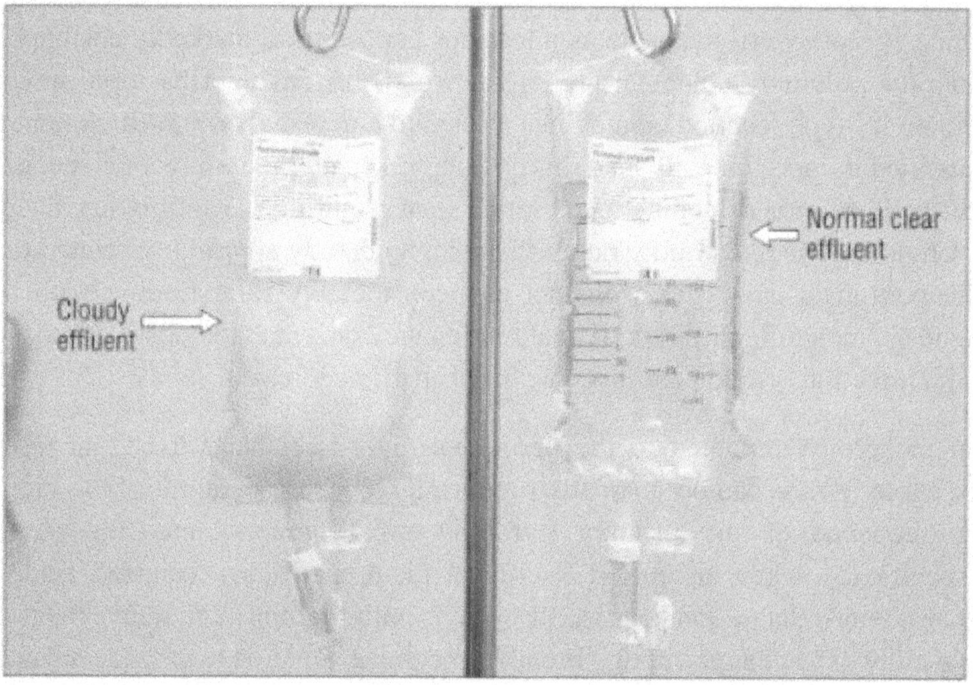

KEY POINT: Peritonitis is diagnosed with any two of three criteria: compatible clinical features, an elevated PMN-predominant effluent white cell count, or a positive culture; empiric treatment should begin immediately once two criteria are met, without awaiting culture confirmation.

Empiric and Organism-Directed Antibiotic Therapy

Initiating Empiric Therapy

Empiric antibiotic therapy, covering both gram-positive and gram-negative organisms given the range of causative pathogens typical of peritoneal dialysis peritonitis, should begin immediately once the diagnostic criteria discussed earlier in this chapter are met, following a unit-specific empiric protocol developed with attention to local organism prevalence and resistance patterns rather than an identical protocol applied uniformly across every geographic region and patient population regardless of local microbiology; a unit's empiric regimen should be reviewed periodically against its own accumulated culture and sensitivity data, adjusting the empiric choice if local resistance patterns have shifted meaningfully since the protocol was last updated.

Governance of a unit's empiric peritonitis protocol, including who holds responsibility for periodic review and update, how frequently that review occurs, and how the accumulated culture and sensitivity data actually feeding that review is compiled and analyzed, deserves the same explicit, structured attention this book has recommended for other recurring clinical protocols throughout its earlier chapters; a protocol technically in existence but never actually revisited against accumulating local data provides only the appearance of evidence-based practice rather than its substance, and a unit's quality improvement infrastructure should treat periodic empiric protocol review as a standing, scheduled responsibility rather than an occasional, informally triggered activity.

Loading doses, where the specific antibiotic and route selected support this approach, are used in many empiric protocols specifically to achieve therapeutic intraperitoneal concentrations more rapidly than a standard maintenance dose alone would allow, reflecting the same urgency this chapter's introduction has emphasized throughout; a delay in achieving adequate antibiotic concentration within the peritoneal cavity, even after the decision to treat has already been made and the first dose administered, still represents a meaningfully longer period of unchecked bacterial proliferation than a loading-dose strategy would allow.

Dwell time also affects intraperitoneal antibiotic exposure meaningfully: an antibiotic instilled into a dialysate fill that dwells for only a brief period before being drained provides less total exposure time at the site of infection than the same antibiotic instilled into a longer-dwelling fill, and prescription adjustments during the acute treatment period, such as extending dwell times specifically to support adequate antibiotic exposure even if this temporarily departs from the patient's usual maintenance dwell schedule, should be considered as part of the overall treatment plan rather than treating the peritonitis-specific antibiotic dosing and the patient's ordinary maintenance dwell schedule as entirely independent, unrelated prescription elements during the acute treatment period.

Route of Antibiotic Administration

Intraperitoneal antibiotic administration, instilling the antibiotic directly into the dialysate rather than delivering it systemically, is generally preferred for peritonitis treatment given the direct, high local concentration this route achieves at the actual site of infection, and most contemporary peritonitis protocols favor intraperitoneal dosing added to each exchange or, in some protocols, a single daily intraperitoneal dose with an extended dwell, over systemic intravenous or oral administration as the primary treatment route for uncomplicated peritonitis confined to the peritoneal cavity itself.

Systemic antibiotic therapy, whether oral or intravenous, becomes the primary or an essential adjunctive route specifically when systemic signs of sepsis are present, when the causative organism or clinical picture suggests a process extending beyond the peritoneal cavity itself, such as the tunnel infection discussed later in this chapter, or when a specific antibiotic's pharmacokinetics make intraperitoneal delivery impractical for adequate systemic and local concentration simultaneously; selecting between these routes, or combining them, should follow the specific clinical picture and organism rather than a single fixed rule applied identically to every patient regardless of presentation severity.

Pharmacokinetic considerations specific to the peritoneal cavity, including reduced antibiotic clearance from the peritoneal space during an actively inflamed peritonitis episode relative to a healthy, uninflamed membrane, can produce higher and more sustained local antibiotic concentrations than would be predicted from a non-inflamed baseline state, a phenomenon sometimes termed the inflamed-membrane effect; while this effect generally works in the treating clinician's favor by supporting adequate local drug exposure, it also means antibiotic dosing established under inflamed conditions may require reassessment as the peritonitis resolves and membrane inflammation subsides, since clearance characteristics at the end of a treatment course may differ meaningfully from those present at its start.

Tailoring Therapy to Culture Results

Once culture and sensitivity results return, typically within forty-eight to seventy-two hours, empiric therapy should be narrowed to target the specific identified organism using the narrowest effective agent the sensitivity profile supports, both to reduce the broader antimicrobial resistance pressure that prolonged broad-spectrum coverage imposes across a unit's patient population and to minimize any unnecessary toxicity or side-effect burden a broader-spectrum agent might carry relative to a more targeted alternative once the actual causative organism is known with confidence.

De-escalation should occur as soon as sensitivity results are available rather than being deferred until the full planned treatment course is nearly complete, since the resistance-selection and toxicity-reduction benefits de-escalation offers accrue over the remaining treatment duration and are therefore greater the earlier de-escalation actually occurs; a unit workflow that flags returned culture results for prompt physician review and prescription adjustment, rather than relying on results being noticed only at the next scheduled patient encounter, supports this timely de-escalation more reliably than depending on individual clinician vigilance to notice a result has returned amid competing clinical demands.

A polymicrobial culture, identifying more than one organism, particularly when that combination includes an enteric organism such as those typically found in bowel flora, should raise specific concern for an underlying bowel-related process, including a possible bowel perforation or other intra-abdominal surgical pathology, discussed further in this chapter's treatment of catheter removal indications, rather than being treated as simply a more complex but otherwise routine peritonitis episode requiring broader antibiotic coverage alone; recognizing this polymicrobial, enteric-organism pattern as a specific trigger for surgical evaluation, rather than antibiotic escalation alone, is a distinct clinical judgment this chapter emphasizes explicitly.

Duration and Monitoring Response

Standard antibiotic duration for uncomplicated peritonitis typically extends for two to three weeks depending on the specific organism identified, with more resistant or difficult-to-clear organisms, including Pseudomonas species and fungal organisms discussed further below, generally requiring the longer end of this range or beyond; treatment duration should be individualized to the specific organism's known clearance characteristics rather than applying a single fixed duration uniformly regardless of the causative pathogen identified.

Clinical response, most directly assessed through serial effluent clarity and repeat cell count at defined intervals during treatment, should show clear improvement within the first several days of appropriate therapy, and a patient failing to show this expected improvement by day three to five of treatment warrants prompt reassessment rather than simply continuing the same regimen for its full planned duration in the hope that improvement will eventually occur; this reassessment should include repeat culture to confirm the organism has not changed or developed resistance during treatment, and consideration of the catheter removal indications developed later in this chapter for a genuinely refractory episode.

CAUTION: Failure to show clear clinical improvement by day three to five of appropriate antibiotic therapy warrants prompt reassessment, including repeat culture, rather than continuing the same regimen for its full planned duration while awaiting eventual improvement.

DIALYSIS RECOGNITION & RESPONSE SYSTEM — Peritonitis Response Arcs

The Pattern: A peritoneal dialysis patient's culture returns polymicrobial with enteric organisms identified.

Stem Signature: More than one organism identified on peritonitis culture, including one or more typically enteric or bowel-flora organisms, in a patient whose clinical presentation may otherwise appear consistent with straightforward peritonitis.

The Decision: Pursue surgical evaluation and abdominal imaging to assess for an underlying bowel-related process such as perforation or another intra-abdominal surgical pathology, rather than treating the finding solely as a more complex peritonitis requiring broader antibiotic coverage alone.

Trap Logic: A polymicrobial culture can be managed as simply a more complicated infection requiring broader-spectrum antibiotics, without recognizing that the specific combination of enteric organisms is a distinct signal pointing toward an underlying surgical abdominal process that antibiotics alone will not resolve.

Response Anchor: A polymicrobial culture with enteric organisms is the trigger for surgical evaluation and abdominal imaging — not simply an indication for broader antibiotic coverage alone.

Exit-Site and Tunnel Infections

Recognizing Exit-Site Infection

Exit-site infection presents with erythema, tenderness, and often purulent drainage confined to the immediate skin surrounding the catheter exit point, generally without extension along the subcutaneous tunnel, and, similarly to the simple exit-site infection discussed for hemodialysis catheters in Chapter 12, often responds to local wound care and topical or oral antibiotic therapy without requiring catheter removal, provided the infection remains genuinely confined to this superficial location and does not progress despite appropriate initial management.

Distinguishing normal, expected exit-site appearance from early infection requires familiarity with a given patient's own baseline exit-site appearance, since some degree of mild, chronic erythema or crusting can represent a patient's normal baseline rather than an active infectious process, and comparing a current examination against prior documented findings, rather than judging the exit site in isolation against a generic population norm, supports more accurate and more consistent recognition of a genuine change warranting treatment.

A twenty-nine-year-old man on continuous ambulatory peritoneal dialysis for six months reports mild redness and slight tenderness at his catheter exit site, noticed during his routine morning care, without any drainage and without the abdominal pain or cloudy effluent that would suggest concurrent peritonitis. Comparing his current appearance against photographs taken at his prior two clinic visits, his care team confirms this represents a genuine change from his established baseline rather than his usual chronic mild erythema, and a swab culture is obtained before initiating topical antibiotic therapy targeting the most likely causative organisms for this presentation. His symptoms resolve over the following week with this local treatment alone, and follow-up culture confirms clearance without any progression to tunnel involvement or peritonitis. This case illustrates the value of a documented baseline exit-site appearance in distinguishing a genuine new infection from a patient's own chronic, stable baseline finding, and the appropriateness of local, non-systemic treatment for an exit-site infection that remains genuinely confined and shows the expected treatment response.

KEY POINT: Comparing a current exit-site examination against a documented prior baseline, rather than judging the site in isolation, distinguishes a genuine new infection from a patient's chronic, stable appearance and guides whether local treatment alone is likely to be adequate.

Tunnel Infection and Its Relationship to Peritonitis

Tunnel infection, extending along the subcutaneous catheter tract beyond the immediate exit site, is both harder to recognize on external examination alone, since the infected segment lies beneath intact skin along much of its course, and considerably more likely to progress to or coexist with frank peritonitis, since the tunnel provides a direct anatomic pathway for organisms to migrate from the exit site toward the peritoneal cavity itself; ultrasound imaging of the tunnel tract, identifying a fluid collection or thickened, edematous tissue along the tract's course, supports this diagnosis when external examination alone is inconclusive.

The deep cuff specifically, positioned within the rectus muscle and therefore not directly visible or palpable on routine examination the way the more superficial cuff and exit site are, represents a particularly difficult segment of the tunnel to assess clinically, and infection localized primarily around this deep cuff can present with comparatively subtle findings on external examination despite representing a genuinely serious infection closely apposed to the peritoneal cavity itself; this is a further reason ultrasound imaging, capable of visualizing the full tunnel course including the deep cuff segment, deserves a relatively low threshold for use whenever tunnel infection is genuinely suspected, rather than being reserved only for cases where external examination has already revealed obvious, unambiguous tunnel involvement.

A patient presenting with peritonitis who also has a currently or recently infected exit site should be evaluated specifically for concurrent tunnel infection as the likely source, since treating the peritonitis component alone with antibiotics while an underlying tunnel infection persists untreated risks early relapse once the antibiotic course concludes; this connection between exit-site findings and a peritonitis presentation is a specific instance of the broader principle that a peritoneal dialysis infection should be evaluated as a potentially interconnected anatomic process rather than assessed as entirely separate, unrelated events simply because they involve different anatomic locations along the same catheter tract.

Confirmed tunnel infection generally requires a longer antibiotic course than a simple exit-site infection alone, reflecting the deeper, less accessible location of the infected tissue and its closer anatomic proximity to the peritoneal cavity, and a tunnel infection that fails to resolve with an appropriately extended antibiotic course, similarly to the refractory peritonitis pattern discussed later in this chapter, generally warrants catheter removal rather than an indefinitely prolonged antibiotic trial, since persistent tunnel infection despite adequate treatment duration reflects the same kind of catheter-level problem that continued antibiotic therapy alone is unlikely to resolve.

Prevention Strategies

Daily exit-site care following a defined protocol, prophylactic topical antibiotic application at the exit site in some protocols specifically shown to reduce Staphylococcus aureus exit-site infection rates, and nasal Staphylococcus aureus carrier screening with decolonization where a carrier state is identified, together constitute the primary evidence-based prevention strategies for exit-site and, by extension, tunnel infection, and a peritoneal dialysis program's infection prevention protocol should incorporate each of these elements as standard practice rather than treating them as optional enhancements applied inconsistently across the patient population.

Patient technique training in exit-site care, reinforced periodically rather than delivered only at initial catheter placement, addresses the reality that technique can drift gradually over months and years of a patient's own self-care routine, and a structured periodic reassessment of a patient's actual exit-site care technique, rather than assuming initial training remains fully retained and correctly applied indefinitely, catches this drift before it contributes to a preventable infection.

Touch contamination during the exchange connection process itself, rather than exit-site or tunnel-related organism migration specifically, is a distinct and important source of peritonitis risk, and reinforcing meticulous hand hygiene and sterile connection technique at every exchange, not only during initial training, addresses this separate risk pathway; some peritonitis episodes attributed presumptively to exit-site or tunnel sources on initial assessment are, on closer review of the specific organism identified and the patient's technique, more consistent with touch contamination during a routine exchange, underscoring that exit-site and tunnel prevention, while essential, do not address every pathway by which peritonitis can develop and should be paired with equally rigorous exchange technique reinforcement.

CLINICAL PEARL: A patient presenting with peritonitis and a concurrent or recent exit-site infection should be evaluated for tunnel infection as the likely underlying source, since treating the peritonitis alone while an untreated tunnel infection persists risks early relapse.

Figure 19.2: Tunnel Infection Extending From an Infected Exit Site

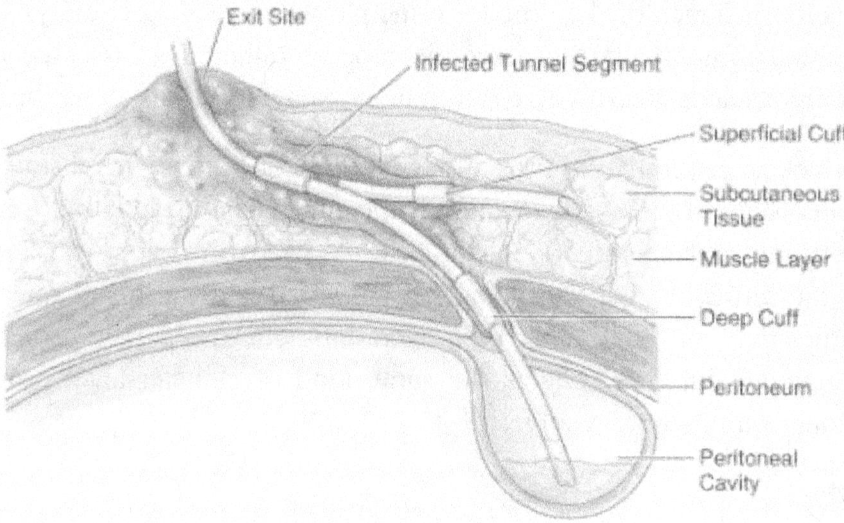

Catheter Removal and Technique Failure

Indications for Catheter Removal

Fungal peritonitis, refractory bacterial peritonitis failing to respond to appropriate antibiotic therapy within an expected timeframe, peritonitis associated with a confirmed tunnel infection that itself fails to resolve with antibiotic therapy alone, and peritonitis arising from a polymicrobial, enteric-organism source suggesting underlying bowel pathology, discussed earlier in this chapter, each generally warrant catheter removal rather than continued salvage attempts, given these presentations' associated risk of severe, difficult-to-clear infection and, in the fungal and bowel-source cases specifically, a natural history poorly responsive to antibiotic therapy alone regardless of how appropriately that therapy is selected and dosed.

Refractory peritonitis, defined as failure to respond adequately to appropriate antibiotic therapy within the timeframe discussed earlier in this chapter, warrants catheter removal once this refractory pattern is confirmed rather than pursuing an extended or repeatedly modified antibiotic course in the hope that a longer or different regimen will eventually succeed where the initial appropriate regimen has already failed to produce the expected improvement; this principle mirrors the same decisive-action-over-prolonged-uncertainty theme this chapter's introduction identified as central to peritonitis management overall, extending it specifically to the decision point at which continued antibiotic-only management should yield to catheter removal.

Fungal peritonitis in particular carries a sufficiently poor prognosis with catheter retention that immediate catheter removal, rather than an antifungal treatment trial with the catheter left in place, is the standard, guideline-supported approach once fungal organisms are confirmed or strongly suspected on culture; this immediate-removal approach for fungal infection specifically stands in contrast to the more graduated, trial-based approach this book has described for many other infectious complications throughout its earlier chapters, reflecting fungal peritonitis's distinctly unfavorable response to catheter-retained management relative to bacterial peritonitis.

Recent or concurrent broad-spectrum antibiotic exposure, whether for a prior bacterial peritonitis episode or for an entirely unrelated indication, is a recognized risk factor for subsequent fungal peritonitis, reflecting the disruption of normal competing bacterial flora that broad-spectrum antibiotic exposure produces; some centers incorporate prophylactic antifungal coverage during any antibiotic course prescribed for bacterial peritonitis specifically to mitigate this recognized risk, an approach supported by some though not universally consistent evidence, and a unit's specific practice in this regard should be guided by its own accumulated experience with fungal peritonitis incidence alongside the broader published literature on this prophylactic approach's net benefit and risk.

Antifungal susceptibility patterns vary meaningfully across different fungal species, and once a fungal organism is identified on culture, infectious disease consultation is generally warranted to guide specific antifungal selection and duration, given the relative rarity of fungal peritonitis in most individual units' experience and the correspondingly greater value of specialist input compared to the more routine bacterial peritonitis management most nephrology teams manage independently on a regular basis without needing this additional specialist involvement.

Technique Failure and Transition Planning

Technique failure, the broader term encompassing a patient's permanent transition away from peritoneal dialysis due to an infectious complication, refractory ultrafiltration failure discussed in Chapter 18, or another peritoneal-dialysis-specific reason, requires the same proactive transition planning discussed in Chapter 18's treatment of the peritoneal-to-hemodialysis transition: initiating hemodialysis vascular access evaluation promptly once catheter removal for infection becomes necessary, rather than waiting until the peritoneal catheter has already been removed and an urgent, unplanned hemodialysis catheter becomes the only immediately available bridge.

A patient undergoing catheter removal for peritonitis, particularly one whose overall clinical trajectory suggests they may wish to return to peritoneal dialysis in the future once the acute infection has fully resolved, benefits from an explicit conversation about this possibility at the time of removal, distinguishing a temporary technique interruption with anticipated future peritoneal dialysis resumption from a permanent technique failure requiring durable hemodialysis access planning; this distinction, while sometimes only clarified with time as the patient's recovery and preferences become clearer, deserves explicit consideration rather than defaulting to an assumption of permanent transition simply because the immediate infectious crisis has necessitated catheter removal.

A structured, standing protocol for initiating hemodialysis vascular access evaluation at the time of any peritoneal catheter removal for infection, applied consistently regardless of whether the transition is ultimately expected to be temporary or permanent, ensures this proactive step occurs reliably rather than depending on an individual clinician remembering to initiate it amid the many other demands an active infectious complication places on the treating team; a patient whose eventual course proves to be a temporary interruption with successful return to peritoneal dialysis has lost little by having this parallel evaluation initiated unnecessarily, while a patient whose course proves to require permanent transition benefits considerably from this evaluation already being underway rather than starting only once the permanent nature of the transition becomes clear.

Recurrent Peritonitis and Catheter Salvage Limits

Recurrent peritonitis, most commonly defined as a repeat episode with the same organism within a defined interval following completion of therapy for a prior episode, suggests either an unresolved underlying source, such as an undertreated tunnel infection or a biofilm the initial antibiotic course failed to fully eradicate from the catheter surface itself, or a catheter increasingly colonized in a way that repeated antibiotic courses are unlikely to resolve durably going forward. A defined limit on the number of recurrent or relapsing episodes tolerated before catheter removal is recommended rather than continued salvage attempts, following a threshold established in unit protocol and informed by published guideline recommendations, protects a patient from an indefinite cycle of repeated antibiotic courses that each carry their own burden and cumulative resistance-selection risk without addressing an underlying catheter-level problem that removal and replacement would resolve more definitively.

Relapsing peritonitis, distinguished from recurrent peritonitis by occurring within a shorter interval and typically involving the identical organism at the identical antibiotic sensitivity profile rather than merely a similar organism type, carries a particularly strong signal toward persistent catheter colonization specifically, since this exact-match pattern is considerably less consistent with a series of genuinely new, independent infections than with a single incompletely treated process recurring from the same unresolved source; this distinction between relapse and recurrence, while sometimes used loosely and interchangeably in casual clinical conversation, carries genuine diagnostic weight that a structured peritonitis tracking system should capture explicitly rather than recording every repeat episode under an undifferentiated single category.

A fifty-two-year-old woman on peritoneal dialysis for five years experiences her third episode of coagulase-negative staphylococcal peritonitis within eight months, each prior episode having initially responded to standard antibiotic therapy before recurring within weeks of treatment completion. Recognizing this pattern as recurrent rather than three unrelated isolated episodes, her nephrology team pursues catheter removal and replacement at a new site rather than a fourth antibiotic trial with the existing catheter retained, reasoning that the repeated relapse pattern despite appropriate prior therapy suggests persistent catheter-level organism colonization, likely within a biofilm the antibiotic courses have been unable to fully eradicate, that continued antibiotic-only management is unlikely to resolve durably. She undergoes catheter removal with a defined antibiotic-free interval before new catheter placement, following which she resumes peritoneal dialysis without further recurrence over the following year. This case illustrates why a recurrent, relapsing infection pattern with the same organism should prompt catheter removal rather than a further antibiotic trial, once that specific recurrent pattern, rather than isolated unrelated episodes, has become clear.

Her care team also reviews her exchange technique and exit-site care in detail during this evaluation, confirming no identifiable technique lapse contributed to the recurrent pattern and supporting their conclusion that persistent catheter-surface biofilm, rather than an ongoing correctable technique issue, best explains her relapsing course; this technique review, performed as a routine component of any recurrent peritonitis evaluation regardless of how confident the clinical team already feels about the underlying explanation, ensures a correctable contributing factor is not overlooked simply because a catheter-level explanation seems most likely at first assessment.

CAUTION: Recurrent peritonitis with the same organism, relapsing shortly after completion of appropriate prior therapy, suggests persistent catheter-level colonization and warrants catheter removal and replacement rather than a further antibiotic trial with the existing catheter retained.

DIALYSIS RECOGNITION & RESPONSE SYSTEM — Peritonitis Response Arcs

The Pattern: A peritoneal dialysis patient experiences a repeat peritonitis episode with the same organism shortly after completing therapy for a prior episode.

Stem Signature: A peritonitis episode identifying the same organism as a prior episode, recurring within weeks of that prior episode's treatment completion, in a pattern now established across two or more such episodes rather than a single isolated recurrence.

The Decision: Recognize this as a recurrent, relapsing infection pattern suggesting persistent catheter-level colonization, and proceed to catheter removal and replacement rather than a further antibiotic trial with the existing catheter.

Trap Logic: Each individual recurrence can be treated as a new, separate episode warranting its own fresh antibiotic trial, without recognizing that the accumulating pattern across multiple recurrences with the same organism points to a catheter-level problem that repeated antibiotic courses alone are unlikely to resolve.

Response Anchor: A recurrent, relapsing pattern with the same organism across multiple episodes is the trigger for catheter removal and replacement — not a further antibiotic trial with the existing catheter retained.

Polymicrobial Culture With Enteric Organisms: Pursue surgical evaluation and abdominal imaging rather than treating the finding solely as an indication for broader antibiotic coverage.

Recurrent Peritonitis With the Same Organism: Recognize the relapsing pattern and proceed to catheter removal and replacement rather than a further antibiotic trial with the existing catheter.

Summary and Key Concepts

Peritonitis is diagnosed with any two of three criteria — compatible clinical features, an elevated PMN-predominant effluent white cell count, or a positive culture — and empiric therapy should begin immediately once two criteria are met, without awaiting culture confirmation.

Intraperitoneal antibiotic administration is generally preferred for uncomplicated peritonitis, with systemic therapy reserved for sepsis, extension beyond the peritoneal cavity, or specific pharmacokinetic considerations; a polymicrobial, enteric-organism culture warrants surgical evaluation for underlying bowel pathology.

Exit-site infection is generally confined and treatable with local care and antibiotics; tunnel infection is harder to recognize externally, more likely to coexist with or precipitate peritonitis, and should be specifically considered in any peritonitis episode with a concurrent or recent exit-site infection.

Fungal peritonitis, refractory bacterial peritonitis, tunnel-infection-associated peritonitis, and polymicrobial enteric-source peritonitis generally warrant catheter removal rather than continued salvage attempts.

Recurrent or relapsing peritonitis with the same organism suggests persistent catheter-level colonization and warrants catheter removal and replacement, with proactive hemodialysis access planning initiated promptly wherever technique failure becomes necessary.

CHAPTER 20: HOME HEMODIALYSIS AND INTENSIVE DIALYSIS REGIMENS

Learning Objectives

Apply patient selection criteria for home hemodialysis and describe the structured training process this modality requires.

Compare short daily and nocturnal home hemodialysis regimens and select between them for an individual patient.

Apply remote monitoring technology and structured troubleshooting protocols to support safe treatment outside the dialysis unit.

Interpret the evidence on clinical outcomes of intensive hemodialysis, including its methodological limitations.

Chapter Overview

Part VI of this book turns to the modalities that depart furthest from the standard, in-center, thrice-weekly hemodialysis framework this book has developed since Chapter 4: home hemodialysis, in its short daily and nocturnal forms, and, in the next chapter, the acute continuous therapies used in critically ill patients. Home hemodialysis returns physiologic and prescription control to the patient and their care partner, extending the self-cannulation and home-based self-care principles introduced in Chapters 10 and 17 into the full scope of an independently performed hemodialysis treatment. This chapter works through who is genuinely suited to this modality, how training actually proceeds, how short daily and nocturnal regimens differ in their physiologic rationale and practical demands, how monitoring and troubleshooting adapt to a setting without immediate clinical staff present, and, finally, what the accumulated outcomes evidence for intensive hemodialysis actually shows and does not show, an evidentiary picture considerably more nuanced than the enthusiasm this modality often generates among its strongest advocates.

Home Hemodialysis Training and Patient Selection

Patient Selection Criteria for Home Hemodialysis

Successful home hemodialysis depends on a combination of factors distinct from the clinical adequacy considerations that dominate modality selection in Chapter 2: adequate cognitive and physical capacity to learn and reliably execute a multi-step technical procedure, a stable home environment with adequate space for equipment and supply storage, and, for most programs, a willing and capable care partner, discussed further in this section, particularly during the initial training and early independent treatment period. Motivation and genuine understanding of the responsibility involved matter as much as raw technical aptitude, since a patient who can technically learn the procedure but lacks the sustained motivation to perform it consistently and safely over months and years is a poorer long-term candidate than one with more modest initial technical confidence but strong, durable commitment to the modality.

No single medical contraindication universally excludes a patient from home hemodialysis candidacy, but several factors warrant careful individualized consideration: significant unaddressed vision or dexterity impairment affecting cannulation and equipment operation, a home environment posing genuine safety concerns such as inadequate electrical or water infrastructure, or a psychiatric or cognitive condition that would compromise reliable, safe self-management. Each of these factors should be assessed on its own specific severity and potential for accommodation or adaptation rather than applied as a categorical exclusion criterion regardless of the individual patient's actual circumstances, since assistive technology, care partner support, and program-specific accommodations can address many of these concerns for a patient who is otherwise strongly motivated toward the modality.

Patients pursuing self-cannulation specifically, discussed in Chapter 10, require a level of comfort with needle insertion that not every otherwise well-suited home hemodialysis candidate possesses initially, and buttonhole technique, also discussed in Chapter 10, is frequently favored for home self-cannulation given its reduced pain and simplified needle placement once an established tract has formed, though its elevated infection risk requires the same rigorous tract-care training discussed in that chapter, now delivered to the patient and care partner rather than to clinical staff performing the cannulation in-center.

A formal, structured psychosocial and functional assessment, performed before training begins rather than relying solely on the referring nephrologist's informal clinical impression, identifies candidacy concerns more systematically than an unstructured referral process alone, and involving social work, occupational therapy where relevant to dexterity or cognitive concerns, and the home training nurse together in this pre-training assessment allows each discipline's specific expertise to inform the overall candidacy determination rather than depending on any single clinician to independently assess every relevant domain.

The Training Process

Home hemodialysis training typically spans several weeks to a few months, delivered by a dedicated home training nurse and progressing through a structured curriculum covering machine operation, water treatment system function where the specific home hemodialysis machine requires one, cannulation technique, recognition and management of common problems, and infection control practices adapted to the home setting; this training pace, considerably longer and more intensive than the general patient education discussed throughout this book for in-center patients, reflects the genuinely higher stakes and skill demands of a patient managing their own treatment without a clinical team physically present at every session.

A graduated independence model, in which the training nurse's direct supervision decreases progressively as the patient and care partner demonstrate consistent competency across each component of the training curriculum, allows training pace to be individualized to the specific patient's learning trajectory rather than compressed into a fixed calendar duration regardless of readiness; a patient or care partner not yet demonstrating reliable competency in a specific skill, such as needle insertion or troubleshooting a specific machine alarm, should not progress to greater independence in that specific domain simply because a predetermined training timeline has elapsed, since doing so risks the patient beginning independent home treatment without genuine mastery of a skill their safety will depend on.

Competency assessment at the conclusion of training, using a structured checklist covering every major skill domain the curriculum addressed, provides an objective confirmation of readiness for independent home treatment rather than relying on the training nurse's informal impression alone, and this same structured assessment tool, reapplied periodically after a patient has been home for some time, supports ongoing competency verification and identifies any skill drift that may have developed since initial training concluded, mirroring the same periodic reassessment principle this book has applied throughout to other skills and prescriptions requiring durable, reliable execution over time.

A defined re-training pathway, available for a patient or care partner whose periodic reassessment reveals meaningful skill drift, or for a patient returning to home hemodialysis after an interruption such as a hospitalization or extended illness, provides a structured route back to independent treatment rather than requiring either an informal, unstructured refresher or a full repeat of the entire initial training curriculum regardless of how much of the original skill set remains genuinely intact; calibrating the intensity of this re-training to the specific skill gaps the reassessment actually identifies, rather than applying a uniform re-training intensity regardless of the specific gap's severity, respects both patient time and program training resources.

The Care Partner Role

A care partner, most commonly a spouse, adult child, or other close family member, plays a role in home hemodialysis that extends beyond simple emotional support: depending on the specific patient's needs and program requirements, the care partner may assist with cannulation, machine setup and breakdown, monitoring during treatment, and emergency response, and formal training for the care partner should therefore mirror the patient's own training in depth and rigor rather than treating the care partner as a secondary participant requiring only basic orientation.

The burden this role places on a care partner, discussed briefly in Chapter 2's treatment of caregiver considerations in modality selection, deserves explicit, ongoing attention rather than being addressed only once at the initial modality decision and then assumed to remain manageable indefinitely; care partner burnout, a recognized phenomenon in the home hemodialysis literature, can develop gradually over months or years of sustained caregiving responsibility, and periodic, direct check-ins with the care partner specifically, separate from the patient's own clinical follow-up, help identify this burnout before it progresses to a point that threatens the sustainability of the home hemodialysis arrangement altogether.

Programs that provide structured respite support, whether through backup in-center treatment availability during a care partner's illness or planned absence, or through connecting patients and care partners with peer support networks of other home hemodialysis families, report better long-term program retention than programs offering training alone without this ongoing structural support; recognizing that a care partner's sustained wellbeing is as integral to a home hemodialysis program's long-term success as the patient's own clinical stability reflects the same person-centered, whole-family consideration this book has applied throughout its treatment of dialysis care more broadly.

KEY POINT: Care partner training should mirror the patient's own training in depth and rigor, and ongoing, direct check-ins with the care partner specifically help identify burnout before it threatens the sustainability of the home hemodialysis arrangement.

Figure 20.1: Home Hemodialysis Training Progression

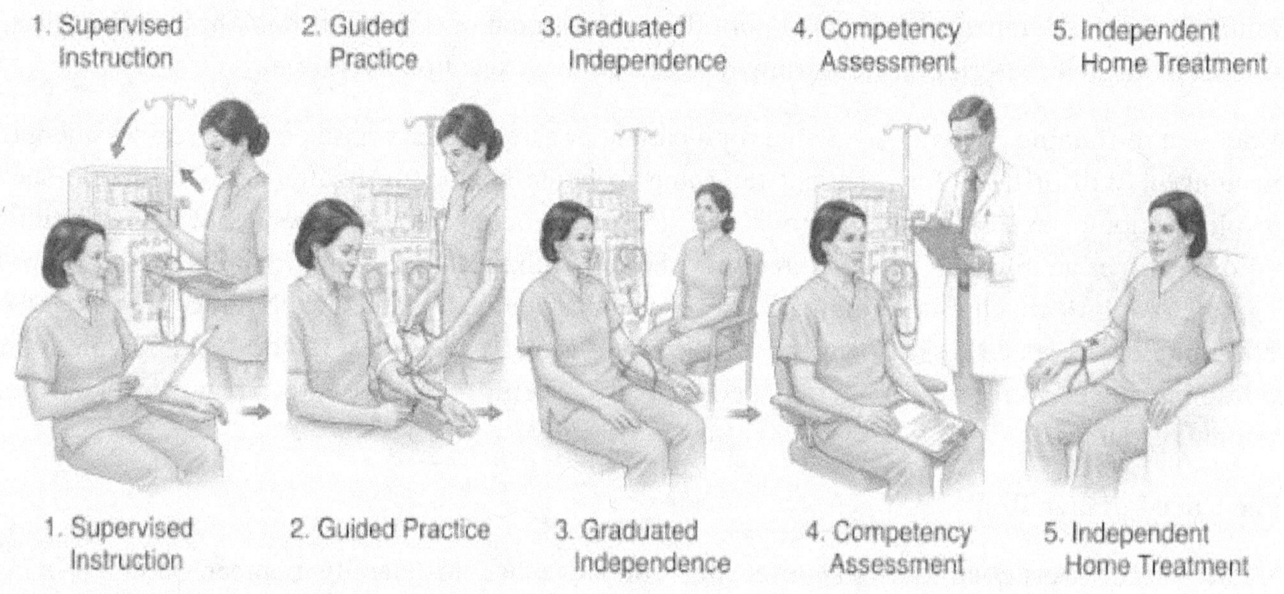

Short Daily and Nocturnal Regimens

Short Daily Hemodialysis

Short daily hemodialysis, typically delivering five to six shorter sessions weekly rather than the standard three longer in-center sessions discussed throughout Part II of this book, distributes the same or a somewhat greater total weekly treatment time across more frequent, shorter individual sessions, reducing the peak-to-trough solute and volume swings the standard thrice-weekly schedule produces and correspondingly reducing the ultrafiltration rate required per session for a given total weekly fluid removal, directly addressing the ultrafiltration-rate-driven hypotension risk discussed extensively in Chapter 13.

This more frequent schedule also shortens the maximum interdialytic interval a patient experiences, eliminating or substantially shortening the extended weekend gap characteristic of standard thrice-weekly treatment, and, as discussed in Chapter 7's treatment of standardized Kt/V, this schedule change itself alters the clinical significance of a given cumulative weekly Kt/V relative to the same total delivered across only three sessions, since the interdialytic peak-and-trough pattern, not solely the cumulative dose, carries independent physiologic consequence.

Total weekly treatment time under a short daily regimen is often comparable to or only modestly greater than standard thrice-weekly treatment, distinguishing short daily hemodialysis's time burden from the more substantial weekly time commitment nocturnal treatment's considerably longer individual sessions represent; this comparatively modest total time increase, distributed across more frequent but shorter individual sessions, is part of why short daily hemodialysis appeals particularly to patients who value the physiologic benefits of more frequent treatment but are unwilling or unable to commit to the substantially longer individual sessions nocturnal treatment requires.

Nocturnal Home Hemodialysis

Nocturnal home hemodialysis extends treatment duration substantially, typically six to eight hours per session performed overnight while the patient sleeps, delivered either thrice weekly or, in its most intensive form, five to six nights weekly; this extended duration allows a considerably lower blood and dialysate flow rate to achieve equivalent or superior total clearance relative to a standard shorter session, since the extended time available compensates for the reduced flow rate, and the correspondingly lower ultrafiltration rate this extended duration permits addresses the hemodynamic instability risk discussed in Chapter 13 as effectively as, or more effectively than, the short daily approach discussed above.

Nocturnal treatment's overnight timing offers the practical advantage of occurring during hours the patient would otherwise be asleep and unavailable for other activities regardless of dialysis, distinguishing it from short daily treatment's daytime or evening time commitment that competes more directly with waking-hour activities including employment; this timing advantage must be weighed against nocturnal treatment's specific safety considerations, discussed further in this chapter's treatment of home monitoring, since a patient asleep during treatment is less able to notice and respond to an evolving problem than a patient awake and alert during a shorter daytime session.

The extended, low-flow-rate profile characteristic of nocturnal treatment also alters middle molecule clearance meaningfully, since the additional dwell-adjacent time this extended session provides supports the kind of protein-bound and middle-molecule clearance discussed in Chapter 4 as depending more heavily on treatment time and frequency than on flow rate alone; patients switching from standard thrice-weekly treatment to nocturnal home hemodialysis frequently report improvement in symptoms such as restless legs and pruritus that Chapter 4 identified as more closely tied to middle-molecule and protein-bound toxin burden than to small-solute clearance alone, providing a plausible mechanistic explanation for some of the quality-of-life improvements discussed later in this chapter.

Selecting Between Regimens

Selection between short daily and nocturnal regimens, and between either of these and remaining on standard in-center thrice-weekly treatment, follows the same individualized, Life-Plan-driven reasoning developed in Chapter 2: a patient's employment schedule, sleep quality and tolerance for overnight equipment operation, transport category discussed in Chapter 16 for any peritoneal dialysis history informing residual physiologic reserve, and personal preference regarding daytime versus overnight time commitment each factor into which regimen, if any intensive home regimen at all, best fits a given patient's circumstances.

A patient with significant residual cardiovascular disease and recurrent intradialytic hypotension despite the standard-schedule prevention strategies detailed in Chapter 13 is a particularly strong candidate for either intensive regimen, given both approaches' shared mechanism of reducing per-session ultrafiltration rate, while a patient primarily motivated by daytime schedule flexibility for employment reasons may find nocturnal treatment's overnight timing specifically appealing in a way a patient more concerned about equipment safety during sleep might not; this individualized matching process, like every other prescription decision in this book, benefits from explicit, structured discussion of the specific patient's priorities rather than defaulting to whichever regimen a given program happens to offer most readily.

Regimen	Typical Frequency	Session Duration	Key Physiologic Advantage
Standard In-Center	Three times weekly	Three to four hours	Established, widely available baseline
Short Daily	Five to six times weekly	Two to three hours	Reduced ultrafiltration rate and shortened interdialytic peaks and troughs
Nocturnal Home	Three to six times weekly	Six to eight hours	Lowest ultrafiltration rate and flow rate for equivalent or superior clearance

CLINICAL PEARL: Both short daily and nocturnal home hemodialysis reduce per-session ultrafiltration rate relative to standard thrice-weekly treatment, making either a reasonable option for a patient with recurrent intradialytic hypotension despite standard-schedule prevention strategies.

Monitoring and Troubleshooting Outside the Dialysis Unit

Remote Monitoring Technology

Contemporary home hemodialysis machines transmit treatment data, including blood flow rate, ultrafiltration rate and volume, and any alarms triggered, to the treating unit remotely, allowing clinical staff to review each home treatment's technical performance without requiring the patient to physically return equipment or manually report every detail, and this remote data stream extends the same trend-based surveillance principle this book has applied throughout to vascular access monitoring and dialysis adequacy assessment into the home setting specifically, where a clinician cannot rely on direct, in-person observation the way they would for an in-center patient.

Video or audio connectivity between the patient's home and the treating unit, available in some but not all home hemodialysis programs, provides a further layer of support beyond passive data transmission, allowing a patient or care partner to reach a live clinician for real-time guidance during an evolving problem rather than relying solely on written troubleshooting materials or a telephone call initiated after a problem has already progressed; programs offering this real-time connectivity report greater patient and care partner confidence in managing home treatment independently than programs relying on data transmission and telephone support alone.

Data security and patient privacy considerations, while not unique to home hemodialysis, take on particular practical importance given the volume and personal nature of the data transmitted from a patient's home environment to the treating unit on a regular basis, and programs should ensure their remote monitoring technology meets applicable data protection standards and that patients understand what data is being transmitted and how it will be used, addressing this consideration explicitly during training rather than treating it as a peripheral technical detail outside the scope of patient education.

Patient Self-Troubleshooting

Structured troubleshooting algorithms, provided to every home hemodialysis patient and care partner as part of training and available as a physical or digital quick-reference during actual treatment, address the specific machine alarms and clinical symptoms a patient is most likely to encounter, distinguishing which specific alarms and symptoms require the patient to stop treatment and call for help immediately from those that can be addressed independently following a defined corrective sequence; this structured approach mirrors the staff-facing troubleshooting protocols discussed throughout Part II and Part III of this book, now adapted for execution by a patient or care partner without formal clinical training.

Recognizing intradialytic hypotension specifically, discussed at length in Chapter 13, deserves particular attention in home patient education, since a patient experiencing evolving hypotension while alone, or with only a care partner present, must recognize and respond to the same early warning signs — nonspecific discomfort, nausea, dizziness — that Chapter 13 emphasized for in-center staff recognition, but must do so without an experienced clinician immediately present to confirm the impression and guide the response; home hemodialysis training therefore places particular emphasis on this specific complication's recognition and self-management given both its relative frequency and the reduced margin for error a home setting without immediate clinical support presents.

Written and video-based troubleshooting reference materials, available for the patient and care partner to consult during an actual treatment rather than relying solely on memory of training content delivered weeks or months earlier, reinforce retention of the specific corrective sequences a given alarm or symptom requires, and periodically updating these reference materials as machine software or protocol details evolve, rather than allowing patients to rely on outdated materials from their original training period, ensures the guidance available at the bedside remains accurate and current throughout a patient's entire home hemodialysis course.

Emergency Protocols for the Home Setting

A clearly defined emergency protocol, specifying exactly when a patient or care partner should call emergency medical services rather than the dialysis unit's own on-call support line, and covering the genuine emergencies discussed in Chapter 15 — suspected air embolism, uncontrolled bleeding from line separation, or cardiac arrest — adapted specifically for execution in a home setting without on-site clinical staff, is an essential component of home hemodialysis training that deserves the same rehearsed, protocol-driven emphasis this book applied to in-center emergency response in Chapter 15.

A forty-eight-year-old man performing nocturnal home hemodialysis for the past year is awakened by his machine's venous pressure alarm and, following his training, checks his access site directly before resetting the alarm, discovering his needle has partially dislodged with visible blood at the site. Following the emergency protocol from his training, he immediately clamps his lines, applies direct pressure to the site, and calls his unit's twenty-four-hour support line, which confirms his response was appropriate and advises him to complete manual hemostasis and discontinue that night's treatment, resuming on his standard schedule the following night after his access is re-examined at his next in-person visit. This case illustrates the value of structured, rehearsed emergency protocol training specifically adapted for the home setting, allowing a patient to respond correctly to a genuine access emergency without a clinician physically present, in a manner directly paralleling the in-center line separation response detailed in Chapter 15.

His unit reviews this event at its subsequent quality meeting, confirming his response followed protocol correctly and using the case as a reinforcing training example for other home patients during their own periodic competency reassessment, illustrating how individual home treatment events, reviewed systematically rather than treated as isolated occurrences relevant only to the specific patient involved, can strengthen training and protocol adherence across a program's entire home hemodialysis population.

CAUTION: Home hemodialysis emergency protocols must specify exactly when a patient or care partner should call emergency medical services rather than the dialysis unit's own support line, covering air embolism, line separation, and cardiac arrest scenarios adapted for a setting without on-site clinical staff.

DIALYSIS RECOGNITION & RESPONSE SYSTEM — Home Therapy Arcs

The Pattern: A home hemodialysis patient's machine alarm indicates a venous pressure abnormality during an unsupervised treatment.

Stem Signature: A venous pressure alarm during home treatment, with the patient or care partner needing to determine independently whether this reflects a benign, correctable issue or a genuine access emergency requiring immediate line clamping and emergency response.

The Decision: Follow the trained troubleshooting sequence: directly inspect the access site for visible dislodgement or bleeding before resetting the alarm, and if a genuine separation or bleeding is confirmed, immediately clamp lines, apply direct pressure, and contact the unit's emergency protocol rather than simply resetting the alarm and continuing treatment.

Trap Logic: A machine alarm during unsupervised home treatment can be reflexively reset without direct site inspection, particularly if the patient is tired or it is the middle of the night during a nocturnal session, risking a missed genuine access emergency that direct inspection would have caught immediately.

Response Anchor: A venous pressure alarm during home treatment warrants direct access site inspection before any alarm reset — not a reflexive reset without first confirming the access itself is secure.

Clinical Outcomes of Intensive Hemodialysis

Cardiovascular and Volume-Related Outcomes

Intensive hemodialysis, whether short daily or nocturnal, has been associated in multiple observational studies and a smaller number of randomized trials with improvements in left ventricular mass, blood pressure control with reduced antihypertensive medication requirement, and phosphate control, plausibly reflecting the more physiologic, continuous-like clearance and volume management pattern intensive schedules provide relative to standard thrice-weekly treatment, echoing the same interdialytic-interval physiologic reasoning developed in Chapter 4 and revisited throughout this chapter.

The Frequent Hemodialysis Network trials, among the most methodologically rigorous randomized evidence available in this area, demonstrated improvement in a composite outcome including left ventricular mass and physical health measures with short daily hemodialysis relative to standard thrice-weekly treatment, though the nocturnal trial within this same research program showed a less consistent pattern of benefit, illustrating that intensive hemodialysis's outcome evidence, while generally favorable, is not uniformly positive across every specific regimen and every specific outcome measure studied.

Phosphate control specifically deserves separate mention given its clinical significance discussed in Chapter 23: intensive hemodialysis's greater cumulative weekly treatment time provides more total phosphate removal than standard thrice-weekly treatment achieves, in some patients sufficient to reduce or eliminate the phosphate binder burden discussed in that chapter, an outcome with direct quality-of-life relevance given the substantial pill burden phosphate binders often impose, independent of the more commonly emphasized cardiovascular outcome measures this section has focused on.

Quality of Life and Patient-Reported Outcomes

Beyond the cardiovascular and biochemical measures discussed above, intensive hemodialysis patients frequently report meaningful improvements in energy level, sleep quality, appetite, and overall functional capacity relative to their prior experience on standard thrice-weekly treatment, and these patient-reported benefits, while less amenable to the objective measurement the cardiovascular outcomes above permit, carry genuine clinical significance in their own right, consistent with the whole-patient, patient-centered outcome framework this book developed for hemodialysis adequacy in Chapter 7 and for peritoneal dialysis adequacy in Chapter 18.

The time burden intensive regimens impose, whether through more frequent short daily sessions or the overnight equipment operation nocturnal treatment requires, represents a genuine cost that must be weighed against these reported benefits for any individual patient, and a patient's own assessment of whether the reported quality-of-life gains justify this time and equipment burden, rather than a population-level average benefit applied uniformly, should guide the ultimately individualized decision of whether to pursue and continue an intensive home regimen.

Employment outcomes specifically, discussed briefly in Chapter 2's treatment of modality-related lifestyle considerations, show a favorable pattern in much of the home hemodialysis literature, with home-based patients, whether on an intensive or standard-frequency home schedule, reporting higher rates of continued employment than in-center patients; this pattern likely reflects both the schedule flexibility home treatment provides and, plausibly, some degree of selection effect similar to that discussed in this chapter's treatment of the broader outcomes evidence, since patients able to sustain employment may also be more likely to successfully complete home hemodialysis training and maintain the modality over time.

Limitations of the Evidence Base

Much of the observational evidence supporting intensive hemodialysis's benefits is subject to the same selection-effect caution this book raised in Chapter 7 regarding hemodialysis dose-escalation evidence more broadly: patients who select and successfully sustain an intensive home regimen may differ systematically from patients who remain on standard in-center treatment in ways beyond the treatment itself, including greater baseline health, motivation, and social support, meaning some portion of the favorable outcomes observed in this population may reflect these underlying differences rather than a direct causal effect of the intensive schedule itself.

Randomized trial evidence, while more methodologically rigorous in principle, has faced its own limitations in this specific research area, including modest sample sizes, challenges in blinding given the fundamentally different treatment experience intensive and standard schedules represent, and, in some trials, results that reached statistical significance for some but not all pre-specified outcomes; clinicians presenting intensive hemodialysis to patients should convey this genuinely nuanced evidence picture honestly, describing the plausible physiologic rationale and the generally favorable, though not uniformly conclusive, outcome evidence, rather than presenting the modality's benefits as more definitively established than the actual evidence base supports.

This honest presentation should not be mistaken for discouraging patients from pursuing intensive hemodialysis; rather, it supports a genuinely informed decision in which a patient understands both the plausible physiologic rationale and real-world reported benefits alongside the evidence's actual limitations, allowing the patient to weigh this information against their own priorities and circumstances in the same shared decision-making framework Chapter 2 developed for modality selection more broadly, rather than either overselling the modality's benefits or, in an overcorrection, understating a generally favorable evidence picture out of excessive caution about its imperfections.

KEY POINT: Intensive hemodialysis outcome evidence is generally favorable but not uniformly conclusive across every trial and outcome measure; clinicians should present this evidence honestly, including its selection-effect and methodological limitations, rather than overstating benefit as more definitively established than the evidence supports.

Figure 20.2: Comparative Interdialytic Solute and Volume Pattern Across Regimens

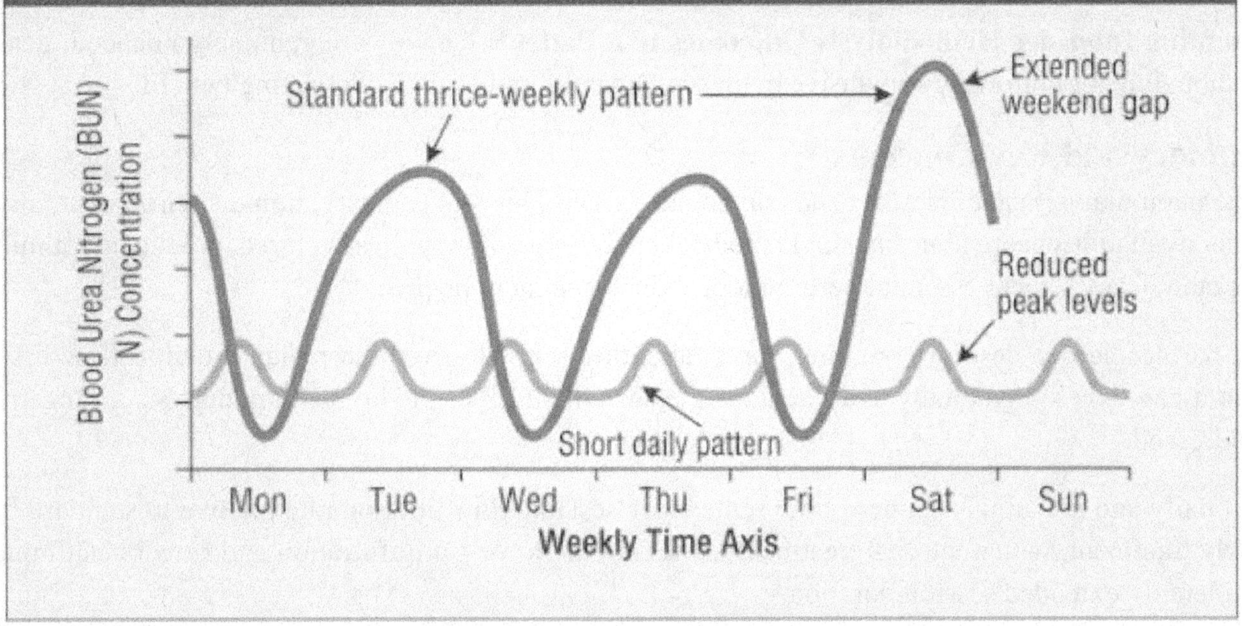

DIALYSIS RECOGNITION & RESPONSE SYSTEM — Home Therapy Arcs

The Pattern: A patient asks whether intensive home hemodialysis will definitely improve their specific clinical outcomes.

Stem Signature: A patient considering a transition to short daily or nocturnal home hemodialysis, seeking a clear, confident answer about whether this transition will improve their specific cardiovascular or quality-of-life outcomes.

The Decision: Present the genuinely nuanced evidence honestly — generally favorable but not uniformly conclusive, subject to selection-effect limitations in much of the observational data — rather than overstating benefit as more definitively established than the evidence actually supports.

Trap Logic: Enthusiasm for a modality with plausible physiologic rationale and generally favorable outcome data can lead to presenting that benefit as more certain and more universally applicable than the actual evidence, including its selection-effect and methodological limitations, genuinely supports.

Response Anchor: Present intensive hemodialysis outcome evidence honestly, including its real limitations — not as a more definitively established benefit than the evidence base actually supports.

A Venous Pressure Alarm During Unsupervised Home Treatment: Directly inspect the access site before resetting the alarm, and follow the emergency protocol immediately if separation or bleeding is confirmed.

Presenting Intensive Hemodialysis Outcomes to a Patient: Convey the genuinely nuanced, generally favorable but not uniformly conclusive evidence honestly, rather than overstating benefit.

Summary and Key Concepts

Home hemodialysis candidacy depends on cognitive and physical capacity, home environment, and care partner availability more than any single medical contraindication, with structured, graduated training and competency assessment essential before independent treatment begins.

Care partner burden deserves ongoing, direct attention separate from the patient's own follow-up, since burnout can develop gradually and threatens the sustainability of the home hemodialysis arrangement if unaddressed.

Short daily and nocturnal regimens both reduce per-session ultrafiltration rate relative to standard thrice-weekly treatment, with nocturnal treatment achieving the lowest ultrafiltration and flow rates through its considerably extended session duration.

Remote monitoring technology and structured, rehearsed troubleshooting and emergency protocols extend this book's trend-based surveillance and protocol-driven emergency response principles into the home setting, where clinical staff are not physically present.

Intensive hemodialysis outcome evidence is generally favorable for cardiovascular, volume-related, and quality-of-life measures, but remains subject to selection-effect and methodological limitations that should be conveyed honestly rather than overstated.

CHAPTER 21: ACUTE KIDNEY INJURY AND CONTINUOUS RENAL REPLACEMENT THERAPY

Learning Objectives

Apply absolute and relative indications for renal replacement therapy in acute kidney injury and assess AKI severity and trajectory.

Distinguish continuous venovenous hemofiltration, hemodialysis, and hemodiafiltration and prescribe an appropriate effluent dose.

Select an appropriate circuit anticoagulation strategy for continuous renal replacement therapy and recognize and respond to filter clotting.

Recognize when transition from continuous to intermittent therapy becomes appropriate and coordinate this transition between the intensive care and nephrology teams.

Chapter Overview

Every chapter to this point in this book has addressed dialysis in the chronic, outpatient context: patients whose kidney failure is an established, ongoing condition managed over months and years. This chapter closes Part VI by turning to a fundamentally different clinical scenario: the critically ill patient with acute kidney injury, often as one component of multi-organ dysfunction, requiring renal replacement therapy delivered continuously over twenty-four hours rather than in the discrete, several-times-weekly sessions this book has otherwise described. Continuous renal replacement therapy shares its underlying physiologic mechanisms, diffusion, convection, and ultrafiltration, with the intermittent hemodialysis detailed in Chapter 4, but its continuous delivery, its typically more hemodynamically fragile patient population, and its intensive care unit setting each introduce considerations distinct enough to warrant this chapter's dedicated treatment. This chapter also marks a transition point in the book's own structure: whereas every earlier chapter addressed the chronic dialysis patient a nephrologist manages over a long-term relationship, this chapter's patient is, in the majority of cases, expected to recover native kidney function and never require chronic dialysis at all, reframing the clinical goal from long-term modality optimization to bridging a patient through an acute physiologic crisis toward anticipated recovery.

This chapter's four sections work through the acute renal replacement pathway in its natural sequence: recognizing when therapy should begin, selecting among the available continuous modality variants and prescribing an adequate dose, managing the circuit anticoagulation this continuous therapy demands, and, finally, recognizing when the patient's improving trajectory supports transitioning back to intermittent therapy or, in the substantial majority of cases, discontinuing renal replacement therapy altogether as native kidney function recovers. Readers should note throughout this chapter how frequently its reasoning echoes principles already established elsewhere in this book for the chronic setting, since continuous renal replacement therapy is best understood not as an entirely separate discipline but as the same underlying physiologic and clinical-decision framework this book has developed throughout, adapted to the acute, critically ill, and typically reversible context this chapter specifically addresses.

Indications for Renal Replacement in Acute Kidney Injury

Absolute Indications

Refractory hyperkalemia unresponsive to medical management, severe metabolic acidosis unresponsive to medical correction, refractory volume overload with pulmonary edema unresponsive to diuretic therapy, and uremic complications including encephalopathy, pericarditis, or bleeding diathesis attributable to uremia, constitute the absolute indications for renal replacement therapy in acute kidney injury, closely paralleling the absolute indications for chronic dialysis initiation developed in Chapter 1, though arising here in the context of an acute, often rapidly evolving critical illness rather than the more gradual chronic kidney disease trajectory that chapter addressed.

Toxin or drug removal, relevant for a defined set of dialyzable substances in the context of severe poisoning or drug overdose, represents a further absolute indication specific to the acute setting without a direct chronic-dialysis parallel, and recognizing which specific toxins are amenable to extracorporeal removal, a determination based on the substance's molecular size, protein binding, and volume of distribution, requires either specific toxicology expertise or consultation with a poison control resource rather than assuming every severe poisoning scenario warrants renal replacement therapy regardless of the specific toxin's actual removability.

Sepsis-associated acute kidney injury, the single most common precipitant of severe AKI requiring renal replacement therapy in the intensive care setting, deserves specific mention given its distinct pathophysiology relative to the more purely ischemic or nephrotoxic AKI mechanisms discussed elsewhere in the nephrology literature: the combination of systemic vasodilation, microvascular dysfunction, and direct inflammatory injury to the tubular epithelium that sepsis produces creates a kidney injury pattern that, while sharing some management principles with other AKI etiologies, also responds to the broader hemodynamic and infectious source control measures the critical care team is simultaneously pursuing, meaning the renal replacement therapy decision in this specific population cannot be considered in isolation from the broader sepsis management occurring concurrently.

Unlike the chronic kidney disease trajectory discussed in Chapter 1, where absolute indications develop gradually and allow at least some anticipatory planning, acute kidney injury's absolute indications can develop within hours in a critically ill patient, and recognizing these indications promptly in this rapidly evolving context depends on the same structured, protocol-driven vigilance this book has emphasized throughout, now applied to a population whose overall clinical instability from other organ system involvement can make an isolated renal indication easier to overlook amid the many other concurrent critical care priorities a multi-organ-failure patient presents.

Relative Indications and Timing Controversy

Beyond the absolute indications above, the appropriate timing of renal replacement initiation in a critically ill patient with acute kidney injury who has not yet developed an absolute indication remains a genuinely debated question in critical care nephrology, with several large randomized trials comparing earlier, more proactive initiation strategies against a more conservative, watchful-waiting approach reserving initiation for the development of an absolute indication or clear clinical deterioration; this evidence base, considered in aggregate, has generally not demonstrated a survival benefit for early initiation over the more conservative approach, a finding that parallels, in the acute setting, the same lack of benefit from early initiation documented for chronic kidney disease progression in the IDEAL trial discussed in Chapter 1.

This evidence has shifted contemporary critical care nephrology practice away from initiating renal replacement therapy preemptively in an oliguric but otherwise metabolically stable patient, instead favoring continued close monitoring with initiation reserved for the development of an absolute indication or clear evidence that spontaneous recovery is not occurring within an expected timeframe; this watchful, symptom-and-trajectory-driven approach mirrors the same shift away from GFR-threshold-driven initiation this book documented in Chapter 1 for the chronic setting, now applied to the acute context with its own distinct time scale measured in hours to days rather than the months to years chronic kidney disease progression typically allows.

This evidence base's application requires some clinical nuance rather than rigid, uniform application regardless of individual patient circumstance: a patient with rapidly accumulating volume overload compromising oxygenation, even without yet meeting a formal absolute indication threshold, may reasonably warrant earlier initiation than a hemodynamically stable patient with similar biochemical values but no comparable respiratory compromise, illustrating that the conservative, watchful approach this evidence supports is a general orientation rather than a rule to be applied without regard for a specific patient's actual trajectory and overall clinical trajectory.

Assessing AKI Severity and Trajectory

Standardized AKI staging criteria, incorporating serum creatinine rise and urine output decline relative to a patient's baseline, classify acute kidney injury severity into defined stages that inform both prognosis and the intensity of monitoring a given patient warrants, and applying this staging consistently, rather than relying on an informal, unstandardized impression of severity, supports more consistent communication across the multidisciplinary critical care team managing a given patient's overall care.

Trajectory, not merely a single staging assessment at one time point, matters as much in the acute setting as the trend-based reasoning this book has emphasized throughout for chronic kidney disease and dialysis prescription monitoring alike: a patient whose creatinine and urine output are stabilizing or improving, even while still meeting criteria for a given AKI stage, presents a different clinical picture and a different renal replacement therapy decision than a patient whose values are actively worsening despite the same nominal staging classification, and this trajectory assessment, requiring serial rather than single-point evaluation, should inform the timing discussion detailed in the previous subsection directly.

A sixty-three-year-old woman with acute kidney injury following major abdominal surgery is oliguric with a rising creatinine on her second postoperative day, meeting a moderate AKI stage by standardized criteria but without any of the absolute indications discussed earlier in this chapter, and with stable hemodynamics on no vasopressor support. Rather than initiating renal replacement therapy based on her staging classification alone, her care team elects close monitoring with serial creatinine and urine output assessment every six hours, alongside conservative fluid management. Over the following thirty-six hours her urine output begins improving and her creatinine trend plateaus and then begins declining, confirming a recovering trajectory that supports continued conservative management without renal replacement therapy, and she is ultimately discharged without ever having required dialysis. This case illustrates the appropriate application of trajectory-based, conservative management for a patient meeting a formal AKI staging threshold but without an absolute indication or a worsening trajectory, avoiding an unnecessary renal replacement therapy initiation that the evidence discussed in this section does not support for this specific clinical picture.

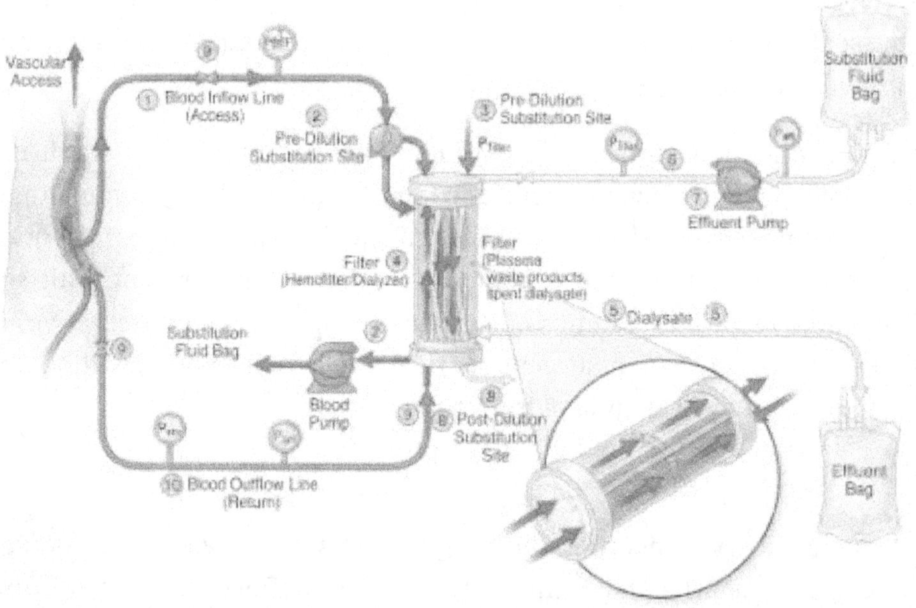

Figure 21.1: CRRT Circuit With Pre- and Post-Dilution Substitution Fluid Sites

KEY POINT: Renal replacement therapy timing in acute kidney injury should be guided by absolute indications and clinical trajectory rather than initiated preemptively based on oliguria or a GFR-equivalent threshold alone, since randomized evidence has not demonstrated benefit from early initiation over a conservative, trajectory-driven approach.

Continuous Venovenous Hemofiltration and Hemodialysis

CVVH: Convective Clearance Mechanism

Continuous venovenous hemofiltration relies entirely on convective clearance, the mechanism detailed in Chapter 4, in which a large volume of plasma water is ultrafiltered across the filter membrane and replaced with a sterile substitution fluid, carrying dissolved solutes out of the blood along with the ultrafiltered water itself rather than relying on a diffusive gradient against a separately flowing dialysate; this purely convective approach achieves middle molecule clearance particularly effectively, following the same convection-favors-larger-molecules principle established in Chapter 4's treatment of hemodiafiltration.

Substitution fluid, replaced either before the filter, termed pre-dilution, or after the filter, termed post-dilution, each carries distinct practical trade-offs: pre-dilution reduces the blood's viscosity and solute concentration entering the filter, reducing clotting risk and extending filter life, but dilutes the blood before clearance occurs, modestly reducing achieved clearance efficiency for a given substitution fluid rate relative to post-dilution, which achieves higher clearance efficiency but at the cost of a more concentrated, viscous post-filter blood more prone to clotting within the filter itself.

Substitution fluid composition, typically a balanced electrolyte solution matched closely to normal plasma composition with a bicarbonate or lactate buffer, must be selected with attention to the specific buffer's metabolic handling: bicarbonate-buffered solutions are generally preferred in patients with significant hepatic dysfunction or lactic acidosis, since lactate-buffered solutions require hepatic conversion to bicarbonate to exert their buffering effect, a conversion that may be impaired in exactly the patients whose critical illness has already compromised hepatic function, potentially blunting the intended buffering benefit in this specific population.

CVVHD and CVVHDF: Adding Diffusive Clearance

Continuous venovenous hemodialysis adds a diffusive component by flowing dialysate countercurrent to blood flow across the filter membrane, following the same countercurrent diffusion principle established in Chapter 4, without the substitution fluid a purely convective approach requires; this diffusive approach is generally simpler to manage from a fluid balance standpoint, since it does not require the substitution fluid volume tracking convective therapies demand, though it achieves comparatively less middle molecule clearance than an equivalent-dose convective approach, mirroring the same diffusion-versus-convection trade-off Chapter 4 established for intermittent hemodialysis.

Continuous venovenous hemodiafiltration combines both diffusive and convective clearance simultaneously, using both dialysate flow and substitution fluid together, and represents the modality of choice in many contemporary intensive care units specifically because it captures the small-solute clearance efficiency of diffusion alongside the middle-molecule clearance advantage of convection, echoing the same combined-mechanism rationale that favors hemodiafiltration in the intermittent hemodialysis setting discussed in Chapter 4; selection among these three modality variants in practice is often driven as much by local unit protocol, equipment availability, and staff familiarity as by patient-specific physiologic considerations, since the clinical outcome differences among the three approaches, where studied, have generally been modest relative to the outcome differences driven by adequate effluent dose delivery discussed next.

A unit's specific modality choice also interacts with practical staffing and equipment considerations distinct from the physiologic rationale discussed above: convective and combined modalities require substitution fluid supply and the associated volume-tracking infrastructure this entails, and a unit's nursing staff must be trained and comfortable with whichever specific modality the unit has standardized around, since inconsistent staff familiarity with an infrequently used modality variant can itself introduce operational risk independent of any physiologic consideration favoring one approach over another.

Prescribing Effluent Dose

Effluent dose, the combined rate of dialysate flow and substitution fluid flow expressed relative to patient body weight, is the primary prescription parameter determining achieved clearance in continuous renal replacement therapy, analogous to the combined role blood flow rate, dialysate flow rate, and treatment time play in intermittent hemodialysis dosing discussed in Chapter 6; a landmark randomized trial comparing higher- and lower-intensity effluent dosing found no additional benefit from a higher intensity once an adequate baseline dose was achieved, a finding directly paralleling the hemodialysis and peritoneal dialysis dose-escalation evidence discussed in Chapters 7 and 18 respectively, and this finding has anchored contemporary effluent dose prescribing around an adequate, evidence-supported target rather than an escalating pursuit of ever-higher clearance.

Actual delivered effluent dose frequently falls short of the prescribed dose in clinical practice, most commonly due to filter downtime from clotting, discussed later in this chapter, treatment interruptions for patient transport or procedures, and other practical delivery gaps inherent to a continuous therapy operating around the clock in a busy intensive care environment; recognizing this common prescription-to-delivery gap, and prescribing with an appropriate margin above the minimum adequate target to accommodate anticipated downtime, helps ensure the actually delivered dose, not merely the prescribed dose on paper, meets the adequacy target this section has established.

CRRT Modality	Primary Clearance Mechanism	Key Practical Consideration
CVVH	Convection (substitution fluid)	Best middle-molecule clearance; requires substitution fluid volume management
CVVHD	Diffusion (dialysate)	Simpler fluid balance tracking; less middle-molecule clearance
CVVHDF	Combined diffusion and convection	Captures both small-solute and middle-molecule clearance advantages

Figure 21.2: AKI Trajectory Patterns Informing the Initiation Decision

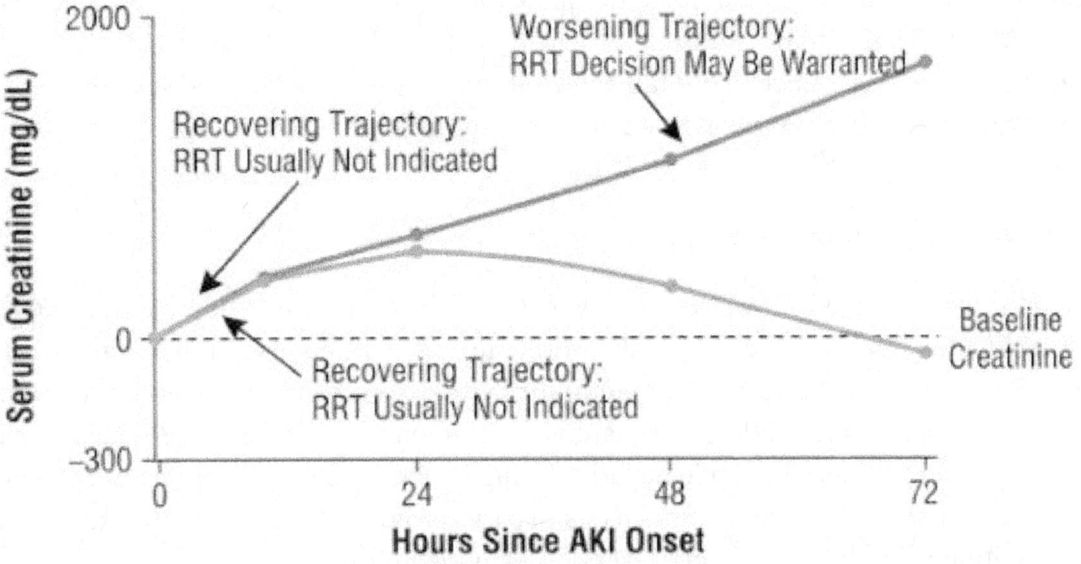

CLINICAL PEARL: Actual delivered effluent dose frequently falls short of the prescribed dose due to filter downtime and treatment interruptions; prescribing with an appropriate margin above the minimum adequate target helps ensure the delivered, not merely prescribed, dose meets adequacy.

Circuit Anticoagulation and Filter Life

Regional Citrate Anticoagulation in CRRT

Regional citrate anticoagulation, introduced in Chapter 8 for intermittent hemodialysis, finds its most extensive and best-established application specifically in continuous renal replacement therapy, where the circuit's continuous, twenty-four-hour operation makes citrate's regional, non-systemic anticoagulant effect particularly valuable given the correspondingly extended duration systemic anticoagulation would otherwise need to be maintained; citrate is now the preferred first-line anticoagulation approach for continuous renal replacement therapy in most contemporary intensive care units, reflecting accumulated evidence showing both superior filter life and reduced bleeding complications relative to systemic heparin in this specific continuous-therapy context.

Monitoring citrate anticoagulation in the continuous therapy context follows the same principles detailed in Chapter 8 — serial post-filter and systemic ionized calcium measurement, with attention to citrate accumulation risk in hepatic dysfunction — but requires more frequent monitoring given the therapy's continuous, twenty-four-hour-a-day operation relative to the discrete, several-hour intermittent hemodialysis treatment session Chapter 8 primarily addressed; standardized citrate protocols, integrated into many contemporary CRRT machines with automated citrate and calcium infusion rate calculation based on blood flow rate, have substantially simplified what was historically a more labor-intensive, manually calculated anticoagulation approach.

Citrate's metabolic effects extend beyond the calcium chelation directly relevant to its anticoagulant mechanism: citrate itself is metabolized to bicarbonate once cleared by the liver, meaning citrate anticoagulation delivers a net alkali load to the patient over the course of continuous therapy, a consideration that should factor into the broader acid-base management plan for a patient already receiving citrate-based anticoagulation, since this alkali contribution adds to whatever acid-base correction the renal replacement therapy itself is separately achieving through its diffusive or convective clearance mechanisms.

Systemic and Anticoagulation-Free Approaches

Systemic heparin anticoagulation, while no longer the preferred first-line approach in most units given citrate's superior filter-life and bleeding-risk profile in the continuous setting, remains a reasonable alternative where citrate is unavailable, contraindicated by severe hepatic dysfunction beyond what standard citrate protocol modifications can safely accommodate, or where specific unit expertise and protocol favor its continued use; systemic heparin dosing in continuous renal replacement therapy follows similar principles to the intermittent hemodialysis heparin protocols discussed in Chapter 8, adjusted for the therapy's continuous rather than discrete-session administration pattern.

Anticoagulation-free continuous renal replacement therapy, appropriate for a patient with a substantial bleeding risk precluding even citrate's largely regional effect, carries a correspondingly higher filter clotting risk than either citrate or systemic heparin, and units employing this approach typically compensate with an increased blood flow rate where the patient's access safely permits it, and heightened staff vigilance for the early clotting signs discussed in the next subsection, accepting more frequent filter changes as a reasonable trade-off against the alternative of anticoagulating a patient whose bleeding risk makes any anticoagulant exposure, however regionally confined, an unacceptable additional risk.

Vascular access adequacy deserves particular attention when anticoagulation-free technique is used, since a well-functioning, high-flow access minimizes the blood stasis within the circuit that most directly predisposes to clotting in the absence of any anticoagulant protection, and a patient on anticoagulation-free CRRT with a suboptimal access, such as a catheter delivering marginal blood flow, may experience filter clotting rates high enough to warrant reconsidering the access itself, following the same access-adequacy evaluation principle this book applied to hemodialysis circuit clotting in Chapter 8, rather than assuming the elevated clotting rate is simply an unavoidable consequence of anticoagulation-free technique alone.

Recognizing and Responding to Filter Clotting

Rising transmembrane pressure, darkening of the blood within the circuit's visible tubing segments, and declining filtrate or effluent flow rate despite unchanged blood flow rate together constitute the characteristic early warning signs of developing filter clotting, and recognizing this pattern early, following the same early-recognition-over-late-detection principle this book has emphasized throughout its treatment of vascular access stenosis in Chapter 11 and hemodialysis circuit clotting in Chapter 8, allows either an anticoagulation adjustment or a planned, elective filter change before the filter clots outright and treatment is unexpectedly interrupted.

Visual inspection of the filter itself, where the specific equipment design allows direct observation of the fiber bundle, can reveal streaking or darkening consistent with developing clot formation even before the pressure and flow parameters discussed above show a clearly abnormal trend, and staff trained to perform this visual check periodically throughout a treatment, rather than relying solely on the machine's automated pressure monitoring, add a complementary layer of early detection paralleling the same visual-plus-instrumented surveillance approach this book recommended for hemodialysis circuit monitoring in Chapter 8.

A filter that clots despite an apparently adequate anticoagulation protocol warrants the same review of the anticoagulation approach itself detailed in Chapter 8 for hemodialysis circuit clotting — whether citrate and calcium infusion rates were properly calibrated, or whether an underlying access-related blood flow limitation is contributing independent of anticoagulation adequacy — rather than simply replacing the filter and continuing with an unmodified protocol that may clot again for the same underlying reason on the replacement filter.

CAUTION: Rising transmembrane pressure and declining effluent flow despite unchanged blood flow rate are early warning signs of filter clotting; recognizing this pattern early allows a planned filter change or anticoagulation adjustment before unexpected treatment interruption occurs.

DIALYSIS RECOGNITION & RESPONSE SYSTEM — Acute Therapy Arcs

The Pattern: A CRRT filter shows a rising transmembrane pressure trend with declining effluent flow.

Stem Signature: A gradual rise in transmembrane pressure accompanied by declining effluent or filtrate flow rate over several hours, with blood flow rate unchanged, in a patient on established anticoagulation for continuous renal replacement therapy.

The Decision: Recognize this as early filter clotting, review whether the current anticoagulation protocol is properly calibrated for this specific patient, and proceed to a planned, elective filter change before the filter clots outright and interrupts treatment unexpectedly.

Trap Logic: A gradually rising pressure trend can be dismissed as an expected feature of a filter simply nearing the end of its typical service life without recognizing that early intervention, whether through anticoagulation adjustment or elective replacement, can extend usable filter life and avoid an unplanned, more disruptive clotting event.

Response Anchor: A rising transmembrane pressure and declining effluent flow trend warrants anticoagulation review and a planned filter change — not simply continued observation until the filter clots outright.

Timing of Transition to Intermittent Therapy

Criteria Supporting Transition

Hemodynamic stabilization sufficient to tolerate the more rapid fluid and solute shifts of intermittent hemodialysis, improving native kidney function evidenced by rising urine output and improving trend in filtration markers, and resolution of the specific acute indication that originally prompted renal replacement therapy initiation together support transitioning from continuous to intermittent therapy, mirroring in reverse the same trajectory-based reasoning this chapter applied earlier to the initiation decision itself.

This transition decision, like the initiation decision discussed earlier in this chapter, benefits from structured, multidisciplinary discussion between the intensive care and nephrology teams rather than being driven by either team unilaterally, since the intensive care team holds the most current information about the patient's overall hemodynamic and multi-organ status while the nephrology team holds the most direct expertise in interpreting the renal-specific trajectory data supporting or arguing against transition readiness.

The Transition Process

Transitioning from continuous to intermittent therapy is typically undertaken gradually rather than as an abrupt single-step change, often beginning with a trial of intermittent hemodialysis while continuous therapy remains available as a fallback should the patient not tolerate the more rapid intermittent fluid and solute shifts adequately; this graduated approach parallels the same graduated-independence principle this book applied to new fistula cannulation in Chapter 10 and to new hemodialysis patient treatment intensity in Chapter 4, extending the general principle that a significant physiologic transition benefits from incremental rather than abrupt implementation wherever the clinical circumstance allows this more gradual approach.

A fifty-nine-year-old man with acute kidney injury from septic shock, having required continuous venovenous hemodiafiltration for eight days, shows progressive hemodynamic stabilization with vasopressor support weaned to a minimal dose, and his urine output has increased substantially over the preceding forty-eight hours alongside an improving creatinine trend. His intensive care and nephrology teams jointly review this trajectory and elect a trial of intermittent hemodialysis, maintaining continuous therapy capability on standby in the event he does not tolerate the transition adequately. His trial intermittent treatment proceeds without significant hemodynamic instability, and his native kidney function continues improving over the following week, ultimately allowing complete discontinuation of renal replacement therapy as his recovery progresses. This case illustrates the collaborative, trajectory-based, and gradually implemented approach to transition this chapter recommends, rather than either an abrupt switch driven by administrative convenience or a reflexive continuation of continuous therapy well past the point his trajectory actually supported transition.

His nephrology team documents this transition explicitly, including the specific trajectory data that supported the decision, in a note accessible to his outpatient follow-up team should he require any nephrology follow-up after hospital discharge, ensuring that his acute kidney injury course and its resolution are communicated clearly to any clinician managing his subsequent care, consistent with the same care-coordination principle this book has applied throughout to transitions between different phases of a patient's overall treatment course.

KEY POINT: Transition from continuous to intermittent renal replacement therapy is best undertaken gradually, with continuous therapy capability retained as a fallback, and decided collaboratively between the intensive care and nephrology teams based on the patient's actual hemodynamic and renal recovery trajectory.

Coordinating Care Between ICU and Nephrology Teams

Structured, regular communication between the intensive care and nephrology teams throughout a patient's continuous renal replacement therapy course, not only at the point transition is being actively considered, supports the kind of shared situational awareness that makes the eventual transition discussion more informed and more timely than it would be if nephrology involvement were limited to periodic, infrequent consultation visits disconnected from the intensive care team's day-to-day bedside observations.

A structured daily or twice-daily review incorporating both teams' perspectives, whether through formal multidisciplinary rounds or a less formal but still consistent structured communication routine, extends the same systemic, workflow-embedded coordination principle this book has applied throughout to Life-Plan revision, prescription review, and vascular access surveillance into the acute, critical care setting specifically, where the rapidly evolving clinical picture makes consistent, frequent communication even more essential than it is in the more stable chronic dialysis context this book's earlier chapters primarily addressed.

DIALYSIS RECOGNITION & RESPONSE SYSTEM — Acute Therapy Arcs

Rising Transmembrane Pressure With Declining Effluent Flow: Review anticoagulation calibration and proceed to a planned, elective filter change before the filter clots outright and interrupts treatment unexpectedly.

Summary and Key Concepts

Absolute indications for renal replacement therapy in acute kidney injury closely parallel the chronic indications developed in Chapter 1; randomized evidence has not demonstrated benefit from early, preemptive initiation over a conservative, trajectory-driven approach.

Continuous venovenous hemofiltration, hemodialysis, and hemodiafiltration differ in their relative reliance on convective versus diffusive clearance, and adequate effluent dose, not escalation beyond an established adequate target, is what the evidence supports.

Regional citrate anticoagulation is now the preferred first-line approach for continuous renal replacement therapy in most units, given its superior filter life and reduced bleeding risk relative to systemic heparin in this continuous-therapy context.

Rising transmembrane pressure with declining effluent flow signals early filter clotting and warrants anticoagulation review and a planned filter change rather than continued observation until outright clotting occurs.

Transition from continuous to intermittent therapy is best undertaken gradually and decided collaboratively between intensive care and nephrology teams based on the patient's hemodynamic and renal recovery trajectory, supported by structured, regular communication throughout the treatment course.

CHAPTER 22: ANEMIA MANAGEMENT IN DIALYSIS PATIENTS

Learning Objectives

Explain the pathophysiology of renal anemia and the contributing factors beyond erythropoietin deficiency alone.

Initiate and titrate erythropoiesis-stimulating agent therapy within current hemoglobin target and safety guidance.

Interpret iron studies in the dialysis population and select between oral and intravenous iron repletion.

Recognize erythropoiesis-stimulating agent hyporesponsiveness and apply a structured evaluation to identify its cause.

Chapter Overview

Part VII of this book turns to the systemic and metabolic complications that accompany long-term dialysis dependence, beginning with anemia, among the earliest and most consistently present of these complications, introduced already in Chapter 1 as a contributor to the fatigue that brings many patients to medical attention as their kidney disease first approaches failure. This chapter develops anemia management in full: the physiologic basis for why kidney failure produces anemia, how erythropoiesis-stimulating agents correct it, how iron status must be assessed and managed alongside these agents, and how to recognize and evaluate the patient whose anemia fails to respond to therapy as expected. As with every other treatment domain this book has addressed, anemia management has evolved away from a single aggressive target pursued uniformly and toward an individualized, risk-aware approach calibrated to each patient's specific circumstances, a theme this chapter revisits explicitly in its treatment of hemoglobin targets and safety.

Pathophysiology of Renal Anemia

Erythropoietin Deficiency as the Primary Mechanism

Erythropoietin, produced primarily by peritubular fibroblast-like cells within the kidney in response to tissue hypoxia, stimulates erythroid progenitor cell proliferation and differentiation within the bone marrow, and progressive nephron loss in chronic kidney disease reduces the kidney's capacity to produce this hormone in proportion to the degree of tissue hypoxia present, producing a relative erythropoietin deficiency that fails to mount the compensatory response an otherwise healthy bone marrow would show given the same degree of anemia-related hypoxic stimulus.

The specific renal cell population responsible for erythropoietin production is particularly vulnerable to the same tubulointerstitial fibrosis and capillary rarefaction that characterizes progressive chronic kidney disease more broadly, meaning the loss of erythropoietin-producing capacity tracks closely with the same structural nephron loss driving a patient's overall decline in kidney function rather than representing an entirely separate, independently regulated process; this structural link explains why erythropoietin deficiency, once established, does not fluctuate substantially with day-to-day variation in a patient's clinical status the way some other hormonal derangements in kidney disease can, but instead follows a more steadily progressive course paralleling the chronic kidney disease trajectory itself. Some capacity for extrarenal erythropoietin production, primarily hepatic, persists even in complete kidney failure, explaining why anemia in dialysis-dependent patients, while often severe, is rarely as profound as would be expected from complete absence of erythropoietin production, and this residual extrarenal contribution, while insufficient alone to maintain adequate erythropoiesis, means erythropoiesis-stimulating agent therapy is supplementing rather than entirely replacing endogenous hormone production in most patients.

This deficiency develops gradually in parallel with the chronic kidney disease trajectory discussed in Chapter 1, typically becoming clinically apparent as anemia in the more advanced stages of chronic kidney disease, though the specific point at which anemia becomes clinically significant varies considerably between patients depending on the rate of decline and other contributing factors detailed in the next subsection; this variability is part of why anemia evaluation and management, discussed later in this chapter, should be individualized to a patient's actual hemoglobin trend and symptom burden rather than triggered by a fixed chronic kidney disease stage applied uniformly.

The clinical consequences of untreated or undertreated renal anemia extend beyond the fatigue most commonly emphasized in patient-facing discussions: reduced tissue oxygen delivery contributes to left ventricular hypertrophy and worsening cardiac function over time, discussed further in Chapter 24, and cognitive function, exercise tolerance, and overall quality of life each show measurable impairment in patients with poorly controlled anemia relative to those whose anemia is adequately managed, underscoring that anemia management, while sometimes treated as a secondary consideration relative to the dialysis prescription itself, carries genuine independent clinical weight deserving the same systematic attention this book has applied to every other chronic complication of kidney failure.

Anemia's contribution to exercise intolerance and reduced physical functioning carries particular relevance for the frailty considerations discussed in Chapter 26, since an older dialysis patient's overall physical reserve and capacity for independent activity depends substantially on adequate tissue oxygen delivery, and a component of what might otherwise be attributed purely to age-related decline or general debility may in fact reflect undertreated or inadequately monitored anemia specifically; this connection supports incorporating anemia status explicitly into the broader frailty assessment framework Chapter 26 developed, rather than evaluating anemia and frailty as entirely separate clinical domains addressed by different specialists without cross-communication.

Contributing Factors Beyond Erythropoietin Deficiency

Iron deficiency, discussed in detail later in this chapter, frequently compounds erythropoietin deficiency in the dialysis population, arising from a combination of reduced dietary intake, impaired gastrointestinal absorption related to the uremic milieu, chronic occult blood loss including the losses associated with the hemodialysis circuit itself and with the more frequent laboratory phlebotomy this population undergoes, and, particularly relevant to the inflammatory state common in dialysis patients, hepcidin-mediated impairment of iron absorption and mobilization from storage sites even when total body iron stores are not frankly depleted.

Chronic inflammation, common in the dialysis population from a combination of the uremic milieu itself, recurrent access-related or other infections discussed throughout this book, and the bioincompatibility considerations discussed in Chapter 5, elevates hepcidin, a hormone that reduces intestinal iron absorption and traps iron within storage cells, producing a functional iron deficiency in which iron is present in the body but not adequately available for erythropoiesis; this distinction between absolute and functional iron deficiency, developed further in this chapter's treatment of iron studies interpretation, has direct implications for whether oral iron, dependent on intestinal absorption, is likely to be effective for a given patient.

Secondary hyperparathyroidism, discussed in Chapter 23, can contribute to anemia through bone marrow fibrosis in severe, longstanding cases, and reduced red blood cell survival, a phenomenon specific to the uremic environment through mechanisms not fully elucidated but well documented empirically, further contributes to anemia independent of erythropoietin production or iron status; recognizing that renal anemia is genuinely multifactorial, rather than attributable to erythropoietin deficiency alone, is essential to understanding why erythropoiesis-stimulating agent therapy alone, without adequate attention to iron status and these other contributing factors, frequently fails to achieve or maintain an adequate hemoglobin response.

The uremic milieu's effect on red cell membrane integrity and deformability, producing the shortened red cell lifespan mentioned above, reflects accumulated uremic toxin exposure acting directly on circulating red cells rather than any deficiency in their initial production, meaning this specific contributing mechanism responds to dialysis adequacy itself, discussed in Chapters 7 and 18, rather than to erythropoiesis-stimulating agent or iron therapy specifically; a patient with persistently inadequate dialysis clearance may show a component of anemia resistant to escalating ESA and iron therapy alone until the underlying adequacy deficit itself is corrected, illustrating a further respect in which anemia management connects directly back to the broader adequacy framework this book developed in earlier chapters rather than functioning as an entirely separate treatment domain.

Vitamin and trace element deficiencies beyond iron, including folate and vitamin B12, warrant consideration as further contributing factors in a dialysis patient with anemia not fully explained by the mechanisms already discussed, particularly given the dietary restrictions and altered nutrient handling this population experiences, and folate losses during hemodialysis treatment itself, similar in principle to the amino acid losses discussed in Chapter 25's treatment of protein-energy wasting, mean folate status deserves periodic attention even though routine folate supplementation is not universally recommended in every dialysis patient regardless of documented deficiency.

Diagnostic Evaluation of Anemia in Kidney Disease

Initial anemia evaluation in a patient with kidney disease includes a complete blood count with red cell indices, iron studies discussed in detail later in this chapter, and, where the clinical picture suggests a cause beyond renal anemia alone, additional evaluation for gastrointestinal blood loss, vitamin B12 or folate deficiency, or a primary hematologic disorder; attributing anemia to kidney disease alone without this basic evaluation risks missing a coexisting, independently treatable cause that erythropoiesis-stimulating agent therapy alone would not adequately address.

A normocytic, normochromic anemia pattern is most typical of uncomplicated renal anemia, and a microcytic pattern should prompt evaluation for iron deficiency or, less commonly, thalassemia trait, while a macrocytic pattern should prompt evaluation for vitamin B12 or folate deficiency rather than being attributed to kidney disease by default; this basic red cell index interpretation, familiar from general internal medicine practice, retains its full diagnostic value in the dialysis population and should not be abandoned simply because a patient's kidney disease provides a ready, if sometimes incomplete, explanation for anemia in isolation.

Reticulocyte count, while sometimes overlooked in routine anemia evaluation, provides useful information about the bone marrow's actual erythropoietic response to whatever stimulus is currently present, and an inappropriately low reticulocyte count relative to the degree of anemia present suggests an underproduction process, consistent with the erythropoietin deficiency and other mechanisms this chapter has emphasized, while an elevated reticulocyte count in the setting of anemia should prompt consideration of ongoing blood loss or hemolysis as a more likely explanation, since these processes would be expected to provoke a compensatory marrow response distinct from the blunted response characteristic of uncomplicated renal anemia.

Erythropoiesis-Stimulating Agent Therapy

ESA Agents and Mechanism of Action

Erythropoiesis-stimulating agents, recombinant formulations designed to replace the deficient endogenous erythropoietin discussed earlier in this chapter, bind the same erythropoietin receptor on marrow erythroid progenitor cells and stimulate their proliferation and differentiation, correcting the anemia's primary mechanism directly; several formulations differ in their specific pharmacokinetics, including circulating half-life, allowing dosing intervals ranging from multiple times weekly to as infrequently as monthly depending on the specific agent selected and the patient's individual response.

Route of administration, whether intravenous or subcutaneous, affects bioavailability and, correspondingly, the dose required to achieve a given hemoglobin response, with subcutaneous administration generally achieving equivalent hemoglobin response at a lower total dose than intravenous administration for the same agent, though intravenous administration is often preferred for hemodialysis patients specifically given its convenient delivery through the existing vascular access already in place during each treatment, illustrating a practical convenience consideration that can outweigh the dose-efficiency advantage subcutaneous administration otherwise offers.

Peritoneal dialysis patients, lacking the routine vascular access intravenous administration during hemodialysis provides, more commonly receive ESA therapy subcutaneously, and this modality-specific difference in typical administration route is worth recognizing explicitly when comparing ESA dose requirements or cost between hemodialysis and peritoneal dialysis populations, since the route difference itself, independent of any underlying difference in erythropoietin deficiency severity between the two populations, contributes to the somewhat lower typical ESA doses often observed in peritoneal dialysis patients relative to hemodialysis patients.

Initiating and Titrating ESA Therapy

ESA therapy is generally initiated once hemoglobin falls below a defined threshold and iron status, discussed in the next section, has been assessed and, where deficient, addressed, since initiating ESA therapy in the setting of untreated iron deficiency predictably produces an inadequate response regardless of the ESA dose used, given iron's essential role as a substrate for the hemoglobin synthesis ESA therapy is attempting to stimulate.

Dose titration follows the hemoglobin trend over successive measurements rather than any single value, with dose increases considered for an inadequate rate of rise and dose reductions or holds considered for a rate of rise exceeding what current guidance considers safe, reflecting the safety considerations discussed in the next subsection; this trend-based titration approach, familiar from this book's treatment of numerous other prescription parameters throughout its earlier chapters, avoids both the undertreatment that reactive, single-value-driven titration risks and the overshoot that overly aggressive, rapid dose escalation can produce.

A defined maximum dose threshold, beyond which continued escalation is reconsidered in favor of the hyporesponsiveness evaluation detailed later in this chapter rather than pursued indefinitely, provides a practical safeguard against the kind of unchecked dose escalation that both fails to resolve an underlying, unaddressed cause and exposes the patient to unnecessary medication burden and cost without corresponding benefit.

Documentation of the specific dose trajectory and hemoglobin response over time, maintained in a format that allows any covering clinician to quickly assess whether a given patient's current dose and response pattern represents stable, adequate control or an evolving hyporesponsiveness pattern, supports the trend-based titration this section emphasizes considerably more effectively than a documentation approach recording only the current dose and most recent hemoglobin value without the historical trend context needed to distinguish these two very different clinical pictures.

Hemoglobin Targets and Safety Considerations

Randomized trials directly testing higher hemoglobin targets against more conservative targets found increased cardiovascular event rates, including stroke, with the higher targets, without a corresponding improvement in patient-reported quality of life sufficient to justify this increased risk, prompting a substantial revision of hemoglobin target guidance away from the more aggressive, near-normal targets earlier practice had pursued and toward a more conservative target range, avoiding both undertreated anemia and the risks this trial evidence associated with aggressive correction.

This evidence parallels, in the anemia-specific context, the same dose-escalation-without-benefit pattern this book has documented repeatedly across other treatment domains: hemodialysis Kt/V in Chapter 7, peritoneal dialysis Kt/V in Chapter 18, and CRRT effluent dose in Chapter 21 each showed no additional benefit from escalation beyond an adequate threshold, and anemia management's hemoglobin target evidence adds cardiovascular harm specifically to this now-familiar pattern, making the case for conservative, evidence-based targets even more directly consequential in this specific domain than in the others where escalation simply failed to help rather than causing documented harm.

The specific stroke risk elevation observed with higher hemoglobin targets is thought to relate to increased blood viscosity and altered platelet function at higher hemoglobin concentrations, mechanisms distinct from the more commonly discussed cardiovascular risk pathways this book has addressed in Chapter 24, and this distinct mechanism underscores that hemoglobin correction, despite its clear benefits at an appropriate target, is not a uniformly protective intervention where more correction is simply better; patients with a prior stroke history or other cerebrovascular risk factors may warrant particular caution regarding the upper end of the target range, an individualization consistent with the risk-stratified approach this book has applied throughout its treatment of every other therapeutic target discussed across its preceding chapters.

KEY POINT: Randomized trials found increased cardiovascular event rates, including stroke, with higher hemoglobin targets, without a corresponding quality-of-life benefit; contemporary practice favors a more conservative target range that avoids both undertreated anemia and the risks aggressive correction has been shown to carry.

Figure 22.1: Erythropoiesis Stimulation Pathway From Kidney to Marrow

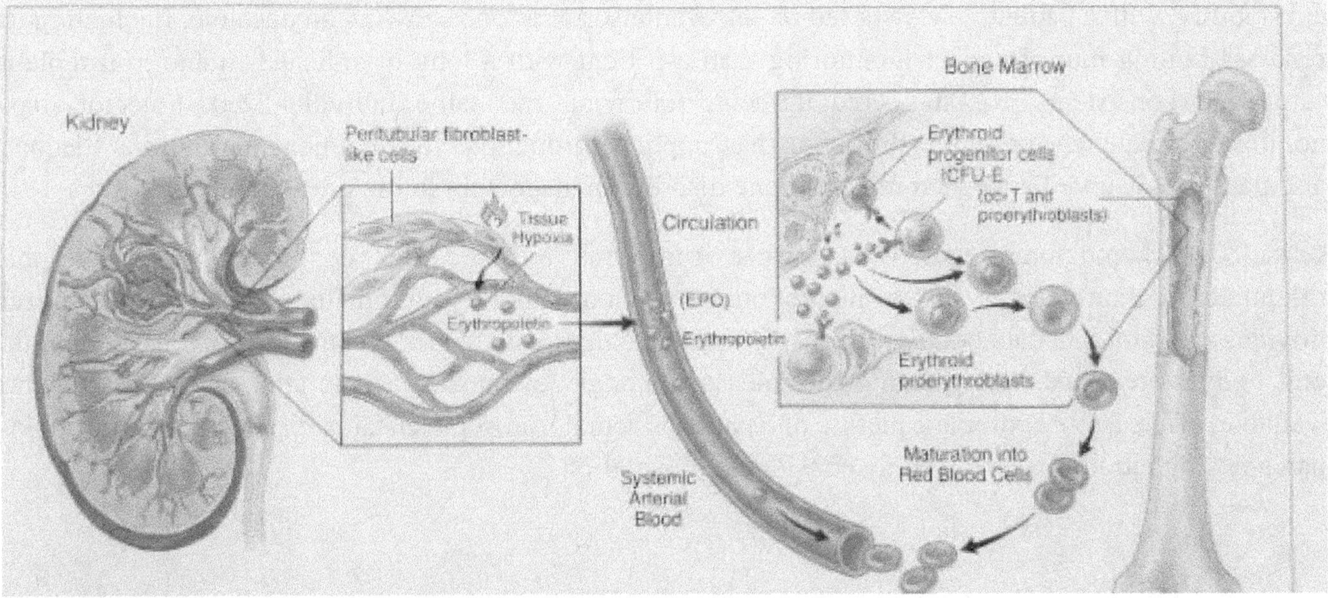

Iron Management and Monitoring

Iron Studies Interpretation in Dialysis Patients

Serum ferritin, reflecting total body iron stores under normal circumstances, is confounded in the dialysis population by its behavior as an acute-phase reactant that rises with inflammation independent of true iron status, meaning a dialysis patient's ferritin level must be interpreted with this inflammatory confounding specifically in mind rather than applying the same reference ranges used in a population without the chronic inflammatory burden this book has described throughout its treatment of the dialysis population.

Assay-to-assay variability in ferritin measurement, reflecting differences in calibration and methodology across different laboratory platforms, adds a further layer of interpretive complexity beyond the inflammatory confounding already discussed, and a patient whose care transitions between laboratories using different ferritin assays may show an apparent change in ferritin trend that reflects this methodological difference rather than a genuine change in iron status; awareness of which specific assay a given laboratory uses, and caution when comparing values across a transition between different laboratories or assay platforms, supports more accurate trend interpretation than assuming every ferritin value is directly comparable regardless of its measurement source.

Transferrin saturation, calculated from serum iron and total iron-binding capacity, provides a complementary measure less confounded by acute inflammation than ferritin alone, and the combination of a low transferrin saturation with a low-to-normal ferritin supports absolute iron deficiency, while a low transferrin saturation with an elevated ferritin, the pattern most consistent with the functional iron deficiency discussed earlier in this chapter, suggests hepcidin-mediated iron sequestration rather than true iron depletion, a distinction with direct implications for the oral-versus-intravenous iron selection discussed in the next subsection.

The frequency of iron studies monitoring should be individualized to a patient's current iron therapy status and stability, with a patient newly started on intravenous iron or one showing an unstable, fluctuating iron trend warranting more frequent monitoring than a patient with a long-established, stable iron repletion status and consistent ESA dose requirement, following the same individualized, trajectory-based monitoring frequency principle this book has applied throughout its treatment of dialysis adequacy, vascular access surveillance, and mineral bone disorder management in the preceding chapters.

Reticulocyte hemoglobin content, a further iron-status measure less confounded by acute-phase inflammation than ferritin and available on many contemporary automated hematology analyzers, provides an additional data point reflecting the iron actually available for recent erythropoiesis rather than total body stores, and incorporating this measure alongside transferrin saturation and ferritin, where available, offers a more complete picture of a patient's actual iron-replete status for ongoing erythropoiesis than any single traditional iron study considered in isolation.

Oral Versus Intravenous Iron Repletion

Oral iron, dependent on intestinal absorption that the hepcidin-mediated mechanism discussed earlier in this chapter specifically impairs, is frequently inadequate to correct iron deficiency in the dialysis population, and several comparative trials have found intravenous iron more effective at achieving target iron parameters and reducing ESA dose requirements than oral iron in hemodialysis patients specifically, reflecting this population's particular predisposition toward the functional iron deficiency pattern oral supplementation is poorly positioned to overcome.

Newer oral iron formulations, designed with improved absorption characteristics or paired with agents intended to counteract hepcidin-mediated absorption blockade, have shown some promise in research settings, though these approaches have not yet displaced intravenous iron as the preferred approach for most dialysis patients with confirmed iron deficiency, and clinicians should remain attentive to this evolving area, consulting current literature rather than relying on a fixed assumption that oral iron is categorically ineffective in every dialysis patient regardless of the specific formulation or adjunctive approach used.

Intravenous iron administration during hemodialysis treatment offers the same practical convenience advantage discussed earlier in this chapter for intravenous ESA administration, using the existing vascular access already in place, and modern intravenous iron formulations permit administration of a larger dose per session with a reduced infusion reaction risk relative to older formulations, though any intravenous iron administration still warrants monitoring for infusion reactions during and immediately following administration, following standard infusion safety practice applicable to any intravenous medication with a recognized, if now uncommon, hypersensitivity risk.

Monitoring and Avoiding Iron Overload

Periodic iron studies monitoring, at an interval determined by unit protocol and individual patient trajectory, guides ongoing intravenous iron dosing decisions and helps avoid the iron overload that repeated dosing without adequate monitoring can produce; iron overload, while historically less emphasized than iron deficiency in dialysis anemia management discussions, carries its own recognized risks including hepatic and cardiac iron deposition in severe, longstanding cases, and a ferritin trend rising progressively despite ongoing supplementation, rather than a single elevated value considered in isolation, should prompt reconsideration of continued iron dosing rather than assuming continued supplementation remains appropriate simply because it has been the established practice for a given patient.

A temporary pause in intravenous iron dosing, rather than an immediate, indefinite discontinuation, is often the appropriate initial response to a rising ferritin trend of uncertain significance, allowing repeat testing after an interval to confirm whether the trend genuinely reflects accumulating overload or instead an inflammation-related transient elevation of the kind this chapter has discussed extensively; this measured, trend-confirming approach avoids both the undertreatment risk of premature discontinuation based on a single elevated value and the overtreatment risk of continuing supplementation through a genuine, sustained overload trend.

CAUTION: A rising ferritin trend despite ongoing intravenous iron supplementation should prompt reconsideration of continued dosing, since iron overload carries its own recognized hepatic and cardiac risks distinct from the iron deficiency this supplementation was originally intended to correct.

Hyporesponsive Anemia and Its Evaluation

Defining and Recognizing ESA Hyporesponsiveness

ESA hyporesponsiveness, defined as failure to achieve or maintain target hemoglobin despite an appropriately escalated ESA dose and adequate iron status, affects a meaningful minority of dialysis patients and should prompt the structured evaluation detailed in this section rather than an open-ended further escalation of ESA dose alone, since further escalation without identifying and addressing an underlying cause both fails to resolve the hyporesponsiveness and exposes the patient to the safety risks associated with higher ESA doses discussed earlier in this chapter.

The specific dose threshold used to trigger formal hyporesponsiveness evaluation varies somewhat across published guidance and individual practice settings, but the underlying principle remains consistent regardless of the exact numeric threshold applied: a patient requiring meaningfully more ESA than would typically be expected to achieve a given hemoglobin response, relative to that patient's own body weight and clinical circumstances, warrants this structured evaluation rather than an assumption that some patients simply require higher doses without further explanation being sought.

Recognizing hyporesponsiveness requires tracking ESA dose alongside hemoglobin response over time, since a patient whose ESA dose has been escalating progressively without a corresponding hemoglobin improvement is showing the hyporesponsiveness pattern this section addresses even if their current hemoglobin remains within an acceptable range, and this trend-based recognition, consistent with the trend-over-single-value principle this book has applied throughout, catches emerging hyporesponsiveness earlier than would recognition based on hemoglobin value alone.

Common Causes of Hyporesponsiveness

Iron deficiency, whether absolute or functional as discussed earlier in this chapter, is the most common and most readily correctable cause of ESA hyporesponsiveness, and should be the first cause excluded or addressed before pursuing the less common causes discussed below; inadequate dialysis adequacy, discussed in Chapters 7 and 18, chronic inflammation or infection from an occult source such as an infected vascular access discussed in Chapters 11 and 12, and secondary hyperparathyroidism discussed in Chapter 23 each represent further recognized contributors to hyporesponsiveness that a structured evaluation should specifically consider.

Less common causes, including a primary hematologic malignancy, chronic blood loss from an unrecognized gastrointestinal or other source, and, rarely, pure red cell aplasia related to anti-erythropoietin antibody development, warrant consideration specifically in a patient whose hyporesponsiveness fails to resolve despite addressing the more common causes above, since pursuing an exhaustive rare-cause evaluation before first excluding the far more common and more readily treatable explanations represents an inefficient sequencing of the diagnostic process this section recommends structuring from most to least likely cause.

Medication review deserves specific attention within this evaluation sequence, since several medication classes, including angiotensin-converting enzyme inhibitors and angiotensin receptor blockers, have been associated with modest ESA hyporesponsiveness in some patients, plausibly through effects on erythropoietin production or erythroid progenitor sensitivity, and while these medications generally retain their important cardiovascular and other indications discussed in Chapter 24, recognizing this potential contribution can inform the overall clinical picture even when discontinuation is not appropriate given the medication's other established benefits for a given patient.

A Structured Evaluation Approach

A structured evaluation sequence, beginning with iron status confirmation and correction, followed by review of dialysis adequacy and vascular access for occult infection, followed by assessment for secondary hyperparathyroidism and inflammatory markers, and, only once these more common causes have been reasonably excluded, evaluation for the rarer hematologic causes discussed above, provides a systematic approach considerably more efficient than an unstructured, ad hoc evaluation pursuing possible causes in no particular order.

Evaluation Step	What to Assess	Rationale for Sequence Position

1. Iron Status	Transferrin saturation, ferritin, reticulocyte hemoglobin content	Most common and most readily correctable cause
2. Dialysis Adequacy	Kt/V trend, residual function	Second most common; directly actionable via prescription review
3. Occult Infection	Vascular access exam, inflammatory markers	Common and often subtle; addressed in Chapters 11-12, 19
4. Secondary Hyperparathyroidism	PTH trend	Recognized contributor per Chapter 23; correctable
5. Rare Hematologic Causes	Peripheral smear, hematology referral	Pursued only after common causes excluded

This sequencing reflects a Bayesian, prevalence-weighted approach to diagnostic evaluation: pursuing the most common and most readily correctable explanations first maximizes the likelihood that each evaluation step yields an actionable finding, while deferring rarer, more resource-intensive evaluations until the more common possibilities have been reasonably excluded avoids the inefficiency and potential patient burden of pursuing an extensive hematologic workup in a patient whose hyporesponsiveness ultimately proves attributable to a straightforward, common cause identifiable earlier in the sequence.

A fifty-five-year-old woman on hemodialysis requires progressively escalating ESA doses over three months without the expected hemoglobin improvement, despite iron studies showing adequate transferrin saturation and ferritin. Following the structured evaluation sequence this chapter recommends, her nephrology team next reviews her dialysis adequacy, finding it within target, and then examines her vascular access, discovering subtle signs of a developing graft infection not yet producing overt systemic symptoms. Treatment of this infection, following the approach detailed in Chapter 11, results in her hemoglobin response normalizing at her prior ESA dose over the following weeks without further escalation required. This case illustrates why hyporesponsiveness evaluation should proceed through a structured sequence considering inflammation and occult infection specifically, rather than assuming iron deficiency must be the explanation whenever iron studies appear reassuring, or resorting to indefinite dose escalation without a structured search for the underlying cause.

Her care team also reviews this case at a subsequent quality meeting, noting that her graft infection had not produced overt systemic symptoms until this evaluation prompted closer examination, and using this experience to reinforce among staff that unexplained ESA hyporesponsiveness should itself be treated as a potential early clue to an otherwise occult infection, prompting access examination even in the absence of more obvious infectious signs such as fever or visible erythema, extending the same subtle-warning-sign vigilance this book has emphasized throughout its treatment of vascular access surveillance in Chapter 11.

Her team also notes in retrospect that her dose escalation pattern, tracked over the preceding three months using the trend-based documentation approach this chapter has recommended, showed a clearly accelerating trajectory rather than a gradual, expected increase, and this accelerating pattern itself, recognized earlier through more attentive trend review, might have prompted the structured evaluation somewhat sooner than the three-month mark at which it was actually initiated; this retrospective observation reinforces the value of actively reviewing dose trajectory shape, not merely whether a dose has increased, since an accelerating rather than steady rate of increase is itself a meaningful signal warranting closer attention.

Aggregate, unit-level tracking of anemia management metrics, including the proportion of patients within target hemoglobin range, average ESA dose, and the frequency of hyporesponsiveness evaluations triggered, provides a population-level quality improvement complement to the individual-patient management this chapter has otherwise emphasized, extending the same population-level surveillance principle this book has applied to peritonitis rates in Chapter 19 and infection prevention benchmarking in Chapter 25; a unit whose aggregate metrics diverge meaningfully from expected benchmarks may benefit from a broader review of its anemia management protocols and practices, similar in principle to the broader practice review this book has recommended whenever an individual clinical pattern suggests a systemic rather than isolated explanation.

CLINICAL PEARL: ESA hyporesponsiveness with reassuring iron studies should prompt evaluation for occult infection, including vascular access infection, and inadequate dialysis adequacy, rather than indefinite further ESA dose escalation without a structured search for the underlying cause.

DIALYSIS RECOGNITION & RESPONSE SYSTEM — Anemia Management Arcs

---

The Pattern: A patient requires progressively escalating ESA doses without the expected hemoglobin response, despite adequate iron studies.

Stem Signature: A rising ESA dose trend over successive treatments without a corresponding hemoglobin improvement, in a patient whose transferrin saturation and ferritin appear adequate on recent testing.

The Decision: Proceed through the structured hyporesponsiveness evaluation sequence — reviewing dialysis adequacy, vascular access for occult infection, and secondary hyperparathyroidism — rather than continuing to escalate ESA dose indefinitely in the absence of an identified explanation.

Trap Logic: Reassuring iron studies can be mistaken for confirmation that no correctable cause of hyporesponsiveness remains, when inflammation from an occult source such as vascular access infection is a common contributor that iron studies alone will not reveal.

Response Anchor: Progressive ESA dose escalation without hemoglobin response, despite adequate iron studies, warrants a structured search for occult inflammation or infection — not continued dose escalation alone.

DIALYSIS RECOGNITION & RESPONSE SYSTEM — Anemia Management Arcs

---

Progressive ESA Dose Escalation Without Response: Proceed through the structured hyporesponsiveness evaluation sequence rather than continuing to escalate dose indefinitely in the absence of an identified explanation.

Summary and Key Concepts

Renal anemia arises primarily from relative erythropoietin deficiency but is frequently compounded by iron deficiency, chronic inflammation with hepcidin-mediated functional iron deficiency, and reduced red cell survival, making it a genuinely multifactorial condition.

ESA therapy should be initiated only after iron status has been assessed and addressed, with dose titrated according to the hemoglobin trend over successive measurements rather than any single value.

Randomized evidence found increased cardiovascular risk with higher hemoglobin targets without a corresponding quality-of-life benefit, supporting a conservative, evidence-based target range over aggressive correction.

Intravenous iron is generally more effective than oral iron in the dialysis population given this population's predisposition toward hepcidin-mediated functional iron deficiency, but requires monitoring to avoid iron overload.

ESA hyporesponsiveness warrants a structured evaluation beginning with iron status, then dialysis adequacy and occult infection, then secondary hyperparathyroidism, before considering rarer hematologic causes, rather than indefinite dose escalation alone.

CHAPTER 23: MINERAL AND BONE DISORDER IN CHRONIC KIDNEY DISEASE

Learning Objectives

Explain the pathophysiology of CKD-mineral and bone disorder, including the FGF23-Klotho axis and progression to secondary hyperparathyroidism.

Apply dietary phosphate control and select among calcium-based and non-calcium-based phosphate binders.

Individualize vitamin D, calcimimetic, and parathyroid hormone target management for a given patient.

Describe vascular calcification mechanisms and renal osteodystrophy subtypes, and integrate mineral management with overall cardiovascular risk.

Chapter Overview

Chronic kidney disease-mineral and bone disorder, abbreviated CKD-MBD, describes the interconnected disturbances in calcium, phosphate, parathyroid hormone, and vitamin D metabolism that develop as kidney function declines, along with their downstream consequences for bone health and vascular calcification. This chapter, following directly from Chapter 22's treatment of anemia as another systemic complication of kidney failure, works through this disorder's pathophysiology from its earliest, most subtle biochemical changes through the phosphate binder and vitamin D and calcimimetic therapies used to manage it, and concludes with the vascular calcification and bone disease consequences that make CKD-MBD management consequential well beyond the biochemical numbers themselves. As with anemia management in the preceding chapter, CKD-MBD management has evolved toward individualized, patient-specific targets rather than a single aggressive correction applied uniformly, and this chapter develops that individualized framework in detail.

Pathophysiology of CKD-Mineral and Bone Disorder

The FGF23-Klotho Axis and Early Phosphate Regulation

Fibroblast growth factor 23, produced by osteocytes in response to rising phosphate load, is among the earliest measurable biochemical changes in chronic kidney disease, rising well before serum phosphate itself becomes overtly elevated on standard laboratory testing; this hormone acts on the kidney, in conjunction with its co-receptor Klotho, to increase urinary phosphate excretion and suppress activation of vitamin D, together maintaining phosphate balance despite declining nephron mass for a considerable period before this compensatory system itself becomes overwhelmed.

FGF23's discovery and characterization over the past two decades has substantially reshaped the conceptual understanding of phosphate homeostasis in chronic kidney disease, shifting emphasis away from a purely kidney-centric model toward a bone-kidney-parathyroid axis in which osteocytes function as active endocrine cells rather than merely passive structural components; this reconceptualization has direct clinical relevance beyond the biochemical mechanism itself, since it suggests that bone health and phosphate homeostasis are more intimately connected than earlier models recognized, a connection this chapter's later treatment of renal osteodystrophy and vascular calcification develops in full.

Klotho expression declines progressively as chronic kidney disease advances, reducing the kidney's responsiveness to FGF23's phosphaturic signal and requiring progressively higher FGF23 concentrations to achieve the same phosphate excretion effect, a compensatory escalation that itself carries recognized adverse consequences, including a direct association between elevated FGF23 and left ventricular hypertrophy independent of phosphate level itself, illustrating that this axis's disturbance carries cardiovascular significance beyond its role in phosphate homeostasis alone.

Because FGF23 elevation precedes overt phosphate abnormality by a considerable margin, some research has explored FGF23 as an early biomarker for CKD-MBD risk stratification well before conventional phosphate, calcium, and PTH testing would flag a concern, though this biomarker approach has not yet translated into routine clinical practice given the assay's limited availability outside research settings and the absence of a clearly established, actionable clinical threshold analogous to the more familiar phosphate and PTH targets this chapter develops throughout.

Progression to Secondary Hyperparathyroidism

As chronic kidney disease progresses further, the FGF23-Klotho compensatory system discussed above becomes insufficient to maintain phosphate balance and adequate active vitamin D levels, and declining active vitamin D directly reduces intestinal calcium absorption while rising phosphate itself directly stimulates parathyroid hormone secretion; the parathyroid gland, chronically stimulated by this combination of declining calcium, declining active vitamin D, and rising phosphate, undergoes progressive hyperplasia and increasingly autonomous hormone secretion, producing the secondary hyperparathyroidism that becomes a defining biochemical feature of advanced chronic kidney disease and, especially, dialysis-dependent kidney failure.

This progressive parathyroid hyperplasia has a specific and clinically important consequence for treatment: a gland that has undergone extensive, longstanding hyperplasia becomes progressively less responsive to medical suppression, whether through vitamin D or calcimimetic therapy discussed later in this chapter, than a gland with more modest, earlier hyperplasia, meaning earlier intervention in the CKD-MBD trajectory generally achieves more durable biochemical control than intervention delayed until parathyroid hyperplasia has already become extensive and, in the most severe cases, developed nodular, monoclonal regions of autonomous hormone secretion largely unresponsive to medical therapy at all.

The transition from diffuse, polyclonal parathyroid hyperplasia to nodular, monoclonal hyperplasia represents a particularly important pathophysiologic threshold, since nodular regions have been shown to express reduced calcium-sensing receptor and vitamin D receptor density relative to diffusely hyperplastic tissue, providing a direct molecular explanation for why these nodular regions respond poorly to both calcimimetic therapy, which acts on the calcium-sensing receptor, and active vitamin D analogs, which act on the vitamin D receptor; recognizing this molecular basis helps explain, rather than simply describe, why earlier intervention in the CKD-MBD trajectory achieves more durable control, since intervening before this nodular transition occurs preserves a parathyroid gland population still responsive to medical suppression.

Parathyroidectomy, surgical removal of some or all of the hyperplastic parathyroid tissue, remains a reasonable and effective option for the subset of patients whose secondary hyperparathyroidism has progressed to this severe, medically refractory stage, and recognizing when medical therapy has genuinely reached its limit, rather than continuing to escalate calcimimetic and vitamin D doses indefinitely in a gland that has become predominantly autonomous, is an important clinical judgment this chapter's later discussion of individualized PTH targets and combination therapy should inform directly.

The CKD-MBD Framework: Biochemistry, Bone, and Calcification

The contemporary CKD-MBD framework explicitly connects three previously more separately considered domains: the biochemical abnormalities in calcium, phosphate, parathyroid hormone, and vitamin D discussed above; the bone histological abnormalities termed renal osteodystrophy, discussed later in this chapter; and the extraskeletal, particularly vascular, calcification that shares overlapping pathophysiology with the bone disease itself, since both processes are governed by related mineralization pathways that can become dysregulated in opposite directions simultaneously, producing a patient with weak, undermineralized bone alongside pathologically calcified vasculature.

This connected framework has direct clinical implications for how CKD-MBD is monitored and managed: a treatment decision addressing the biochemical abnormalities in isolation, without considering its potential effect on bone health and vascular calcification, risks improving one domain at the expense of another, a tension explored throughout this chapter's treatment of specific phosphate binder and vitamin D therapy choices and developed most fully in this chapter's final section connecting mineral management explicitly to overall cardiovascular risk.

KEY POINT: FGF23 rises well before serum phosphate becomes overtly elevated, and progressive parathyroid hyperplasia becomes less responsive to medical suppression over time, meaning earlier intervention in the CKD-MBD trajectory generally achieves more durable biochemical control than delayed intervention.

Figure 23.1: The FGF23-Klotho-Parathyroid Hormone Axis in CKD Progression

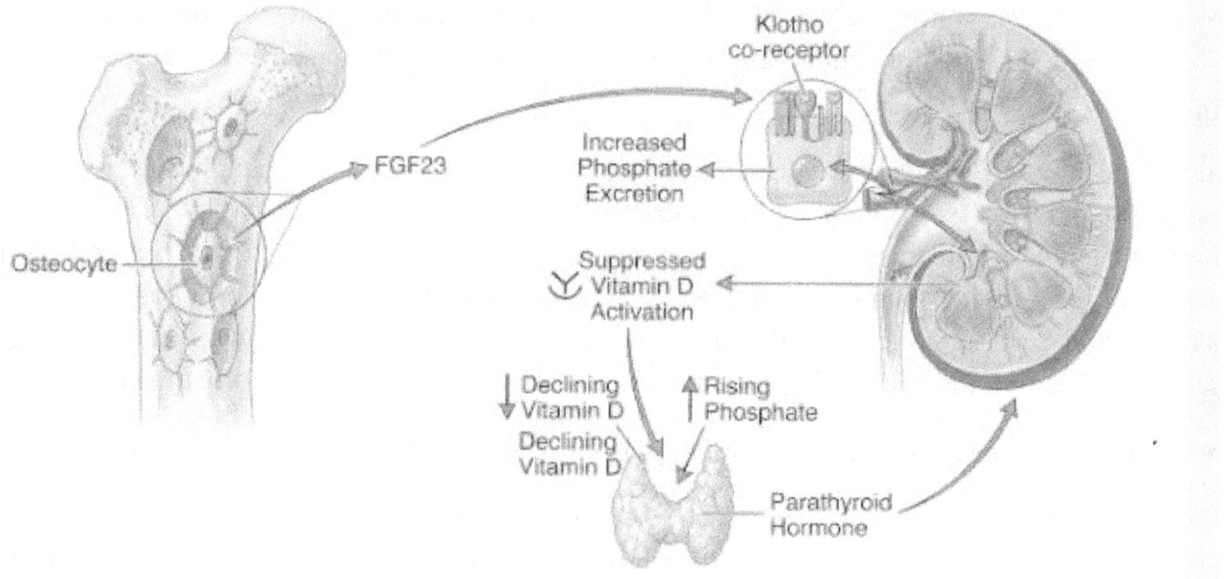

Phosphate Binders and Dietary Phosphate Control

Dietary Phosphate Sources and Patient Education

Dietary phosphate exists in two functionally distinct forms with markedly different intestinal absorption characteristics: organic phosphate, naturally present in protein-rich foods and absorbed at a variable, generally incomplete rate depending on the specific food source, and inorganic phosphate, added to many processed and packaged foods as a preservative or flavor enhancer and absorbed at a considerably higher, near-complete rate regardless of the food's overall nutritional profile; patient education distinguishing these two forms, rather than treating all dietary phosphate as equivalent, allows more effective dietary counseling than a generic instruction to simply reduce protein intake, which would unnecessarily restrict a nutritionally important food category while potentially overlooking the more concentrated, more completely absorbed inorganic phosphate hidden in processed food additives.

Reading food labels specifically for phosphate-containing additives, identifiable by their chemical names rather than the word phosphate necessarily appearing explicitly, is a practical skill this book's patient education throughout has emphasized should be taught explicitly rather than assumed to be intuitive, and a dietitian with specific training in this distinction, working directly with patients on practical label-reading and food selection strategies, achieves more effective phosphate control through dietary counseling alone than general verbal advice to avoid high-phosphate foods without this specific, actionable guidance.

Restaurant and convenience food consumption, common across the general population and no less common among dialysis patients balancing treatment schedules against work and family obligations, presents a particular phosphate control challenge given the difficulty of verifying additive content in food prepared outside a labeled retail package, and practical counseling addressing this specific real-world eating pattern, rather than assuming all dietary counseling occurs in the context of home-prepared, label-readable food, better serves patients whose actual eating patterns include a meaningful proportion of food from these less transparent sources.

Plant-based versus animal-based protein sources also differ meaningfully in phosphate bioavailability despite sometimes similar total phosphate content on a nutrient composition table, since phosphate bound within phytate in plant-based foods is less completely absorbed by the human digestive tract, which lacks substantial phytase activity, relative to the more readily bioavailable phosphate in animal-based protein sources; this distinction offers a further practical dietary counseling consideration beyond the organic-versus-inorganic distinction already discussed, particularly relevant for a patient incorporating more plant-based protein sources into their diet for other health or personal reasons.

Calcium-Based Phosphate Binders

Calcium-based phosphate binders, taken with meals to bind dietary phosphate within the gut lumen before it can be absorbed, are effective and inexpensive but carry a recognized risk of contributing to positive calcium balance and, correspondingly, to the vascular calcification discussed later in this chapter, particularly when used at higher doses or in combination with active vitamin D therapy that independently increases intestinal calcium absorption; this calcium-load consideration has driven a shift in many contemporary practice settings toward limiting total calcium-based binder dose and favoring non-calcium-based alternatives, discussed next, particularly for patients with evidence of vascular calcification or low bone turnover already present.

Timing of calcium-based binder administration relative to meals matters practically for effectiveness: a binder taken well before or after a meal, rather than with the meal itself, has little phosphate to bind at the time it is present in the gut and passing through, and patient education on this specific timing point, seemingly a minor practical detail, directly affects whether a prescribed binder actually achieves its intended phosphate-binding effect in practice.

Calcium acetate and calcium carbonate, the two most commonly used calcium-based binder formulations, differ somewhat in their elemental calcium content and phosphate-binding capacity per unit dose, and a patient switching between these two specific formulations, whether for cost, tolerability, or formulary reasons, should have their prescribed dose adjusted accordingly rather than assuming a simple one-to-one tablet substitution provides equivalent phosphate binding, since this assumption could result in either inadequate phosphate control or an unintended increase in total calcium exposure depending on the direction of the substitution.

Non-Calcium-Based Phosphate Binders

Non-calcium-based phosphate binders, including sevelamer and lanthanum carbonate among others, avoid the calcium load calcium-based binders impose while achieving comparable phosphate-binding efficacy, and comparative studies have shown reduced vascular calcification progression with non-calcium-based binders relative to calcium-based binders in several though not all study populations, supporting their preferential use in patients at elevated calcification risk, including those with pre-existing vascular calcification evident on imaging obtained for other clinical indications.

Cost and pill burden considerations favor calcium-based binders in some patients and practice settings, since non-calcium-based alternatives are generally more expensive and, for some specific formulations, require a larger number of tablets to achieve comparable phosphate-binding capacity; selecting among available binders therefore requires weighing calcification risk, cost, insurance coverage, and pill burden together for an individual patient rather than applying a single preferred binder uniformly across an entire practice's patient population regardless of these individualizing factors.

Adherence considerations deserve particular attention in binder selection given the substantial pill burden phosphate binders of any category typically impose, often requiring multiple tablets with every meal across an entire day, and a patient's actual, honestly reported adherence pattern, rather than an assumption of full adherence based on the prescribed regimen alone, should inform interpretation of phosphate control that appears inadequate despite an apparently appropriate binder prescription; exploring adherence barriers directly and non-judgmentally, following the same person-centered approach this book has applied throughout its treatment of medication and dietary adherence, often reveals a more actionable explanation than assuming the prescribed binder regimen itself is simply insufficient.

Binder Category	Example Agents	Key Advantage	Key Consideration
Calcium-Based	Calcium carbonate, calcium acetate	Inexpensive, effective	Positive calcium balance risk; limit total dose
Sevelamer	Sevelamer carbonate	No calcium load; some LDL-lowering effect	Higher cost; larger pill burden in some formulations
Lanthanum	Lanthanum carbonate	No calcium load; effective at lower pill burden	Higher cost; long-term tissue deposition monitored

Vitamin D and Parathyroid Hormone Management

Native and Active Vitamin D Therapy

Native vitamin D, either ergocalciferol or cholecalciferol, requires two sequential hydroxylation steps to become fully active, the first in the liver and the second in the kidney, and this second, kidney-dependent activation step is progressively impaired as kidney function declines, meaning native vitamin D supplementation alone becomes progressively less effective at raising active vitamin D levels as chronic kidney disease advances, even when the more commonly measured storage form of vitamin D shows adequate or even robust correction with supplementation.

Active vitamin D analogs, including calcitriol and other synthetic analogs designed to retain vitamin D receptor activation while reducing some of calcitriol's intestinal calcium and phosphate absorption effects, bypass this impaired renal activation step directly, suppressing parathyroid hormone secretion through direct vitamin D receptor activation on the parathyroid gland itself; these agents carry their own risk of increasing intestinal calcium and, to a lesser degree depending on the specific analog, phosphate absorption, requiring the same calcium-balance and vascular calcification considerations discussed earlier in this chapter to inform dosing and monitoring.

Selective vitamin D receptor activators, designed to preferentially activate vitamin D receptors on the parathyroid gland relative to those in the intestine, aim to suppress PTH with proportionally less intestinal calcium and phosphate absorption increase than older, less selective analogs, though this selectivity is relative rather than absolute, and calcium and phosphate monitoring remains essential even when using an agent marketed for its selective activation profile, since clinically meaningful calcium and phosphate absorption increases can still occur, particularly at higher doses.

Calcimimetics

Calcimimetic agents, acting on the calcium-sensing receptor on parathyroid cells to increase its sensitivity to circulating calcium and thereby suppress parathyroid hormone secretion through a mechanism entirely distinct from vitamin D receptor activation, offer a complementary or alternative approach to secondary hyperparathyroidism management specifically advantageous in that they suppress parathyroid hormone without the calcium and phosphate absorption increase active vitamin D analogs carry, and in some formulations may modestly lower rather than raise serum calcium, an advantage for a patient whose calcium level or vascular calcification risk argues against further active vitamin D dose escalation.

Combination therapy, using both a calcimimetic and an active vitamin D analog at more modest individual doses than either agent would require used alone, allows the complementary suppressive mechanisms to work together, often achieving better parathyroid hormone control at a lower cumulative calcium and phosphate burden than escalating either single agent alone to achieve the same degree of suppression, illustrating a combination-therapy principle with parallels to the multimodal prevention bundles this book has recommended in other treatment domains, including the intradialytic hypotension prevention strategy detailed in Chapter 13.

Gastrointestinal side effects, including nausea, represent the most common tolerability concern with calcimimetic therapy, and dose titration beginning at a lower starting dose with gradual escalation as tolerated, rather than initiating at a higher target dose immediately, improves overall treatment tolerability and adherence; a patient who discontinues calcimimetic therapy prematurely due to poorly managed initial gastrointestinal side effects loses the therapeutic benefit this agent could otherwise provide, making this practical titration consideration as clinically consequential as the mechanistic rationale for the agent's use in the first place.

Individualizing PTH Targets

Contemporary parathyroid hormone target guidance favors a range rather than a single numeric target, and, importantly, favors trending PTH over time rather than reacting to any single measurement, reflecting both PTH's substantial intra-individual assay and biological variability and the recognition, paralleling this book's treatment of hemodialysis and peritoneal dialysis adequacy in Chapters 7 and 18, that a single aggressive target pursued uniformly does not necessarily produce better outcomes than an individualized range accounting for a patient's specific bone turnover status and overall clinical picture.

Age and life expectancy considerations, paralleling the frailty-adjusted, individualized reasoning this book applied to older dialysis patients in Chapter 26, warrant explicit incorporation into PTH target setting: an older patient with limited life expectancy may derive less net benefit from aggressive PTH suppression aimed primarily at preventing fracture and vascular calcification consequences that typically manifest over years to decades, relative to a younger patient with a longer anticipated treatment horizon over which these cumulative benefits would have more time to accrue, supporting a more individualized rather than uniform approach to target-setting across a dialysis unit's full age spectrum of patients.

Over-suppression of parathyroid hormone, whether through excessive active vitamin D or calcimimetic dosing, risks adynamic bone disease, a low-turnover state discussed further in this chapter's treatment of renal osteodystrophy subtypes, in which bone becomes unable to adequately buffer calcium and phosphate loads, paradoxically worsening rather than improving the vascular calcification risk this chapter's mineral management is ultimately intended to reduce; this risk of over-suppression is a direct argument against treating a lower PTH as uniformly better and for the individualized, range-based target approach this subsection recommends.

CAUTION: Over-suppression of parathyroid hormone risks adynamic bone disease, a low-turnover state that paradoxically worsens vascular calcification risk; a lower PTH is not uniformly better, and an individualized, range-based target should guide therapy rather than pursuing maximal suppression.

Vascular Calcification and Renal Osteodystrophy

Mechanisms of Vascular Calcification

Vascular calcification in chronic kidney disease proceeds through an active, cell-mediated process rather than passive mineral deposition alone: vascular smooth muscle cells undergo phenotypic transformation toward an osteoblast-like state under the influence of elevated phosphate, uremic toxins, and the mineral and hormonal disturbances discussed throughout this chapter, actively depositing calcium-phosphate mineral within the vessel wall in a manner mechanistically analogous to normal bone formation occurring in the distinctly wrong location.

This active mechanism explains why vascular calcification, once thought to be an inevitable, irreversible consequence of aging accelerated by kidney disease, is now understood as a potentially modifiable process responsive to the same mineral management interventions detailed throughout this chapter, and why the phosphate binder selection, vitamin D and calcimimetic dosing, and PTH target individualization this chapter has developed all carry direct relevance to vascular calcification risk rather than being relevant to bone health alone in isolation from the vascular consequences this section addresses.

Matrix Gla protein and fetuin-A, endogenous circulating calcification inhibitors whose activity depends on adequate vitamin K status and whose levels or function may be reduced in chronic kidney disease, represent a further mechanistic layer in vascular calcification pathophysiology beyond the direct phosphate and mineral effects already discussed, and this inhibitor-deficiency pathway has generated research interest in vitamin K supplementation as a potential adjunctive calcification-prevention strategy, though this approach remains investigational rather than an established standard of care recommendation at this time, and clinicians should distinguish this promising but still-developing research direction from the well-established phosphate binder and PTH management strategies this chapter has already detailed as current standard practice.

Coronary artery calcification scoring, obtained through dedicated cardiac computed tomography imaging, provides a quantitative, reproducible measure of this calcification burden that can be tracked over time in patients at particular risk, though routine, universal screening with this specific imaging modality is not currently recommended given cost and radiation exposure considerations relative to its incremental value beyond the clinical risk factors and biochemical trends this chapter has already emphasized; selective use in patients whose overall risk profile or clinical trajectory raises specific concern remains a reasonable, individualized application of this imaging tool rather than a routine, universal screening recommendation.

Renal Osteodystrophy Subtypes

Renal osteodystrophy encompasses a spectrum of bone histological abnormalities ranging from high-turnover disease, most commonly osteitis fibrosa related to longstanding, poorly controlled secondary hyperparathyroidism, through low-turnover adynamic bone disease, discussed earlier in this chapter as a risk of PTH over-suppression, to mixed patterns combining features of both; bone biopsy remains the definitive diagnostic method for distinguishing these subtypes but is invasive and infrequently performed in routine practice, meaning clinical management often proceeds based on the broader biochemical and clinical picture rather than histological confirmation in most patients.

A seventy-year-old woman on hemodialysis for six years with a PTH suppressed well below her target range following aggressive calcimimetic and active vitamin D therapy develops new bone pain and is found to have a rising alkaline phosphatase inconsistent with her low PTH, prompting her nephrology team to suspect adynamic bone disease from over-suppression rather than the high-turnover disease her biochemical trend alone might otherwise suggest. Her calcimimetic and vitamin D doses are reduced to allow PTH to rise back into her individualized target range, and her bone pain improves over the following months as her bone turnover normalizes. This case illustrates why PTH suppression should be targeted to an individualized range rather than pursued maximally, and why new symptoms in a patient with a very low PTH should prompt consideration of adynamic bone disease specifically rather than assuming a low PTH is uniformly reassuring.

CLINICAL PEARL: New bone pain or fracture in a patient with a markedly suppressed PTH should prompt consideration of adynamic bone disease from over-suppression, rather than assuming a low PTH value is uniformly reassuring for bone health.

Integrating Mineral Management With Overall Cardiovascular Risk

Because vascular calcification contributes directly to the cardiovascular disease burden discussed in Chapter 24, and because several of this chapter's specific management decisions, including calcium-based binder use and active vitamin D dosing, carry direct calcification-risk trade-offs, CKD-MBD management should be considered an integral component of a patient's overall cardiovascular risk management rather than a separate, biochemistry-focused domain addressed in isolation from the cardiovascular considerations Chapter 24 develops in full.

A structured periodic review integrating phosphate, calcium, PTH, and vitamin D trends alongside any available vascular calcification imaging and the patient's overall cardiovascular risk profile provides a more complete basis for mineral management decisions than reviewing biochemical values in isolation, extending the same whole-patient, integrated assessment principle this book has applied throughout to hemodialysis and peritoneal dialysis adequacy in Chapters 7 and 18 and to anemia management in Chapter 22.

DIALYSIS RECOGNITION & RESPONSE SYSTEM — Mineral Bone Disorder Arcs

The Pattern: A patient with markedly suppressed PTH develops new bone pain or an unexpected fracture.

Stem Signature: New bone pain, an unexpected fracture, or a rising alkaline phosphatase inconsistent with a very low PTH, in a patient receiving aggressive calcimimetic or active vitamin D therapy that has suppressed PTH well below the individualized target range.

The Decision: Consider adynamic bone disease from PTH over-suppression as the explanation, reduce calcimimetic and vitamin D dosing to allow PTH to rise back into the individualized target range, and monitor for symptomatic improvement rather than assuming the low PTH value is reassuring.

Trap Logic: A very low PTH can be interpreted as a treatment success, when in fact over-suppression itself produces adynamic bone disease with its own distinct symptom burden and paradoxically worsened vascular calcification risk relative to a PTH maintained within the individualized target range.

Response Anchor: New bone pain or fracture with a markedly suppressed PTH warrants considering adynamic bone disease and reducing suppressive therapy — not reassurance that a low PTH value reflects successful treatment.

New Bone Pain or Fracture With Markedly Suppressed PTH: Consider adynamic bone disease from over-suppression and reduce suppressive therapy to allow PTH to rise back into the individualized target range.

Summary and Key Concepts

FGF23 rises early in chronic kidney disease as a compensatory phosphaturic signal, and progressive Klotho decline and parathyroid hyperplasia drive secondary hyperparathyroidism as this compensation becomes insufficient.

Dietary phosphate education should distinguish organic from inorganic, additive-based phosphate given their markedly different absorption rates, and phosphate binder selection should weigh calcification risk, cost, and pill burden together for an individual patient.

Active vitamin D and calcimimetics suppress parathyroid hormone through distinct mechanisms and can be combined to achieve better control at lower cumulative calcium and phosphate burden than escalating either agent alone.

PTH targets should be individualized to a range and trended over time rather than reacted to as a single value, since over-suppression risks adynamic bone disease that paradoxically worsens vascular calcification risk.

Vascular calcification proceeds through an active, cell-mediated process responsive to mineral management interventions, and CKD-MBD management should be integrated with overall cardiovascular risk assessment rather than treated as a separate biochemical domain.

CHAPTER 24: CARDIOVASCULAR DISEASE AND FLUID MANAGEMENT IN DIALYSIS PATIENTS

Learning Objectives

Describe the cardiovascular risk burden in the dialysis population, including traditional and uremia-specific risk factors.

Apply volume assessment methods and dry weight determination as an ongoing, periodically reassessed process.

Distinguish volume-dependent from volume-independent hypertension and individualize antihypertensive management accordingly.

Recognize heart failure phenotypes and pericardial disease patterns specific to kidney failure and integrate cardiology and nephrology care.

Chapter Overview

Cardiovascular disease is the leading cause of death in the dialysis population, exceeding infection, malignancy, and every other cause combined in most epidemiologic accounts of dialysis mortality. This chapter, following anemia in Chapter 22 and mineral and bone disorder in Chapter 23, addresses the cardiovascular complications that these two preceding chapters have already shown to be mechanistically intertwined with kidney failure's broader systemic burden, drawing together threads this book has introduced piecemeal across many earlier chapters, including intradialytic hemodynamic instability in Chapter 13, vascular calcification in Chapter 23, and access-related high-output cardiac effects in Chapter 11, into a single, integrated cardiovascular framework. This chapter works through the population's distinctive risk burden, the volume assessment and dry weight determination process that sits at the center of both hemodynamic stability and long-term cardiovascular risk, hypertension management adapted to this population's specific physiology, and the heart failure and pericardial disease patterns kidney failure produces.

Cardiovascular Risk Burden on Dialysis

Epidemiology of Cardiovascular Disease in Dialysis

Cardiovascular mortality in dialysis-dependent patients substantially exceeds that of an age- and sex-matched general population, with the relative risk increase most pronounced in younger dialysis patients, whose cardiovascular mortality can approach that of a general population several decades older; this age-independent excess risk reflects the accelerated cardiovascular aging kidney failure appears to impose, a phenomenon incompletely explained by traditional cardiovascular risk factors alone and increasingly attributed to the uremia-specific mechanisms detailed in the next subsection.

This excess risk is present even before dialysis initiation, detectable across the chronic kidney disease trajectory discussed in Chapter 1, and progresses rather than resolves once dialysis begins, indicating that dialysis itself, despite correcting the uremic and volume derangements that would otherwise be fatal, does not fully arrest the cardiovascular injury processes chronic kidney disease has already set in motion; this observation has shaped a research and clinical focus on earlier cardiovascular risk modification throughout the chronic kidney disease trajectory rather than deferring cardiovascular attention until dialysis dependence has already developed.

Cardiovascular mortality risk also varies meaningfully by dialysis vintage, the duration a patient has been treated, with the highest relative risk often observed in the earliest months following dialysis initiation, a period during which the physiologic adjustment to treatment itself, alongside whatever acute illness may have precipitated urgent initiation in some patients, compounds the more chronic cardiovascular risk this chapter otherwise addresses; recognizing this early, vintage-dependent risk elevation supports particularly close cardiovascular monitoring and volume management attention during a patient's first several months of dialysis dependence specifically.

Traditional and Uremia-Specific Risk Factors

Traditional cardiovascular risk factors, including diabetes, hypertension, dyslipidemia, and smoking, remain highly prevalent in the dialysis population and contribute to cardiovascular risk through the same atherosclerotic mechanisms operating in the general population, but traditional risk factor burden alone does not fully explain the magnitude of excess cardiovascular risk this population carries, motivating substantial research attention toward uremia-specific mechanisms operating largely independent of, or synergistically with, these traditional factors.

Vascular calcification, discussed at length in Chapter 23, chronic volume overload and the left ventricular hypertrophy it produces, chronic inflammation from the uremic milieu and recurrent access-related or other infections discussed throughout Part III of this book, and the intradialytic hemodynamic stress and myocardial stunning discussed in Chapter 13 together constitute a uremia-specific cardiovascular injury pathway operating alongside, and interacting with, the traditional risk factors familiar from general cardiovascular medicine; this dual-pathway model, traditional plus uremia-specific, is essential to understanding why cardiovascular risk reduction strategies proven effective in the general population, such as intensive statin therapy, have shown more limited benefit in randomized trials conducted specifically in the dialysis population, since a treatment targeting only the traditional, atherosclerotic pathway leaves the uremia-specific pathway's contribution to risk entirely unaddressed.

Lipid management specifically illustrates this dual-pathway complexity: while dyslipidemia remains a traditional risk factor of clear relevance, the specific lipid abnormalities characteristic of advanced kidney disease differ somewhat from the pattern typical of the general population, and statin trials conducted specifically in dialysis populations have generally shown more modest cardiovascular benefit than the same agents demonstrate in non-dialysis populations, a finding that has shaped more selective, individualized statin use in this population rather than uniform, guideline-driven prescription based solely on traditional lipid targets extrapolated from general population evidence.

Sudden Cardiac Death in the Dialysis Population

Sudden cardiac death accounts for a disproportionate share of cardiovascular mortality in the dialysis population relative to the general population, and its risk shows a distinctive temporal pattern clustering around the dialysis treatment itself and the interdialytic interval surrounding it, particularly the extended weekend gap discussed in Chapter 20's treatment of intensive hemodialysis schedules, implicating the rapid electrolyte and volume shifts this book has described throughout Part II as direct contributors to this specific, acutely fatal outcome rather than sudden cardiac death occurring randomly with respect to the treatment cycle.

This treatment-cycle-linked pattern connects directly to several of this book's earlier chapters: the hyperkalemia-related arrhythmia risk detailed in Chapter 15, the dialysate potassium individualization principles developed in Chapter 6, and the intensive hemodialysis schedule modifications discussed in Chapter 20 that reduce the peak-to-trough electrolyte and volume swings implicated in this sudden cardiac death pattern; recognizing sudden cardiac death as substantially treatment-cycle-related, rather than an unpredictable, unrelated event, reframes several of this book's earlier prescription and scheduling discussions as cardiovascular risk reduction strategies in their own right, not merely as measures addressing intradialytic symptoms or adequacy alone.

Autonomic dysfunction, common in the dialysis population and related to both the uremic milieu and the structural cardiac changes this chapter has documented, further compounds sudden cardiac death risk by impairing the normal compensatory heart rate and vascular tone responses that would otherwise help buffer against the rapid electrolyte and volume shifts of treatment, and assessment of heart rate variability, while not yet a routine clinical test in most dialysis practice settings, has shown research promise as a potential risk-stratification tool identifying patients at particularly elevated sudden cardiac death risk who might benefit from especially close monitoring around the treatment cycle.

KEY POINT: Sudden cardiac death risk clusters around the dialysis treatment cycle and the extended interdialytic interval, implicating rapid electrolyte and volume shifts directly and reframing dialysate potassium individualization and intensive scheduling as cardiovascular risk reduction strategies in their own right.

Figure 24.1: Temporal Clustering of Sudden Cardiac Death Around the Dialysis Cycle

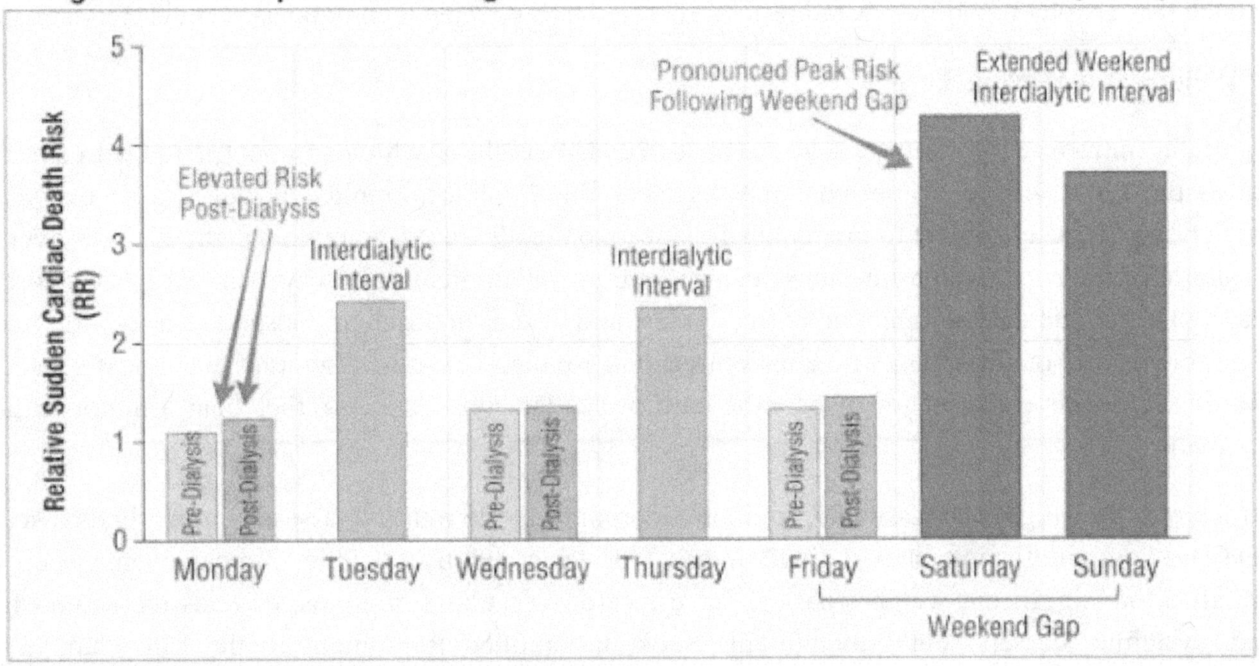

Volume Assessment and Dry Weight Determination

Clinical and Objective Volume Assessment Methods

Volume assessment in the dialysis population, introduced in Chapter 4 and revisited throughout this book's treatment of intradialytic hypotension in Chapter 13 and peritoneal dialysis volume management in Chapter 18, combines physical examination findings including jugular venous pressure, peripheral edema, and pulmonary auscultation with objective adjuncts including bioimpedance spectroscopy and point-of-care ultrasound assessment of inferior vena cava characteristics, and this chapter's cardiovascular framing adds a further dimension to why this assessment matters: chronic volume overload, beyond its acute symptomatic consequences, drives the left ventricular hypertrophy and hypertension that constitute major independent contributors to the cardiovascular mortality this chapter's opening section documented.

Natriuretic peptide levels, while used more cautiously in the dialysis population than in patients with normal kidney function given reduced renal clearance elevating baseline levels independent of volume status, can still provide useful trend information when interpreted against a given patient's own established baseline rather than the general population reference ranges these assays were originally validated against, offering a further complementary data point alongside the clinical and imaging-based assessment methods already discussed.

Lung ultrasound, assessing B-line count as a marker of pulmonary interstitial fluid, has emerged as a further point-of-care volume assessment tool with growing evidence supporting its use in the dialysis population, offering a complementary window into volume status distinct from the cardiac-focused inferior vena cava assessment already discussed, and incorporating this technique where available and where staff have received appropriate training adds a further data point to the multi-method assessment approach this chapter recommends rather than relying on any single technique as sufficient in isolation.

Dry Weight as a Moving Target

Dry weight, introduced in Chapter 4 as the post-dialysis weight at which a patient is judged euvolemic, requires the same scheduled, periodic reassessment this book has applied throughout to every other prescription parameter subject to gradual drift, since a patient's true euvolemic weight changes over time with alterations in nutritional status, muscle mass, and overall clinical trajectory; a dry weight set correctly a year ago is not guaranteed to remain correct today, and the cardiovascular consequences of a dry weight that has drifted out of alignment with a patient's actual euvolemic status, discussed in the next subsection, make this reassessment a matter of genuine cardiovascular consequence rather than a minor technical adjustment.

A structured dry weight reassessment protocol, incorporating the multiple assessment methods discussed in the previous subsection at a defined interval or triggered by specific clinical events such as a hospitalization, significant weight change, or new cardiovascular symptoms, extends the same trigger-based, systemic reassessment principle this book has applied throughout to the Life-Plan, dialysis prescriptions, and vascular access surveillance into the specific domain of dry weight determination.

Consequences of Chronic Volume Mismanagement

A dry weight set too high leaves a patient in a state of chronic volume overload between treatments, contributing directly to the hypertension, left ventricular hypertrophy, and cardiovascular morbidity this chapter's opening sections have documented, often without the patient necessarily reporting overt symptoms on a day-to-day basis, since chronic, gradually accumulated overload can be considerably less symptomatic than the acute volume shifts this book has discussed in other contexts, making this consequence easy to under-recognize in the absence of the deliberate, scheduled assessment the previous subsection recommends.

A dry weight set too low, conversely, produces the recurrent intradialytic hypotension discussed extensively in Chapter 13, with its own independent cardiovascular consequences including the myocardial stunning and progressive cardiac injury that chapter documented; recognizing which of these two failure modes, chronic overload or chronic underfilling, a given patient's specific presentation reflects, rather than assuming volume overload is always the more likely explanation for any cardiovascular symptom, is essential to selecting the correct corrective direction for dry weight adjustment.

Muscle mass changes over time, whether from the protein-energy wasting discussed in Chapter 25 or from the frailty-related sarcopenia discussed in Chapter 26, directly affect the accuracy of a dry weight target that has not been recently reassessed, since a patient's true euvolemic weight declines as muscle mass declines even if fat mass and overall volume status remain otherwise stable, meaning a fixed dry weight target that fails to account for this muscle mass trajectory will gradually become inappropriately high relative to the patient's actual, evolving body composition, producing the chronic volume overload this section has already identified as a significant, often under-recognized cardiovascular risk.

CAUTION: Chronic volume overload from a dry weight set too high is often less symptomatic day-to-day than acute volume shifts, making it easy to under-recognize without deliberate, scheduled reassessment; a dry weight set too low produces its own distinct cardiovascular consequences through recurrent intradialytic hypotension.

Hypertension Management in the Dialysis Population

Volume-Dependent Versus Volume-Independent Hypertension

Volume-dependent hypertension, driven directly by the chronic volume overload discussed in the previous section, responds primarily to correcting dry weight and ultrafiltration adequacy rather than to antihypertensive medication escalation, and a patient whose hypertension responds substantially to a dry weight correction confirms this volume-dependent mechanism directly, while a patient whose blood pressure remains elevated despite confirmed euvolemia at an appropriately reassessed dry weight demonstrates a volume-independent component requiring the pharmacologic and other approaches discussed in this section.

Distinguishing these two hypertension patterns matters practically because treating volume-dependent hypertension with escalating antihypertensive medication alone, without addressing the underlying volume excess, both fails to address the root cause and risks the intradialytic hypotension discussed in Chapter 13 as antihypertensive medication effect compounds with the ultrafiltration-related volume shifts of treatment itself; this distinction is a specific application of the same trap-logic pattern this book has developed throughout, in which a downstream symptom is treated directly without first addressing an upstream, more fundamental cause the symptom is actually signaling.

Antihypertensive Medication Selection and Timing

Antihypertensive medication selection in the dialysis population should account for dialyzability, since some agents are substantially removed during hemodialysis treatment and may require dosing adjustment or timing around the treatment schedule to maintain consistent blood pressure control, while agents minimally cleared by dialysis provide more consistent, treatment-independent blood pressure coverage; this dialyzability consideration, an application of the same pharmacokinetic reasoning this book applied to symptom-management medication selection in Chapter 3, should inform both agent selection and dosing schedule for a dialysis-dependent patient specifically.

Medication timing relative to the dialysis treatment itself, discussed briefly in Chapter 13's treatment of intradialytic hypotension risk factors, deserves explicit attention here from the complementary hypertension-management perspective: a short-acting antihypertensive taken shortly before a scheduled treatment may compound intradialytic hypotension risk, as Chapter 13 detailed, while the same medication timed to a different point in the interdialytic interval may provide effective blood pressure control without this compounding risk, illustrating that medication timing, not merely selection and dose, is a genuine prescription variable in this population's hypertension management.

A structured medication timing chart, mapping each patient's specific antihypertensive regimen against their individual dialysis schedule and noting the rationale for each medication's specific timing, provides a practical, reviewable record supporting consistent implementation of this timing-aware prescribing approach across a unit's nursing and physician staff, extending the same structured, documented approach this book has recommended throughout for other individualized prescription parameters rather than relying on this timing rationale being retained only in an individual prescriber's memory.

Intradialytic Blood Pressure Patterns

Intradialytic hypertension, a paradoxical rise in blood pressure during treatment affecting a meaningful minority of patients rather than the more common hypotensive pattern this book has emphasized throughout Chapter 13, is associated with its own distinct adverse outcome profile and appears mechanistically related to endothelial dysfunction and volume-independent vasoconstrictive responses rather than the plasma-refilling-related mechanisms underlying intradialytic hypotension, representing a genuinely distinct clinical entity rather than simply the opposite end of a single hemodynamic instability spectrum.

Recognizing this pattern specifically, rather than assuming any intradialytic blood pressure abnormality must reflect the hypotension this book has discussed at greater length, matters because the appropriate response differs substantially: intradialytic hypertension does not respond to the ultrafiltration reduction and fluid administration measures Chapter 13 recommends for hypotension, and may in some cases actually worsen with these interventions if the underlying mechanism is genuinely volume-independent rather than related to inadequate fluid removal.

KEY POINT: Intradialytic hypertension is a distinct clinical entity from the more common intradialytic hypotension, with a different underlying mechanism and a correspondingly different management approach; it does not respond to, and may worsen with, the ultrafiltration and fluid measures used for hypotension.

Heart Failure and Pericardial Disease in Kidney Failure

Heart Failure With Preserved and Reduced Ejection Fraction in Dialysis

Heart failure with preserved ejection fraction, reflecting the diastolic dysfunction discussed in Chapter 13 as a major contributor to intradialytic hypotension risk, is the more common heart failure phenotype in the dialysis population, driven by the combination of hypertension, left ventricular hypertrophy, and chronic volume and pressure loading this chapter has documented throughout; this phenotype's management centers substantially on the volume and blood pressure control measures this chapter has already developed, since the diastolic dysfunction itself has fewer specific pharmacologic treatment options than the more extensively studied reduced ejection fraction phenotype.

Heart failure with reduced ejection fraction, while less common than the preserved ejection fraction phenotype in this population, still occurs at elevated frequency relative to the general population and benefits from the same guideline-directed medical therapy proven effective in heart failure more broadly, though several standard heart failure medications require dose adjustment or careful monitoring given reduced renal clearance or the hyperkalemia risk certain agent classes carry in a population already predisposed to potassium derangement, discussed extensively in Chapters 6 and 15.

Mineralocorticoid receptor antagonists, an increasingly important component of guideline-directed heart failure therapy in the general population, warrant particular caution in the dialysis population given their hyperkalemia risk in patients with minimal or absent residual urinary potassium excretion, and while some trial evidence supports their cautious use in carefully selected, closely monitored dialysis patients with reduced ejection fraction heart failure, this use requires closer potassium surveillance than would be typical in a patient with preserved native kidney function, following the same enhanced monitoring principle this book has applied throughout to medications carrying population-specific risk in kidney failure.

Uremic and Dialysis-Associated Pericarditis

Uremic pericarditis, introduced in Chapter 1 as an absolute indication for urgent dialysis initiation, can also occur in a patient already established on dialysis, termed dialysis-associated pericarditis, typically reflecting inadequate dialysis clearance or another intercurrent factor rather than the pre-initiation uremic toxin accumulation Chapter 1 addressed; recognizing this presentation in an established dialysis patient should prompt the same urgency Chapter 1 emphasized for the pre-initiation context, including assessment for tamponade physiology and consideration of intensified dialysis, since the underlying inflammatory process and its tamponade risk are shared between the two clinical scenarios regardless of whether the patient has already been established on dialysis.

A pericardial friction rub or new pleuritic chest pain in an established dialysis patient, rather than being attributed reflexively to a non-cardiac cause given the patient's already-established dialysis status, should prompt the same diagnostic evaluation Chapter 1 detailed, including echocardiography to assess effusion size and hemodynamic significance, since dialysis-associated pericarditis, while less common than the pre-initiation presentation, carries the same tamponade risk and the same urgency this book's earlier treatment of the condition established.

Integrating Cardiology and Nephrology Care

Given this chapter's demonstration that cardiovascular disease in the dialysis population arises from a combination of traditional and uremia-specific mechanisms, effective management requires genuine collaboration between cardiology and nephrology rather than either discipline managing cardiovascular risk in isolation from the other's specific expertise; a structured, regular communication pathway between a patient's nephrology and cardiology teams, rather than infrequent, siloed consultation, supports the kind of integrated management this chapter's whole-patient framework requires.

A sixty-one-year-old man on hemodialysis for three years with longstanding hypertension poorly controlled despite escalating antihypertensive therapy is referred for cardiology evaluation given new exertional dyspnea. Rather than further escalating his antihypertensive regimen alone, his nephrology team first reassesses his dry weight, applying the structured reassessment protocol detailed earlier in this chapter, and identifies that his estimated dry weight has not been formally reassessed in over a year despite a documented decline in his muscle mass over that period suggesting his true euvolemic weight has likely fallen. A trial dry weight reduction, implemented gradually and monitored closely for tolerance, results in substantial improvement in his blood pressure control and resolution of his exertional dyspnea without requiring further antihypertensive escalation, and his cardiology evaluation, completed in parallel, confirms preserved ejection fraction with findings consistent with hypertensive heart disease rather than an independent primary cardiac process. This case illustrates why volume-dependent hypertension should be actively considered and addressed through dry weight reassessment before escalating antihypertensive medication, and how collaborative nephrology-cardiology evaluation, pursued in parallel rather than sequentially, provided a more complete and more efficient path to this patient's actual underlying explanation.

His care team documents this outcome explicitly in his chart, including the specific dry weight reassessment findings that prompted the successful adjustment, ensuring that any future clinician reviewing his case understands the reasoning behind his current target rather than encountering only the numeric value without the clinical context that established it.

CLINICAL PEARL: Poorly controlled hypertension despite escalating antihypertensive therapy should prompt dry weight reassessment specifically, since volume-dependent hypertension responds to correcting the underlying volume excess rather than to further medication escalation alone.

DIALYSIS RECOGNITION & RESPONSE SYSTEM — Cardiovascular Risk Arcs

---

The Pattern: A patient's hypertension remains poorly controlled despite escalating antihypertensive medication.

Stem Signature: Persistently elevated blood pressure despite progressive antihypertensive dose escalation, in a patient whose dry weight has not been formally reassessed recently despite a plausible reason, such as declining muscle mass or weight change, to suspect it may no longer reflect true euvolemic status.

The Decision: Reassess dry weight using the structured, multi-method assessment approach this chapter details, and pursue a trial dry weight adjustment if reassessment suggests the current target no longer reflects true euvolemia, rather than continuing to escalate antihypertensive medication alone.

Trap Logic: Poorly controlled hypertension can prompt reflexive antihypertensive escalation without considering that the underlying driver may be volume-dependent, a mechanism that medication escalation alone will not resolve and that specifically responds to dry weight correction instead.

Response Anchor: Poorly controlled hypertension despite escalating medication warrants dry weight reassessment — not continued antihypertensive escalation alone without first considering a volume-dependent explanation.

DIALYSIS RECOGNITION & RESPONSE SYSTEM — Cardiovascular Risk Arcs

Poorly Controlled Hypertension Despite Escalating Medication: Reassess dry weight using a structured, multi-method approach and pursue a trial adjustment rather than continuing medication escalation alone.

Summary and Key Concepts

Cardiovascular mortality in the dialysis population substantially exceeds that of an age-matched general population, reflecting both traditional risk factors and uremia-specific mechanisms including vascular calcification, chronic volume overload, inflammation, and intradialytic hemodynamic stress.

Sudden cardiac death risk clusters around the dialysis treatment cycle and the extended interdialytic interval, reframing dialysate potassium individualization and intensive scheduling as direct cardiovascular risk reduction strategies.

Dry weight requires scheduled, periodic reassessment as a moving target, since both chronic overload and chronic underfilling carry distinct, independently significant cardiovascular consequences.

Volume-dependent hypertension should be distinguished from volume-independent hypertension and addressed through dry weight correction rather than antihypertensive escalation alone, and intradialytic hypertension is a distinct entity from intradialytic hypotension requiring a different management approach.

Heart failure with preserved ejection fraction is the more common phenotype in dialysis patients, uremic and dialysis-associated pericarditis carries the same tamponade urgency regardless of prior dialysis status, and integrated cardiology-nephrology care supports more complete management than either discipline acting in isolation.

CHAPTER 25: NUTRITION, INFECTION, AND HEPATITIS C IN THE DIALYSIS POPULATION

Learning Objectives

Define protein-energy wasting and apply nutritional assessment tools to distinguish malnutrition from inflammation in kidney failure.

Apply dietary protein, potassium, and phosphate recommendations individualized to hemodialysis and peritoneal dialysis.

Explain the dialysis population's elevated infection risk and apply recommended vaccination and infection prevention practices.

Describe hepatitis C prevalence, transmission risk, and direct-acting antiviral treatment in the dialysis population.

Chapter Overview

This chapter closes Part VII of this book, bringing together three domains that, while distinct in their specific clinical content, share a common thread: each reflects a systemic vulnerability that dialysis dependence imposes beyond the kidney failure itself. Protein-energy wasting, a nutritional syndrome distinct from simple undernutrition, affects a substantial proportion of dialysis patients and predicts mortality independent of other risk factors this book has discussed. Infection risk, elevated across nearly every category this book has addressed from vascular access in Part III to peritonitis in Chapter 19, warrants its own dedicated treatment of the population-level prevention strategies, vaccination, and infection control practices that reduce this elevated baseline risk. Hepatitis C, historically a major nosocomial risk within dialysis units specifically, has been transformed by direct-acting antiviral therapy from a chronic, largely unmanageable condition into a curable one, reshaping both the clinical and infection-control landscape this chapter addresses in its final section.

Readers arriving at this point will have now completed the full systemic and metabolic complication framework this book has developed across Part VII's four chapters: anemia in Chapter 22, mineral and bone disorder in Chapter 23, cardiovascular disease in Chapter 24, and now nutrition, infection, and hepatitis C here, each addressing a distinct clinical domain while sharing this book's consistent emphasis on individualized, trend-based assessment over uniform, one-size-fits-all management applied without regard for a specific patient's actual circumstances and trajectory.

Protein-Energy Wasting and Nutritional Assessment

Defining Protein-Energy Wasting in Kidney Failure

Protein-energy wasting describes a syndrome of depleted protein and energy stores in kidney failure driven by a combination of reduced dietary intake, often related to the uremic anorexia discussed in Chapter 1, chronic inflammation that independently promotes muscle catabolism, metabolic acidosis that similarly promotes protein breakdown, and the dialysis procedure itself, which removes amino acids and other nutrients alongside the uremic toxins it is intended to clear; this multifactorial origin distinguishes protein-energy wasting from simple caloric undernutrition, since addressing dietary intake alone, without addressing the inflammatory and metabolic contributors, frequently fails to reverse the syndrome.

Metabolic acidosis's specific contribution to protein-energy wasting deserves particular emphasis given its correctability: chronic, undertreated metabolic acidosis directly stimulates skeletal muscle protein degradation through activation of the ubiquitin-proteasome pathway, and correcting acidosis through adequate dialysis clearance, discussed in Chapters 7 and 18, or through oral bicarbonate supplementation where appropriate, addresses this specific catabolic driver directly rather than requiring nutritional intervention alone to overcome a metabolic process actively working against nutritional repletion efforts.

Protein-energy wasting is strongly and independently associated with mortality in the dialysis population, a finding replicated across numerous cohort studies and holding even after adjustment for the comorbidities that might otherwise be presumed to explain this association, underscoring that nutritional status deserves the same systematic, proactive attention this book has applied to every other major complication domain rather than being treated as a secondary concern addressed only once more overtly symptomatic problems have been managed.

The dose-response relationship between severity of protein-energy wasting and mortality risk, with even modest degrees of wasting associated with measurably increased risk relative to well-nourished patients, argues against a binary, present-or-absent conceptualization of this syndrome in favor of the same graded, trend-based severity assessment this book has applied throughout to other chronic complications, and this graded relationship supports intervening at the earliest identifiable signs of nutritional decline rather than reserving intervention for only the most severe, advanced presentations of protein-energy wasting.

Nutritional Assessment Tools and Markers

Serum albumin, while widely used as a nutritional marker given its ready availability on routine laboratory panels, is substantially confounded by inflammation, which independently suppresses hepatic albumin synthesis regardless of a patient's actual nutritional intake, meaning a low albumin in an inflamed patient does not necessarily indicate primary malnutrition and, conversely, a normal albumin does not exclude genuine nutritional compromise in a patient without significant concurrent inflammation; this confounding, familiar from this book's treatment of albumin as an imperfect adequacy marker in Chapters 7 and 18, applies with equal force to its use as a nutritional marker specifically.

The subjective global assessment, a structured clinical examination and history tool incorporating weight change, dietary intake history, gastrointestinal symptoms, functional capacity, and physical examination findings including muscle wasting and subcutaneous fat loss, provides a nutritional assessment less confounded by inflammation than albumin alone, and its routine, periodic application, rather than reliance on laboratory markers alone, supports more accurate identification of genuine protein-energy wasting; normalized protein catabolic rate, introduced in Chapter 7 as a byproduct calculation from routine hemodialysis adequacy blood work, provides a further, low-burden data point reflecting a patient's actual recent dietary protein intake.

Bioimpedance analysis, discussed in Chapter 24 primarily as a volume assessment tool, also provides body composition information, including estimated lean body mass and fat mass, that complements the subjective global assessment and biochemical markers already discussed, and this dual utility, volume status alongside body composition, makes bioimpedance a particularly efficient assessment tool where available, since a single measurement session can inform both the cardiovascular volume management discussed in Chapter 24 and the nutritional assessment this chapter addresses, rather than requiring separate, redundant assessment processes for these two related but distinct clinical purposes.

Serial tracking of these assessment measures over time, rather than a single evaluation at one point, allows a gradual nutritional decline to be recognized before it progresses to severe, more difficult-to-reverse protein-energy wasting, extending the same trend-based recognition principle this book has applied consistently throughout its treatment of dialysis adequacy, anemia management, and mineral bone disorder; a structured, scheduled nutritional reassessment interval, incorporating subjective global assessment alongside the relevant laboratory markers, should be built into routine dialysis unit workflow rather than performed only reactively once a patient's decline has already become clinically obvious through weight loss or overt physical wasting.

The Inflammation-Malnutrition Connection

The malnutrition-inflammation-atherosclerosis complex, a framework connecting protein-energy wasting to the chronic inflammatory state and accelerated cardiovascular disease discussed in Chapter 24, illustrates that nutritional status in kidney failure cannot be considered in isolation from the broader inflammatory and cardiovascular picture this book has developed throughout Part VII; a patient with protein-energy wasting frequently shows evidence of this interconnected complex rather than nutritional compromise as an isolated, independent finding, and management should address the inflammatory drive, where an identifiable and treatable source such as an occult infection exists, alongside direct nutritional support rather than pursuing nutritional intervention alone.

Recognizing an occult inflammatory source, including the vascular access infection and peritonitis sources this book has discussed extensively in Parts III and V, as a potential contributor to a patient's declining nutritional status extends the same structured, source-seeking evaluation this book recommended for ESA hyporesponsiveness in Chapter 22, since inflammation's effects on erythropoiesis and on nutritional status share overlapping mechanisms and often warrant a similar diagnostic approach when either presents without an obvious explanation.

This interconnection also has practical implications for how a unit organizes its multidisciplinary care: a dietitian working in isolation from the broader nephrology team, without visibility into a patient's recent infection history, dialysis adequacy trend, or inflammatory markers, is poorly positioned to distinguish primary dietary noncompliance from this broader inflammatory picture, whereas a dietitian integrated into regular multidisciplinary review, with access to this same clinical information the treating nephrologist reviews, can contribute more effectively to identifying which specific mechanism best explains a given patient's nutritional decline.

KEY POINT: Protein-energy wasting reflects a multifactorial syndrome connecting inflammation, metabolic acidosis, and reduced intake rather than simple caloric undernutrition alone; declining nutritional markers should prompt evaluation for an occult inflammatory source rather than dietary counseling alone.

Figure 25.1: The Malnutrition-Inflammation-Atherosclerosis Complex

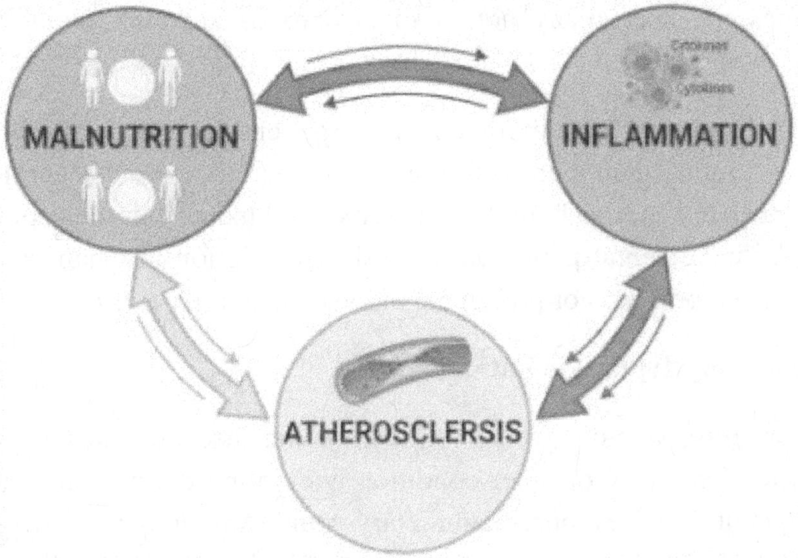

Dietary Management Across Modalities

Protein Requirements in Hemodialysis and Peritoneal Dialysis

Dietary protein requirements in dialysis-dependent patients exceed those recommended for the general population, reflecting both the amino acid losses dialysis itself imposes, discussed earlier in this chapter, and the elevated catabolic demands the uremic and inflammatory state places on protein metabolism; peritoneal dialysis patients require correspondingly higher protein intake than hemodialysis patients given the additional protein losses through the peritoneal membrane discussed in Chapter 16, a modality-specific distinction that should inform dietary counseling rather than applying an identical protein target across both modalities without this adjustment.

Practical protein target translation into actual food choices requires dietitian involvement given the potassium and phosphate considerations that accompany many high-protein foods, discussed earlier in this chapter and in Chapter 23 respectively, since a patient given only an abstract gram-based protein target without concrete food-level guidance may struggle to translate that target into an actual eating pattern that simultaneously meets protein needs while respecting individualized potassium and phosphate considerations, underscoring why this chapter has emphasized dietitian involvement as essential rather than optional throughout its treatment of dietary management.

Potassium and Fluid Restriction Individualization

Potassium restriction guidance should be individualized to a patient's actual predialysis potassium trend and residual kidney function discussed throughout this book, rather than applying a uniform restriction to every dialysis patient regardless of individual biochemical trajectory; a patient with substantial residual kidney function and consistently normal predialysis potassium may tolerate a considerably more liberal potassium intake than a patient with minimal residual function and recurrent hyperkalemia, and applying an unnecessarily restrictive diet to the former patient risks the same protein-energy wasting this chapter's opening sections addressed, since many potassium-rich foods are also valuable protein and nutrient sources.

Fluid restriction, similarly, should be individualized to a patient's actual interdialytic weight gain pattern and residual urine output rather than a uniform volume restriction applied regardless of these individual factors, and this individualized approach mirrors the same incremental, residual-function-aware reasoning this book developed for incremental peritoneal dialysis prescription in Chapter 17, now applied to the dietary fluid guidance a hemodialysis or peritoneal dialysis patient receives.

Nutritional Support for the Hyporexic Patient

A patient with poor appetite, whether from uremic anorexia discussed in Chapter 1, medication side effects, or an underlying depressive or other condition warranting the mental health attention this book has emphasized throughout, requires more than dietary counseling alone: identifying and addressing the specific underlying cause of reduced appetite, where identifiable, alongside oral nutritional supplementation and, in more severe or refractory cases, more intensive nutritional support, provides a more complete approach than dietary advice alone directed at a patient whose fundamental barrier is reduced appetite rather than inadequate nutritional knowledge.

Oral nutritional supplements, formulated specifically for the dialysis population's altered electrolyte and fluid tolerance relative to general population supplement formulations, provide a practical intervention for a patient with inadequate dietary intake despite appropriate underlying-cause evaluation and management, and involving a renal dietitian specifically, rather than a general nutrition consultation without this population-specific expertise, ensures supplementation recommendations account for the phosphate, potassium, and fluid considerations this chapter and Chapter 23 have both emphasized.

A sixty-eight-year-old man on hemodialysis for two years shows progressive weight loss and declining albumin over three months, initially attributed to dietary noncompliance and addressed with repeated dietary counseling alone without improvement. A more structured evaluation, incorporating subjective global assessment and a review for occult inflammatory sources following this chapter's recommended approach, identifies no infectious source but does reveal significant depressive symptoms accompanied by profound anorexia that the patient had not previously disclosed. Referral for mental health evaluation and treatment, alongside continued nutritional support, results in gradual improvement in both his mood and his nutritional trajectory over the following months. This case illustrates why declining nutritional status warrants evaluation for the full range of contributing factors this chapter has discussed, including mental health conditions affecting appetite, rather than assuming dietary noncompliance or an inflammatory process must be the explanation whenever dietary counseling alone fails to reverse a nutritional decline.

Nutrient	General Population Guidance	Dialysis-Specific Consideration
Protein	Standard population intake	Increased requirement; higher still in peritoneal dialysis given membrane losses
Potassium	No specific restriction typically needed	Individualized to residual function and predialysis trend, not uniformly restricted
Fluid	No specific restriction typically needed	Individualized to interdialytic weight gain and residual urine output
Phosphate	No specific restriction typically needed	Individualized per Chapter 23, distinguishing organic from inorganic additive sources

Infection Risk and Vaccination in Dialysis Patients

Immune Dysfunction in Kidney Failure

Kidney failure produces a state of both immune activation and immune deficiency simultaneously, a seemingly paradoxical combination in which chronic inflammation, discussed throughout this chapter and Chapter 22, coexists with impaired neutrophil function, reduced lymphocyte responsiveness, and blunted vaccine response relative to the general population; this combined dysfunction explains both the elevated infection risk this population carries and the comparatively reduced, though still clinically meaningful, protection vaccination provides relative to the protection the same vaccines afford in immunocompetent individuals.

This immune dysfunction compounds the more mechanical infection risk factors this book has discussed throughout, including the vascular access breach discussed in Part III and the peritoneal catheter breach discussed in Part V, meaning a dialysis patient's elevated infection risk reflects both an impaired host defense and multiple recurring opportunities for pathogen entry, a combination that argues for layering multiple complementary prevention strategies, discussed throughout this section, rather than relying on any single intervention alone.

Uremic toxin accumulation itself directly impairs neutrophil oxidative burst and phagocytic capacity, mechanisms distinct from but additive to the chronic inflammatory state already discussed, and this direct toxin-mediated immune impairment provides a further rationale, beyond the mechanical infection-risk factors this book has emphasized throughout Parts III and V, for why adequate dialysis clearance itself, discussed in Chapters 7 and 18, contributes to infection risk reduction as a byproduct of its primary uremic toxin removal function, extending the connection this chapter has drawn between dialysis adequacy and the broader systemic complications Part VII addresses.

Lymphocyte subset abnormalities, including reduced naive T-cell populations and accelerated immune senescence relative to age-matched individuals without kidney failure, have been documented in the dialysis population and may partly explain why this population's infection risk and vaccine hyporesponsiveness persist despite otherwise adequate nutritional status and dialysis adequacy, suggesting that immune dysfunction in kidney failure reflects a genuine, only partially reversible consequence of the uremic environment rather than a fully correctable downstream effect of the other complications this book has addressed throughout Part VII.

Recommended Vaccinations and Timing

Hepatitis B vaccination, using the higher-dose formulation specifically recommended for the dialysis population given this population's blunted vaccine response discussed above, along with influenza, pneumococcal, and other routinely recommended adult vaccinations following current national guidance, together constitute the core vaccination program every dialysis unit should implement systematically rather than relying on opportunistic, inconsistent vaccination during otherwise unrelated clinical encounters.

Vaccination timing relative to dialysis treatment itself deserves specific attention: administering vaccines toward the end of a hemodialysis session, rather than at the start, avoids the theoretical though likely modest concern of the treatment itself affecting vaccine antigen distribution, and a structured vaccination tracking system, integrated into a unit's routine workflow rather than dependent on individual clinician memory, ensures each patient's vaccination status remains current and that due vaccinations are administered promptly rather than delayed indefinitely amid the many other demands a busy dialysis unit's clinical workflow presents.

Infection Prevention Practices in the Dialysis Unit

Hand hygiene, surface disinfection between patients, and appropriate personal protective equipment use collectively constitute the foundational infection prevention practices every dialysis unit should apply consistently, and these practices carry particular importance in the dialysis unit's specific shared treatment environment, where multiple patients receive treatment in close physical proximity, often with shared equipment surfaces, over an extended treatment session that provides considerable opportunity for pathogen transmission if these basic practices are not applied rigorously and consistently.

Structured surveillance for infection clusters across a unit's patient population, extending the same clustering-assessment principle this book developed for water treatment contamination in Chapter 5 and pyrogenic reactions in Chapter 14, helps identify a unit-level infection control lapse before it produces a larger outbreak, and this surveillance should specifically track bloodborne pathogen status, discussed in the next section, given the particular consequences a bloodborne pathogen transmission event within a dialysis unit can carry.

KEY POINT: Kidney failure produces combined immune activation and immune deficiency, blunting vaccine response while elevating infection risk; hepatitis B vaccination uses a higher-dose formulation specifically for this population, and structured tracking ensures vaccination status remains current.

Hepatitis C and Bloodborne Pathogen Management

Hepatitis C Epidemiology and Transmission in Dialysis

Hepatitis C prevalence in the dialysis population has historically exceeded general population rates substantially, reflecting nosocomial transmission risk within the shared dialysis treatment environment before contemporary infection control practices, including the dedicated equipment and isolation approaches discussed later in this section, became standard; transmission risk within a dialysis unit relates primarily to breaches in standard infection control practice, including inadequate equipment disinfection between patients or lapses in injection and medication handling technique, rather than the hemodialysis procedure itself carrying inherent transmission risk when standard precautions are properly applied.

Contemporary hepatitis C prevalence in dialysis units has declined substantially in regions with well-established infection control practice and, more recently, with curative antiviral treatment reducing the population of chronically infected patients able to serve as a transmission source, though prevalence remains elevated relative to the general population in many settings, particularly reflecting the population's historical exposure before contemporary blood product screening and infection control practices were established.

Genotype distribution among dialysis patients with chronic hepatitis C generally mirrors the genotype distribution in the broader general population within a given geographic region, since transmission within the dialysis setting does not preferentially select for any particular genotype, and this consideration matters primarily for treatment regimen selection, discussed in the next subsection, since some direct-acting antiviral regimens are genotype-specific while others offer pangenotypic coverage suitable regardless of the infecting genotype.

Screening and Direct-Acting Antiviral Treatment

Routine periodic hepatitis C screening, following current national guidance for screening interval and method, identifies both new transmission events warranting the unit-level investigation discussed in the next subsection and previously undetected chronic infection warranting the antiviral treatment discussed below, and this routine, scheduled screening, rather than testing only when a specific clinical concern arises, provides the surveillance foundation the clustering-based infection detection this chapter has emphasized throughout depends on.

Direct-acting antiviral therapy has transformed hepatitis C from a chronic, largely unmanageable condition into a curable one, with cure rates exceeding those achieved with older interferon-based regimens by a substantial margin and with a considerably more favorable side-effect profile, and this transformation has direct relevance to a dialysis patient's kidney transplant candidacy, discussed in Chapter 27, since successful hepatitis C treatment removes what was historically a significant barrier to transplant listing for an affected patient; treating hepatitis C promptly upon diagnosis, rather than deferring treatment, therefore carries relevance extending well beyond the hepatitis C infection itself into a patient's broader long-term care trajectory.

Dosing considerations for direct-acting antiviral agents in the dialysis population have evolved alongside the broader treatment landscape, with several contemporary regimens now suitable for use without dose adjustment across the full range of kidney function, including dialysis dependence, removing what was historically a more significant treatment barrier when earlier-generation regimens required more substantial modification or were contraindicated in advanced kidney disease; consulting current, regularly updated treatment guidance rather than relying on older regimen-specific knowledge is particularly important in this rapidly evolving treatment area.

Isolation Practices and Unit-Level Prevention

Dedicated machines and, in some unit protocols, dedicated treatment areas for hepatitis C-positive patients, historically a more universally applied practice, have been reconsidered in some contemporary settings given improved infection control practice and the declining chronic infection prevalence direct-acting antiviral treatment has produced, though many units continue this dedicated-equipment approach as an additional layer of protection beyond standard infection control practice alone, particularly during any period of active investigation following a newly identified infection or suspected transmission event.

Universal precautions applied consistently and rigorously to every patient regardless of known bloodborne pathogen status, rather than relaxed vigilance for patients believed to be uninfected, remain the foundational infection control practice underlying all of this section's more specific recommendations, since a patient's bloodborne pathogen status at any given moment reflects only the most recent screening result and cannot fully exclude a very recent, not-yet-detectable infection, meaning consistent universal precaution application protects against transmission risk that status-based, differential precaution intensity alone would not fully address.

A confirmed new hepatitis C infection in a previously negative dialysis patient should prompt immediate investigation for a shared unit-level source, following the same clustering-investigation approach this book has applied to water treatment contamination in Chapter 5 and peritonitis in Chapter 19, reviewing infection control practice, equipment sharing, and medication handling technique across the unit rather than assuming the new infection reflects an isolated, unexplained event unrelated to the shared treatment environment.

A dialysis unit identifies a new hepatitis C infection in a patient who had tested negative at routine screening one year prior, with no identified outside exposure risk on careful history. Recognizing this as a potential unit-level transmission event, the unit's infection control team immediately reviews recent infection control practice, equipment disinfection logs, and medication preparation technique across the unit, and screens all other patients treated on the same machine and in the same treatment area during the preceding months. This investigation identifies a lapse in medication vial handling technique by a staff member new to the unit, promptly corrected through retraining, and no additional cases are identified among the screened patients. This case illustrates the appropriate response to a new hepatitis C diagnosis in a previously negative dialysis patient: treating it as a potential sentinel event for a broader unit-level infection control lapse, warranting immediate, structured investigation, rather than an isolated, unexplained occurrence requiring no further unit-level action.

CAUTION: A new hepatitis C infection in a previously negative dialysis patient should prompt immediate investigation for a shared unit-level source, reviewing infection control practice and screening other patients on the same equipment, rather than being treated as an isolated, unexplained event.

DIALYSIS RECOGNITION & RESPONSE SYSTEM — Systemic Complication Arcs

---

The Pattern: A dialysis patient develops a new hepatitis C infection after a previously negative screening result.

Stem Signature: A newly positive hepatitis C test in a patient who had previously tested negative at routine screening, without a clearly identified outside exposure risk on careful history.

The Decision: Treat this as a potential sentinel event for a unit-level infection control lapse, immediately reviewing infection control practice and screening other patients treated on the same equipment or in the same area during the relevant period, rather than treating the case as isolated.

Trap Logic: A new infection in a single patient can be treated as an isolated, unexplained clinical event without pursuing the broader unit-level investigation that would reveal a shared, correctable infection control lapse potentially affecting other patients as well.

Response Anchor: A new hepatitis C infection in a previously negative patient warrants immediate unit-level investigation and screening of other patients on the same equipment — not treatment as an isolated, unexplained occurrence.

DIALYSIS RECOGNITION & RESPONSE SYSTEM — Systemic Complication Arcs

---

A New Hepatitis C Infection in a Previously Negative Patient: Treat as a potential sentinel event for a unit-level infection control lapse, reviewing practice and screening other patients on the same equipment rather than treating the case as isolated.

Summary and Key Concepts

Protein-energy wasting reflects a multifactorial syndrome connecting inflammation, metabolic acidosis, and dialysis-related nutrient losses rather than simple undernutrition, and declining nutritional markers should prompt evaluation for an occult inflammatory source.

Dietary protein, potassium, and fluid guidance should be individualized to modality, residual kidney function, and actual biochemical trend rather than applying uniform restrictions across the entire dialysis population.

Kidney failure produces combined immune activation and immune deficiency, and a layered approach combining higher-dose vaccination, structured tracking, and rigorous unit-level infection prevention addresses this population's elevated infection risk.

Direct-acting antiviral therapy has transformed hepatitis C into a curable condition with direct relevance to future transplant candidacy, supporting prompt treatment upon diagnosis rather than deferral.

A new hepatitis C infection in a previously negative dialysis patient should prompt immediate investigation for a shared unit-level source, extending the same clustering-based investigation principle this book has applied to other shared-environment infection risks.

CHAPTER 26: DIALYSIS IN PEDIATRIC, GERIATRIC, AND PREGNANT PATIENTS

Learning Objectives

Apply pediatric-specific growth, modality, and transition-of-care considerations in dialysis management.

Assess frailty in older dialysis patients and adapt modality and prescription decisions accordingly.

Apply an intensified dialysis prescription and monitoring approach for a pregnant dialysis-dependent patient.

Adapt the Life-Plan shared decision-making framework across pediatric, geriatric, and pregnant populations, including family involvement and equity considerations.

Chapter Overview

Part VIII, this book's final part, addresses populations whose dialysis care requires adaptation beyond the general adult framework this book has developed across its preceding twenty-five chapters. This chapter addresses three such populations together: children, whose growth and development impose considerations entirely absent from adult care; older, often frail adults, whose dialysis decision-making must weigh treatment burden against benefit differently than a younger, more physiologically resilient patient; and pregnant dialysis-dependent patients, a genuinely rare but increasingly viable clinical scenario given evolving intensified dialysis approaches. Though clinically distinct, these three populations share a common thread this chapter develops explicitly in its final section: each requires a more deliberately adapted application of the Life-Plan and shared decision-making framework Chapter 2 established for the general adult population, rather than treating that framework as a fixed protocol applied uniformly regardless of a patient's specific developmental stage, physiologic reserve, or life circumstance.

Pediatric Dialysis Considerations

Growth and Developmental Considerations

Growth failure, a consequence of chronic kidney disease and dialysis dependence largely specific to the pediatric population, reflects the combined effects of chronic metabolic acidosis, secondary hyperparathyroidism and the mineral bone disorder framework discussed in Chapter 23, protein-energy wasting discussed in Chapter 25, and growth hormone resistance that develops in the uremic state, together producing a growth trajectory that, left unaddressed, falls progressively further behind healthy peers over the course of a child's dialysis-dependent years; this growth impact carries lifelong consequence in a way no equivalent concern exists for an adult patient beginning dialysis after growth has already concluded, making growth monitoring and its underlying contributors a distinctly pediatric priority this book's adult-focused chapters have not directly addressed.

Recombinant growth hormone therapy, used specifically to address this growth impairment where dietary, metabolic, and mineral bone disorder optimization alone prove insufficient, requires careful monitoring and specialized pediatric nephrology expertise beyond what this book's general adult framework provides, and a pediatric patient's overall management should be directed by a center with this specific expertise rather than adapted informally from adult-focused protocols and experience alone, given the materially different growth-related priorities and treatment considerations this population presents.

Final adult height achieved despite optimal contemporary management still frequently falls somewhat short of genetic height potential in children who spent significant developmental years with chronic kidney disease or dialysis dependence, and this residual growth deficit, even after growth hormone therapy and other optimization measures, should be discussed honestly with families as part of realistic expectation-setting, following the same candid, evidence-based communication approach this book has applied throughout to prognostic discussions, rather than implying that optimal management guarantees fully normalized adult height in every case.

Modality Selection in Pediatric Patients

Peritoneal dialysis is frequently preferred as the initial modality for younger children specifically, given the technical challenges hemodialysis vascular access presents in small children with correspondingly small vessels, and given peritoneal dialysis's more physiologically gentle, continuous clearance pattern that avoids the hemodynamic stress of intermittent hemodialysis in a child whose cardiovascular reserve may be more limited than an adult's; this modality preference parallels, in the pediatric context, the same access-feasibility and hemodynamic-tolerance reasoning this book developed in Chapter 2 for adult modality selection, now weighted more heavily toward peritoneal dialysis given pediatric vascular access's specific technical challenges.

Home-based care, whether peritoneal dialysis or, in older children and adolescents, home hemodialysis discussed in Chapter 20, is particularly valued in pediatric nephrology given its capacity to minimize school and normal childhood activity disruption relative to frequent in-center treatment, and family training for pediatric home dialysis follows the same structured, graduated training principles Chapter 20 developed for adult home hemodialysis, now adapted to train parents or other caregivers rather than the patient directly performing self-care, given a young child's inability to independently manage their own treatment.

Vascular access planning in children who do progress to hemodialysis, whether as an older adolescent or a younger child for whom peritoneal dialysis has become unsuitable, requires particular attention to vessel preservation given the multi-decade access needs a child beginning dialysis young may eventually face, extending the same vein-preservation principle this book emphasized in Chapter 9 with even greater urgency given a pediatric patient's potentially much longer subsequent lifetime of vascular access needs relative to a patient beginning dialysis later in adult life.

Transition to Adult Care

Transition from pediatric to adult nephrology care, typically occurring during adolescence or early adulthood, represents a distinct clinical process warranting its own structured, deliberate planning rather than an abrupt handoff at an arbitrary age threshold, since a young adult transitioning from a pediatric care model, often involving substantial parental involvement in treatment management, to an adult care model expecting greater patient autonomy and self-management, requires a graduated transition period building this autonomy progressively rather than expecting immediate, complete self-sufficiency at the moment of transfer.

This transition process shares structural similarities with the graduated independence training this book developed for home hemodialysis in Chapter 20, now applied to the broader transfer of overall care responsibility rather than a single technical skill set, and a structured transition program, ideally beginning well before the actual transfer of care occurs, addresses not only the practical skills of self-management but the psychosocial adjustment to assuming greater responsibility for one's own chronic disease management that this transition represents; poor transition planning is a recognized contributor to gaps in care and clinical deterioration during this vulnerable period, underscoring that transition itself deserves the same deliberate, structured attention this book has applied to every other significant care transition addressed throughout its chapters.

Educational and vocational planning, integrated into the transition process alongside the medical self-management skills already discussed, recognizes that a young adult transitioning to adult nephrology care is simultaneously navigating other major life transitions, including higher education or early career entry, and coordinating transition timing with these other significant life events, where feasible, rather than treating the medical transition as occurring in isolation from a patient's broader life trajectory, supports better overall adjustment during this genuinely demanding period of simultaneous transitions.

KEY POINT: Growth failure, largely specific to pediatric dialysis, reflects combined metabolic, mineral, and growth hormone resistance mechanisms, and transition from pediatric to adult care requires deliberate, graduated planning rather than an abrupt handoff at an arbitrary age threshold.

Figure 26.1: Graduated Transition From Pediatric to Adult Nephrology Care

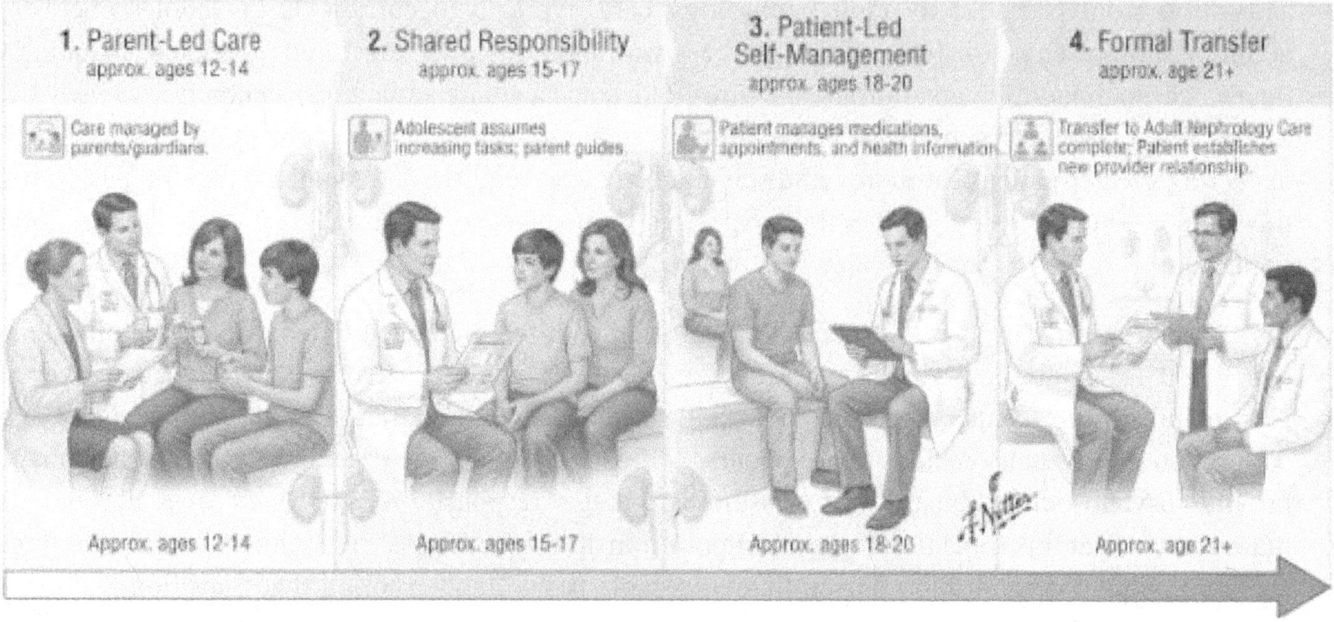

Geriatric Dialysis Considerations and Frailty

Frailty Assessment in Older Dialysis Patients

Frailty, a clinical syndrome of reduced physiologic reserve across multiple organ systems distinct from chronological age alone, affects a substantial proportion of the older dialysis population and predicts mortality, hospitalization, and functional decline independent of age or traditional comorbidity measures, meaning two patients of identical age can carry meaningfully different treatment tolerance and prognosis depending on their specific frailty status; structured frailty assessment, using a validated tool incorporating measures such as grip strength, gait speed, and unintentional weight loss, provides an objective basis for this distinction rather than relying on informal clinical impression alone.

Serial frailty reassessment, rather than a single evaluation performed only at dialysis initiation, allows recognition of a patient whose frailty status changes over their dialysis course, whether improving with adequate nutritional and anemia management following the frameworks Chapters 22 and 25 developed, or declining despite these interventions, and this trend-based reassessment supports ongoing recalibration of prescription intensity and overall care goals as a patient's actual physiologic reserve evolves, extending the same trend-over-single-value principle this book has applied consistently throughout its treatment of every other chronic assessment domain.

Frailty assessment at the point of dialysis initiation decision-making, discussed in Chapter 1's treatment of absolute and relative indications, adds a further dimension to that decision beyond the biochemical and symptomatic indications this book has emphasized throughout: a frail older patient's expected benefit from dialysis initiation, and their expected tolerance of the treatment burden dialysis imposes, may differ substantially from a non-frail patient of the same chronological age and similar biochemical indication severity, supporting the individualized, whole-patient decision-making this book has emphasized throughout rather than a uniform indication threshold applied regardless of frailty status.

Modality and Prescription Adaptations for Frail Patients

A frail patient's dialysis prescription often benefits from adaptations similar in principle to the incremental peritoneal dialysis approach discussed in Chapter 17: a reduced initial treatment intensity, whether shorter hemodialysis sessions or a less intensive peritoneal dialysis regimen, may better match a frail patient's physiologic tolerance than a standard full-intensity prescription, with intensity increased only as tolerated rather than initiating at standard intensity and hoping the patient adapts to a burden that may exceed their actual physiologic reserve from the outset.

Transportation burden, treatment-related fatigue, and the practical challenges frailty imposes on attending regular in-center treatment sessions deserve explicit consideration in modality selection for this population, and home-based modalities, whether peritoneal dialysis or home hemodialysis, may offer meaningful advantages for a frail patient specifically by reducing the transportation and waiting-room burden in-center treatment imposes, provided adequate caregiver support, discussed further in this chapter's treatment of family involvement, is available to support the technical demands home-based care requires.

Cognitive Impairment and Dialysis Decision-Making

Cognitive impairment, common in the older dialysis population and sometimes exacerbated by the uremic milieu itself in a manner partially reversible with adequate dialysis clearance, complicates both informed decision-making about dialysis initiation and continuation and the practical self-management tasks home-based modalities require, and formal cognitive screening, incorporated into the broader frailty and geriatric assessment this section has developed, identifies this consideration explicitly rather than leaving it to informal clinical impression alone.

A patient with significant cognitive impairment identified through this screening warrants involvement of a surrogate decision-maker in the shared decision-making process this book has emphasized throughout, following the same principles this book applied to conservative and palliative kidney management decision-making in Chapter 3, and recognizing when cognitive impairment has progressed to a degree that meaningfully affects a patient's capacity for informed dialysis decision-making, rather than assuming full decisional capacity by default in every older patient regardless of cognitive status, is an essential component of ethically sound care for this population.

CAUTION: Frailty assessment should inform dialysis initiation, prescription intensity, and modality selection decisions in older patients, and formal cognitive screening should identify patients for whom surrogate decision-maker involvement is warranted, rather than assuming full decisional capacity by default.

Pregnancy in Dialysis-Dependent Patients

Fertility and Pregnancy Rates in Dialysis

Fertility is substantially reduced in dialysis-dependent women, reflecting the uremic milieu's suppressive effects on the hypothalamic-pituitary-ovarian axis, and pregnancy in this population, while rare, occurs more frequently than earlier clinical experience suggested and has become an increasingly viable prospect for a well-selected patient given the intensified dialysis prescription and monitoring approaches discussed in this section; a patient expressing interest in pregnancy should have this specifically discussed as part of her overall Life-Plan and reproductive health counseling rather than pregnancy being presumed categorically impossible or inappropriate simply because she is dialysis-dependent.

Contraceptive counseling deserves equal attention alongside pregnancy-desire counseling, since an unplanned pregnancy in a dialysis-dependent woman not already receiving the intensified prescription and multidisciplinary preparation this section describes carries even greater risk than a planned, prepared pregnancy, and proactive contraceptive discussion, addressing the reduced but not absent fertility this population experiences, ensures that a patient not currently desiring pregnancy has appropriate contraceptive support rather than assuming reduced fertility provides adequate protection against unplanned conception on its own.

Successful pregnancy outcomes in dialysis-dependent women have improved substantially with contemporary intensified dialysis protocols relative to earlier-era outcomes achieved with standard thrice-weekly treatment, though pregnancy in this population remains high-risk, with elevated rates of preterm delivery, low birth weight, and other obstetric complications relative to the general population even under optimized, intensified dialysis management, and this risk profile should be discussed candidly and thoroughly as part of the reproductive counseling and shared decision-making this section develops.

Intensified Dialysis Prescription During Pregnancy

Intensified hemodialysis, typically increasing treatment frequency to a daily or near-daily schedule during pregnancy, represents the standard contemporary approach to dialysis prescription in this population, extending the same intensive hemodialysis principles discussed in Chapter 20 to their most aggressive clinical application, and this intensification aims to more closely approximate the continuous solute and volume clearance native kidney function would otherwise provide throughout pregnancy, minimizing the uremic exposure that has been associated with adverse fetal outcomes in earlier-era experience with less intensive dialysis prescriptions during pregnancy.

Volume management during pregnancy requires particular attention given the physiologic volume expansion and altered fluid dynamics pregnancy itself produces, superimposed on the volume management principles this book developed in Chapter 24; dry weight, discussed extensively in that chapter as a moving target requiring periodic reassessment even in the non-pregnant population, requires considerably more frequent reassessment during pregnancy given the rapid, ongoing physiologic changes pregnancy imposes over a comparatively short timeframe, and a fixed dry weight determined early in pregnancy will not remain accurate throughout its course.

Maternal and Fetal Monitoring

Maternal and fetal monitoring during a dialysis-dependent pregnancy requires close collaboration between nephrology and maternal-fetal medicine specialists, extending the same integrated, multidisciplinary care principle this book emphasized for nephrology-cardiology collaboration in Chapter 24, now applied to a pregnancy-specific multidisciplinary team; this collaboration should be established early, ideally before or immediately upon confirmation of pregnancy, rather than nephrology and obstetric care proceeding in parallel without the structured, regular communication this genuinely high-risk clinical scenario demands.

Blood pressure management during pregnancy requires selecting antihypertensive agents with an established pregnancy safety profile, since several agents commonly used in the general dialysis population discussed in Chapter 24 carry specific contraindications during pregnancy, and this medication reconciliation should be performed proactively upon pregnancy confirmation rather than continuing a pre-pregnancy antihypertensive regimen without this specific safety review.

KEY POINT: Intensified, near-daily hemodialysis during pregnancy minimizes uremic exposure and has substantially improved pregnancy outcomes relative to standard thrice-weekly treatment, but dry weight requires considerably more frequent reassessment given pregnancy's rapid physiologic changes.

Shared Decision-Making Across Special Populations

Adapting the Life-Plan Framework for Special Populations

The Life-Plan framework developed in Chapter 2 for the general adult population requires deliberate adaptation, not abandonment, for each of the three populations this chapter has addressed: a pediatric patient's Life-Plan must anticipate the pediatric-to-adult care transition discussed earlier in this chapter, a frail older patient's Life-Plan must weigh treatment burden against benefit with the frailty-specific considerations this chapter has developed, and a pregnant patient's Life-Plan must accommodate the temporary, intensive prescription escalation pregnancy requires; in each case, the underlying Life-Plan principle of individualized, trajectory-aware planning remains constant even as its specific application differs substantially across these populations.

Recognizing which population-specific considerations apply to a given patient, and adapting the general Life-Plan framework accordingly rather than applying either the general adult framework unmodified or an entirely separate, disconnected approach for each special population, reflects the same both-general-and-individualized reasoning this book has applied consistently throughout its treatment of prescription, adequacy, and complication management across every earlier chapter.

Family and Surrogate Involvement

Family involvement in dialysis decision-making and, for home-based modalities, in actual treatment delivery, takes on particular importance across all three populations this chapter addresses: parents for pediatric patients, adult children or other caregivers for frail older patients, and partners or family members supporting a pregnant patient through an intensified, more demanding treatment schedule; this family involvement should be actively supported and structured, following the same care partner training and burnout-prevention principles this book developed for home hemodialysis in Chapter 20, rather than assumed to occur adequately without explicit programmatic attention and support.

A fourteen-year-old girl with chronic kidney disease approaching dialysis dependence is being prepared, alongside her parents, for the eventual transition to adult nephrology care she will face in several years, and her pediatric nephrology team begins structured transition planning well in advance, gradually shifting responsibility for appointment scheduling, medication management, and eventually treatment-related decision-making from her parents toward the patient herself as she progresses through adolescence, following the graduated independence model this chapter recommends. By the time she formally transfers to adult care at age nineteen, she has already developed substantial self-management competency and confidence, and her transition proceeds smoothly without the care gaps or clinical deterioration sometimes seen with less structured transition processes. This case illustrates the value of beginning transition planning well before the actual transfer of care occurs, building autonomy progressively rather than expecting an abrupt shift in responsibility at the moment of transfer itself.

CLINICAL PEARL: Structured transition planning for pediatric patients approaching adult care should begin well before the actual transfer occurs, gradually building patient self-management competency rather than expecting an abrupt shift in responsibility at the moment of transfer.

Equity Considerations in Special Population Care

Access to the specialized resources this chapter has discussed, including pediatric nephrology expertise, structured frailty assessment tools, and maternal-fetal medicine collaboration for pregnant patients, varies considerably across different geographic and healthcare system settings, and recognizing this variation as a genuine equity concern, rather than assuming every patient has equal access to the specialized, population-adapted care this chapter recommends, is essential to honestly characterizing the care gap that can exist between what this chapter describes as best practice and what is actually achievable for a given patient in a given setting.

Where specialized resources are not locally available, structured referral pathways to a regional center with the relevant expertise, combined with telehealth-supported collaborative care models where feasible, can partially bridge this gap, and proactively identifying which special-population considerations a given patient's local care setting can and cannot adequately address, rather than discovering this gap only once a clinical need has already arisen, supports more timely referral and better-coordinated care across these settings.

Language and cultural considerations further compound the equity concerns this section has raised, since the specialized, often lengthy discussions this chapter's populations require, including transition planning conversations, frailty and goals-of-care discussions, and reproductive counseling, depend heavily on effective communication, and ensuring adequate interpreter services and culturally responsive counseling approaches are genuinely available, rather than assumed to be adequate without direct verification, is essential to delivering the individualized, shared decision-making care this chapter's framework describes equitably across a diverse patient population.

DIALYSIS RECOGNITION & RESPONSE SYSTEM — Special Population Arcs

The Pattern: A dialysis-dependent patient falls into one of this chapter's special populations — pediatric, frail older adult, or pregnant.

Stem Signature: A patient whose developmental stage, frailty status, or pregnancy status introduces considerations beyond the general adult dialysis framework this book has developed throughout its preceding chapters.

The Decision: Adapt the Life-Plan and shared decision-making framework explicitly to this population's specific considerations — growth and transition planning, frailty-adjusted prescription and decision-making, or intensified pregnancy-specific prescription and multidisciplinary monitoring — rather than applying the general adult framework unmodified.

Trap Logic: A special population's dialysis care can be managed using the general adult framework unmodified, without recognizing the specific adaptations this chapter has detailed, risking outcomes and care processes poorly matched to that population's actual needs and circumstances.

Response Anchor: A patient in one of this chapter's special populations warrants explicit adaptation of the Life-Plan framework to their specific considerations — not the general adult framework applied unmodified.

DIALYSIS RECOGNITION & RESPONSE SYSTEM — Special Population Arcs

A Patient in a Special Population (Pediatric, Frail Older Adult, or Pregnant): Adapt the Life-Plan and shared decision-making framework explicitly to this population's specific considerations rather than applying the general adult framework unmodified.

Summary and Key Concepts

Pediatric dialysis care must address growth failure, favors peritoneal dialysis and home-based modalities for younger children, and requires deliberate, graduated transition planning to adult care beginning well before the actual transfer occurs.

Frailty, distinct from chronological age alone, should be formally assessed and should inform dialysis initiation, prescription intensity, and modality decisions in older patients, alongside cognitive screening to identify patients warranting surrogate decision-maker involvement.

Pregnancy in dialysis-dependent patients, while high-risk, has become increasingly viable with intensified, near-daily dialysis prescriptions and requires considerably more frequent dry weight reassessment and close nephrology-obstetric collaboration.

The Life-Plan framework requires deliberate adaptation, not abandonment, for each special population, with family and surrogate involvement actively supported and structured rather than assumed to occur adequately without explicit attention.

Access to specialized special-population resources varies considerably across care settings, and proactively identifying local care gaps supports more timely referral and better-coordinated care than discovering these gaps only once a clinical need has already arisen.

CHAPTER 27: KIDNEY TRANSPLANT EVALUATION AND PERIOPERATIVE DIALYSIS CONSIDERATIONS

Learning Objectives

Apply the components of transplant candidacy evaluation, including medical, cardiovascular, cancer, and psychosocial assessment.

Compare living and deceased donor pathways and apply preemptive transplantation principles.

Manage perioperative dialysis needs, delayed graft function, and early immunosuppression-dialysis interactions.

Apply long-term post-transplant monitoring principles and manage the transition back to dialysis after graft failure.

Chapter Overview

This final chapter closes the book by addressing kidney transplantation, the treatment that offers the greatest survival and quality-of-life benefit of any kidney replacement option for an appropriately selected candidate, and the outcome toward which this book's Life-Plan framework, introduced in Chapter 2, has pointed for many patients throughout their dialysis course. Transplant evaluation, living and deceased donor pathways, the perioperative dialysis management this book's nephrology-focused readership will most directly participate in, and the long-term follow-up and graft failure management that brings some patients back to dialysis after a period of transplant function, together complete this book's treatment of the full kidney replacement therapy spectrum introduced in Chapter 1. This chapter also closes a narrative arc running throughout this book: the Life-Plan is not merely a modality-selection framework for choosing among dialysis options, but a genuinely comprehensive planning structure that includes transplantation as a central, often preferred destination, and the hepatitis C treatment discussed in Chapter 25, the vein-preservation principles discussed in Chapter 9, and the residual function preservation strategies discussed throughout this book's peritoneal dialysis chapters all connect directly to transplant candidacy in ways this chapter makes explicit.

This chapter, and this book, close with the same underlying philosophy that has run throughout: kidney failure care is not a single, static treatment decision made once and then executed unchanged indefinitely, but a genuinely lifelong, evolving trajectory requiring ongoing, individualized, trend-based attention across every domain this book has addressed, from the initial Life-Plan discussion in Chapter 2 through modality selection, prescription management, complication prevention and response, and, for many patients, transplant evaluation and, for some, the return to dialysis after a transplant's eventual failure. The proactive, anticipatory planning principle this book has applied consistently, whether to vascular access creation, dry weight reassessment, anemia and mineral bone disorder management, or the transplant evaluation timing this chapter emphasizes, reflects a single, unifying clinical philosophy: recognizing where a patient's trajectory is heading, and acting before an urgent, unplanned crisis forces a reactive response, consistently produces better outcomes than waiting for problems to fully develop before addressing them.

Transplant Candidacy Evaluation

Medical Evaluation Components

Transplant candidacy evaluation begins with a comprehensive medical assessment establishing that a patient's overall health status supports both the surgical procedure itself and the sustained immunosuppression a transplant requires, including assessment of infection risk, prior malignancy history, and the cardiovascular and cancer screening detailed in the next subsection; this evaluation, typically coordinated by a dedicated transplant center rather than the referring dialysis unit alone, draws on the patient's full clinical history this book's earlier chapters have addressed, including their dialysis adequacy trend, vascular access history, and any complications from the systemic and metabolic domains discussed throughout Part VII.

Hepatitis C status, discussed in Chapter 25, deserves specific mention in this evaluation context given direct-acting antiviral therapy's transformation of what was historically a significant transplant candidacy barrier into a fully treatable, often curable condition; a patient with untreated chronic hepatitis C discovered during transplant evaluation should be referred promptly for antiviral treatment as detailed in Chapter 25, since successful treatment removes this barrier and allows transplant evaluation to proceed, illustrating directly how this book's earlier chapters connect forward into the transplant evaluation process this chapter now develops.

Cardiovascular and Cancer Screening

Cardiovascular risk assessment, drawing directly on the cardiovascular disease framework developed in Chapter 24, forms a central component of transplant evaluation given the elevated baseline cardiovascular risk this book has documented throughout the dialysis population and the additional physiologic stress the transplant surgery itself imposes; a candidate with significant, unaddressed cardiovascular disease may require cardiac intervention or risk factor optimization before transplant listing proceeds, following the same integrated cardiology-nephrology collaboration principle Chapter 24 recommended for cardiovascular management more broadly.

Age-appropriate cancer screening, following standard general population screening guidelines supplemented by any additional screening specific to a candidate's individual risk factors, identifies malignancy that would require treatment and an appropriate disease-free interval before transplantation, since post-transplant immunosuppression can accelerate recurrence or progression of an unaddressed or inadequately treated malignancy; this screening should be completed as part of the evaluation process itself rather than deferred until after listing, since a malignancy diagnosis discovered after listing may require the candidate to be temporarily removed from the waiting list until appropriate treatment and observation intervals have been completed.

Dialysis-specific malignancy risk factors, including the modestly elevated risk of certain cancers observed in the long-term dialysis population relative to the general population, plausibly related to the chronic immune dysfunction discussed in Chapter 25, warrant incorporation into a candidate's individualized screening plan beyond standard age-based general population guidelines alone, and a transplant center's evaluation protocol should account for this population-specific risk elevation rather than applying general population screening intervals and thresholds without this dialysis-specific consideration.

Psychosocial Evaluation and Waitlist Management

Psychosocial evaluation, assessing a candidate's support system, mental health status, substance use history, and demonstrated capacity for the medication adherence sustained immunosuppression requires, forms an essential component of transplant evaluation given the serious consequences medication nonadherence carries for graft survival; this evaluation should be conducted with the same person-centered, non-judgmental approach this book has emphasized throughout its treatment of mental health and psychosocial considerations, identifying and addressing modifiable barriers to adherence rather than using psychosocial findings solely as grounds for exclusion without first exploring whether structured support could address an identified concern.

Once listed, a candidate's status requires ongoing maintenance, including periodic re-evaluation of medical fitness for transplant and continued dialysis care meeting the adequacy and complication-management standards this book has developed throughout its preceding chapters, since a candidate whose overall health deteriorates significantly while awaiting transplant may require reassessment of continued listing appropriateness; maintaining excellent, comprehensive dialysis care throughout the waiting period, rather than treating waitlisted status as reducing the importance of ongoing dialysis quality, both serves the patient's immediate wellbeing and preserves their ongoing transplant candidacy.

KEY POINT: Untreated hepatitis C, discovered during transplant evaluation, should prompt prompt referral for direct-acting antiviral treatment rather than being treated as a fixed barrier, since successful treatment removes this historically significant obstacle to transplant candidacy.

Figure 27.1: The Kidney Replacement Therapy Life-Plan Across a Lifelong Trajectory

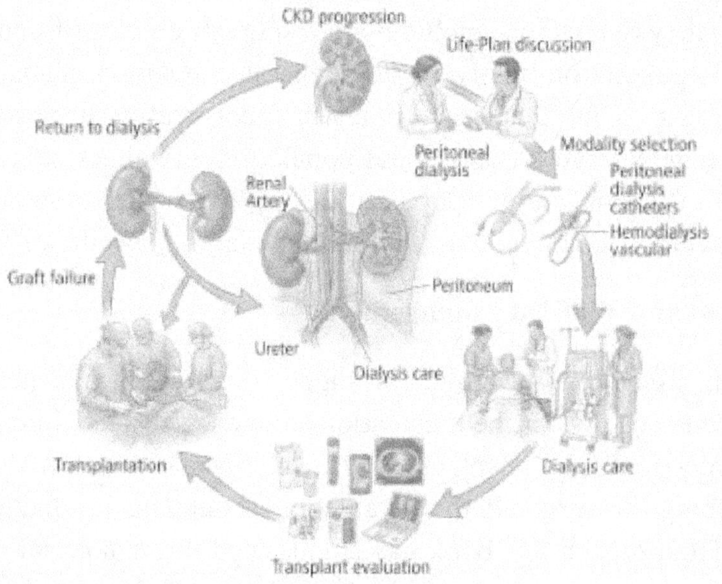

Living Versus Deceased Donor Considerations

Living Donor Evaluation and Advantages

Living donor transplantation offers several advantages over deceased donor transplantation, including generally superior long-term graft survival, a planned rather than emergent surgical timing that allows optimal recipient preparation, and, most significantly for the Life-Plan framework this book has developed throughout, the potential for preemptive transplantation before dialysis initiation becomes necessary at all, discussed further in this section; identifying a potential living donor early in a patient's chronic kidney disease trajectory, ideally as part of the same Life-Plan discussion Chapter 2 recommended initiating well before dialysis becomes necessary, maximizes the opportunity for this preferred pathway.

Living donor evaluation, conducted with the same rigor as recipient evaluation and with particular attention to ensuring the donor's decision is genuinely voluntary and adequately informed of both the surgical risks and the long-term implications of living with a single kidney, follows established protocols designed to protect donor welfare as a priority independent of, though obviously connected to, the recipient's own transplant candidacy evaluation discussed in the previous section.

Long-term donor follow-up, extending years beyond the donation itself, has become an increasingly emphasized component of comprehensive living donor programs, tracking donor kidney function, blood pressure, and overall health over time to build the evidence base informing future donor counseling and to identify and address any late donor complications promptly, reflecting an evolving recognition that donor welfare responsibility extends well beyond the immediate perioperative period into a genuinely long-term follow-up commitment paralleling, in spirit, the same longitudinal, trend-based monitoring philosophy this book has applied throughout to dialysis patients themselves.

Deceased Donor Allocation and Waiting Time

Deceased donor allocation follows established, structured criteria incorporating waiting time, immunologic compatibility, and other factors specific to a given allocation system's particular policies, and waiting times vary considerably by geographic region and blood type, meaning a candidate's realistic expected waiting time should be discussed openly as part of the Life-Plan and shared decision-making framework this book has emphasized throughout, allowing a patient to make informed decisions about dialysis modality and overall care planning with a realistic understanding of their likely transplant timeline rather than an overly optimistic or pessimistic assumption not grounded in their specific circumstances.

Registration at multiple transplant centers, where permitted by a given allocation system's specific policies, can meaningfully reduce a candidate's effective waiting time by accessing multiple donor pools simultaneously, and this option should be discussed with candidates for whom it may offer meaningful benefit, extending the same proactive, informed patient engagement principle this book has applied throughout its treatment of shared decision-making.

Preemptive Transplantation

Preemptive transplantation, receiving a transplant before dialysis initiation becomes necessary, offers superior outcomes relative to transplantation after a period of dialysis dependence, reflecting both the avoidance of dialysis-associated cardiovascular and other complications this book has documented throughout and, plausibly, a healthier overall candidate profile at the time of transplantation; this outcome advantage provides a further, concrete rationale for the early Life-Plan and transplant evaluation initiation this book has recommended since Chapter 2, ideally identifying transplant candidacy and, where applicable, a potential living donor well before the absolute or relative dialysis initiation indications discussed in Chapter 1 are reached.

A patient whose chronic kidney disease trajectory suggests dialysis initiation is likely within the coming one to two years, following the trajectory-based planning principle Chapter 1 developed, should have transplant evaluation initiated at this point specifically to maximize the opportunity for preemptive transplantation, rather than deferring transplant evaluation until after dialysis has already begun; this timing recommendation is among the most directly actionable applications of this book's overall Life-Plan philosophy, translating the abstract principle of early, proactive planning into a specific, evidence-supported clinical recommendation with meaningful outcome consequences.

CLINICAL PEARL: Preemptive transplantation, before dialysis initiation, offers superior outcomes relative to post-dialysis transplantation; transplant evaluation should begin when a patient's trajectory suggests dialysis initiation within one to two years, not deferred until after dialysis has already begun.

Perioperative Dialysis Management

Dialysis Immediately Before Transplant Surgery

A dialysis-dependent patient receiving a deceased donor transplant, typically on short notice given the unpredictable timing of organ availability, often requires a dialysis treatment shortly before surgery to optimize volume and electrolyte status for the procedure, and coordinating this preoperative treatment within the compressed timeframe deceased donor transplantation typically allows requires close communication between the transplant surgical team and the patient's usual dialysis unit or the transplant center's own dialysis facilities, extending the same structured, multidisciplinary coordination principle this book emphasized for CRRT transition planning in Chapter 21 to this distinct but structurally similar coordination challenge.

Potassium status specifically warrants careful attention in this preoperative dialysis session, since surgical stress and anesthesia can independently affect potassium handling, and a patient entering transplant surgery with a potassium level at the upper end of an acceptable range carries less margin before reaching a level of concern than one whose preoperative dialysis has achieved a more comfortably normal level, following the same individualized, trend-aware potassium management principle this book developed in Chapters 6 and 15.

Delayed Graft Function and Early Post-Transplant Dialysis

Delayed graft function, in which the newly transplanted kidney does not immediately produce adequate urine output and clearance, occurs more commonly following deceased donor transplantation, particularly with an extended cold ischemia time, than following living donor transplantation, and a patient experiencing delayed graft function may require continued dialysis in the immediate post-transplant period while awaiting graft function recovery, applying the same absolute and relative indication framework Chapter 1 and Chapter 21 developed for dialysis initiation, now applied to this specific transitional post-transplant scenario.

Distinguishing delayed graft function, which typically resolves over days to weeks as the graft recovers from the ischemic insult of the transplant process itself, from other causes of post-transplant graft dysfunction, including acute rejection or a surgical or vascular complication, requires the same structured, multidisciplinary evaluation this book has emphasized throughout, and dialysis support during this evaluation and recovery period should be managed with attention to preserving any residual native kidney function the patient may retain and avoiding unnecessary vascular access trauma to a fistula or graft that may ultimately no longer be needed once graft function recovers, following the vein-preservation principles developed in Chapter 9.

Immunosuppression Initiation and Dialysis Interactions

Immunosuppressive medication initiation, typically beginning at the time of transplant surgery itself, requires attention to dialyzability and dosing adjustment for several agent classes, particularly relevant for a patient still requiring dialysis support during delayed graft function, since some immunosuppressive agents are meaningfully cleared by dialysis and require dose timing or adjustment relative to the treatment schedule, following the same dialyzability-aware medication management principle this book applied to antihypertensive medication selection in Chapter 24.

Close collaboration between the transplant team managing immunosuppression and the nephrology or dialysis team providing any concurrent dialysis support during this early post-transplant period is essential, since medication level monitoring, dose adjustment, and dialysis timing decisions each affect the others in ways that require coordinated, rather than independently managed, decision-making across both teams during this transitional period.

Therapeutic drug monitoring for calcineurin inhibitors and other narrow-therapeutic-index immunosuppressive agents requires particular attention to the timing of blood sampling relative to both medication dosing and any concurrent dialysis session, since a trough level drawn without proper attention to this timing relationship can produce a misleading result that either prompts an unnecessary dose adjustment or fails to detect a genuine dosing problem, and standardized institutional protocols specifying exact sampling timing relative to both dosing and dialysis schedule reduce this source of measurement error considerably more effectively than relying on ad hoc timing coordination for each individual sample.

CAUTION: Delayed graft function requiring continued post-transplant dialysis support should be managed with attention to preserving vascular access that may no longer be needed once graft function recovers, and immunosuppression dosing requires coordination with dialysis timing given several agents' meaningful dialyzability.

Post-Transplant Follow-Up and the Failed Transplant Return to Dialysis

Long-Term Post-Transplant Monitoring

Long-term post-transplant monitoring, incorporating regular graft function assessment, immunosuppression level monitoring, and surveillance for the cardiovascular disease, infection risk, and malignancy risk that persist, and in some respects intensify, under sustained immunosuppression, extends many of this book's earlier disease-specific frameworks into the post-transplant context: the cardiovascular risk assessment principles from Chapter 24, the infection prevention and vaccination principles from Chapter 25, and the vigilant, trend-based surveillance philosophy this book has applied consistently throughout its treatment of every chronic complication domain.

A transplant recipient's ongoing relationship with a nephrology team, whether the same team that managed their pre-transplant dialysis care or the transplant center's own dedicated post-transplant nephrology service, should maintain the same structured, proactive monitoring approach this book has emphasized throughout rather than assuming a successful transplant eliminates the need for the vigilant, trend-based clinical attention this book's every chapter has recommended for the pre-transplant dialysis population.

Recurrent native disease, particularly relevant for a patient whose original kidney failure arose from a condition with recognized recurrence potential in the transplanted kidney, warrants disease-specific monitoring beyond the general graft function surveillance already discussed, and a transplant recipient's original diagnosis, established well before transplantation during the initial evaluation and workup discussed throughout this book's earlier chapters, should inform this disease-specific monitoring plan rather than being treated as historical information no longer relevant once transplantation has occurred.

Recognizing Graft Failure

Graft failure, whether from chronic rejection, recurrent native disease affecting the transplanted kidney, or another cause, presents with a gradually rising creatinine and declining estimated glomerular filtration rate following a trajectory conceptually similar to the native chronic kidney disease progression detailed in Chapter 1, and the same trajectory-based Life-Plan reasoning that chapter developed for native kidney disease applies directly to a failing transplant, now anticipating a likely eventual return to dialysis, or, for a well-selected candidate, evaluation for a repeat transplant, rather than treating graft failure as an entirely novel clinical scenario disconnected from this book's foundational Chapter 1 framework.

Early identification of a declining transplant trajectory, through the same structured, scheduled monitoring detailed in the previous subsection, allows the same anticipatory planning benefits Chapter 1 documented for native kidney disease progression: timely vascular access planning following the vein-preservation principles from Chapter 9, transplant re-evaluation where appropriate, and the same avoidance of an urgent, unplanned dialysis initiation this book has emphasized as a preventable and consequential failure mode throughout its treatment of the chronic kidney disease trajectory.

Returning to Dialysis After Transplant Failure

A patient returning to dialysis after transplant failure often carries a distinct psychological burden beyond the clinical considerations this book has otherwise emphasized, having experienced a period of life without dialysis dependence and now facing its return, and this emotional dimension deserves explicit acknowledgment and support, extending the same person-centered, whole-patient consideration this book has applied throughout its treatment of the initial dialysis initiation decision in Chapters 1 through 3, now recognizing that a return to dialysis carries its own distinct psychological weight warranting equally thoughtful attention.

A forty-two-year-old woman who received a preemptive living donor transplant eight years ago from her sister now shows a gradually rising creatinine over the preceding year, consistent with chronic graft dysfunction, and her nephrology team, recognizing this trajectory early through the structured monitoring this chapter recommends, initiates vascular access planning proactively following the same vein-preservation principles this book emphasized in Chapter 9, well before her graft function reaches a level requiring urgent dialysis initiation. She is also evaluated for repeat transplant candidacy and, given her excellent overall health and strong social support, is placed on the waiting list while her graft continues to provide partial function. Her eventual transition to hemodialysis, when it becomes necessary, proceeds with an already-matured fistula in place, avoiding the urgent catheter-based initiation this book has identified throughout as a preventable, consequential failure mode. This case illustrates how the Life-Plan framework this book introduced in Chapter 2 applies with equal force to a failing transplant as to native chronic kidney disease progression, and how proactive planning, extended across this book's entire arc from initial modality selection through transplant evaluation and, where necessary, back to dialysis, serves a patient's interests at every stage of a genuinely lifelong kidney disease journey.

CLINICAL PEARL: A declining transplant trajectory should trigger the same proactive Life-Plan reasoning this book applied to native chronic kidney disease progression, including timely vascular access planning, rather than waiting until urgent dialysis initiation becomes unavoidable.

DIALYSIS RECOGNITION & RESPONSE SYSTEM — Transplant Transition Arcs

The Pattern: A kidney transplant recipient shows a gradually rising creatinine consistent with chronic graft dysfunction.

Stem Signature: A gradual, sustained rise in creatinine and decline in estimated glomerular filtration rate over successive follow-up visits in a transplant recipient, without an acute, reversible cause identified on evaluation.

The Decision: Apply the same trajectory-based Life-Plan reasoning developed in Chapter 1 for native chronic kidney disease progression: initiate proactive vascular access planning and repeat transplant candidacy evaluation well before dialysis becomes urgently necessary, rather than waiting until graft failure is complete.

Trap Logic: A declining transplant trajectory can be monitored passively without proactive access or repeat-transplant planning, on the assumption that transplant failure is a distinct clinical scenario unlike native kidney disease progression, when in fact the same anticipatory planning principle applies with equal force and equal benefit.

Response Anchor: A declining transplant trajectory warrants the same proactive Life-Plan and vascular access planning this book applies to native kidney disease progression — not passive monitoring until dialysis becomes urgently unavoidable.

DIALYSIS RECOGNITION & RESPONSE SYSTEM — Transplant Transition Arcs

A Declining Transplant Trajectory: Apply the same trajectory-based Life-Plan reasoning as native chronic kidney disease progression, initiating proactive vascular access and repeat transplant planning well before dialysis becomes urgently necessary.

Summary and Key Concepts

Transplant candidacy evaluation encompasses medical, cardiovascular, cancer, and psychosocial assessment, with untreated hepatitis C now a readily addressable rather than fixed barrier given direct-acting antiviral therapy.

Living donor transplantation offers superior outcomes and the possibility of preemptive transplantation before dialysis initiation, which itself confers better outcomes than post-dialysis transplantation, making early transplant evaluation a direct, actionable application of this book's Life-Plan philosophy.

Perioperative dialysis management requires coordinated attention to preoperative optimization, delayed graft function support with vascular access preservation, and immunosuppression-dialysis timing interactions.

Long-term post-transplant monitoring extends this book's cardiovascular, infection, and trend-based surveillance frameworks into the post-transplant context, and graft failure follows a trajectory-based course to which the same Life-Plan reasoning developed for native kidney disease applies directly.

A patient returning to dialysis after transplant failure benefits from the same proactive vascular access and psychosocial support this book has emphasized throughout, completing the full circle of this book's Life-Plan framework across the entire arc of a lifelong kidney disease journey.

THE DIALYSIS RESPONSE MASTER INDEX

The Dialysis Response Master Index consolidates every Pattern Recognition instance built into the Rhythm Layer across all twenty-seven chapters of this handbook into a single, indexed reference navigator, organized here by Part and chapter for rapid lookup during clinical practice. Each entry distills its chapter's full Pattern, Stem Signature, Decision, Trap Logic, and Response Anchor structure into a compact, scannable form: the presenting clinical picture, the decisive action it calls for, and the correct response distilled into a single anchor statement. This Index is a pure reference navigator — it contains no questions, no drills, no item bank, and no answer key of any kind. Entries are cross-referenced by chapter number so the reader can return to the full clinical discussion, case, and supporting evidence whenever more depth is needed. The Index is organized to be scanned quickly at the bedside, on call, or before a shift, in the same spirit as the pattern atlases and decision libraries used throughout contemporary clinical reference publishing.

Part I — Foundations of Kidney Replacement Therapy

Chapter 1: Chronic Kidney Disease Progression and the Decision to Initiate Kidney Replacement Therapy

A patient with known chronic kidney disease presents with a creatinine substantially higher than their established trend — Rapid rise in creatinine over days to a few weeks, often accompanied by a clear precipitant such as a new nephrotoxic medication, a diarrheal illness, contrast exposure, or a change in diuretic dosing; urine output may be preserved or reduced. DECISION: Evaluate for and remove reversible contributors — hold nephrotoxins, correct volume depletion, rule out obstruction with renal ultrasound — before accepting the new creatinine as the patient's chronic baseline or accelerating the initiation timeline on the basis of it. Do not stage a new baseline off a single creatinine value obtained during an acute illness; recheck after the precipitant has resolved.

A patient with advanced chronic kidney disease develops pleuritic chest pain — Sharp chest pain worsened by inspiration and lying flat, a pericardial friction rub on auscultation, and, in more severe cases, jugular venous distension with a narrowed pulse pressure suggesting tamponade physiology. DECISION: Treat this as uremic pericarditis until proven otherwise in a patient with this degree of kidney impairment, obtain an echocardiogram to assess effusion size and hemodynamic significance, and initiate urgent dialysis — uremic pericarditis is an absolute indication for urgent start regardless of the numeric GFR. A pericardial friction rub in a patient approaching kidney failure is an absolute indication for urgent dialysis initiation, not a finding to manage symptomatically.

A patient with relative indications for initiation and a mature, ready access — Diuretic-resistant volume overload without frank pulmonary edema, mild asterixis without confusion, and stable rather than rapidly worsening electrolytes, in a patient whose vascular or peritoneal access has already been created and assessed as usable. DECISION: Proceed with a scheduled, non-emergent initiation using the prepared access rather than defaulting to urgent catheter placement, preserving the modality and access pathway already established under the patient's Life-Plan. Relative indications with a ready access support a scheduled start; only absolute indications, or relative indications with no usable access, justify an urgent, unplanned one.

A patient approaching kidney failure who has not yet been referred for access or modality education — GFR in the G4 range or a trajectory projecting kidney failure within one to two years, with no vascular or peritoneal access referral yet placed and no modality education yet delivered. DECISION: Refer for access evaluation and begin modality education now, at G4, rather than waiting for G5 or for symptoms to appear — fistula maturation and informed modality choice both require a runway measured in months. Begin access referral and modality education at G4, not G5 — waiting for symptoms forfeits the runway that makes a scheduled, patient-chosen start possible.

Chapter 2: The ESKD Life-Plan: Modality Selection and Patient-Centered Care

A patient's clinical trajectory has diverged from the modality plan constructed at an earlier visit — A transplant evaluation is discontinued, a peritoneal membrane develops declining ultrafiltration capacity, or a functional decline makes a previously chosen home modality newly impractical — in a patient whose Life-Plan has not been revisited since it was originally written. DECISION: Trigger a scheduled Life-Plan review rather than allowing the original plan to continue by default; reassess modality trajectory and revise the Access Needs plan to match the patient's current, not historical, circumstances. A major clinical transition is itself the trigger for Life-Plan review — do not wait for the plan to visibly fail before reconsidering it.

A patient presents persistent, unresolved ambivalence after standard modality education — The patient has received balanced comparative information across two or more encounters, finds each option's outcome data reassuring, but remains unable to commit to a modality, often citing the daily demands of each option as similarly intimidating in the abstract. DECISION: Escalate from verbal comparative education to concrete, experiential resources — a home assessment, a peer-patient conversation, or a hands-on equipment demonstration — rather than repeating the same comparative statistics a further time. Repeated verbal education rarely resolves ambivalence that concrete, experiential exposure to the modality's daily reality can resolve in a single encounter.

A patient is identified with advanced kidney disease only at the point of an unplanned hospitalization, with no prior Life-Plan of any kind — Uremic symptoms prompting hospital presentation, no established nephrology follow-up, no modality education, and no vascular or peritoneal access in place at the time an absolute or relative indication for initiation is identified. DECISION: Place a central venous catheter as an explicitly temporary bridge, and begin modality education and permanent access evaluation in parallel within the same hospitalization, rather than completing the full Life-Plan conversation before any access decision is made. Treat every late-referred catheter as a bridge with an active permanent-access plan attached from day one, not as a default long-term solution.

A peritoneal dialysis patient shows early signs of declining membrane function on routine testing — A peritoneal equilibration test shows transition toward a higher transporter category, accompanied by declining ultrafiltration despite escalating dextrose concentration, in a patient with no active hemodialysis access. DECISION: Initiate hemodialysis access evaluation now, in parallel with any transplant re-evaluation, so that a mature access is available before peritoneal ultrafiltration failure becomes clinically limiting, rather than waiting for outright technique failure to trigger access creation reactively. A rising transporter category with declining ultrafiltration is the trigger to begin the next access in the Life-Plan sequence — not a cue to simply escalate the current prescription further.

Chapter 3: Conservative and Palliative Kidney Management

A patient with advanced kidney disease is being assessed for conservative kidney management candidacy — Advanced age with significant frailty, high comorbidity burden, and a low estimated survival benefit from dialysis on a validated prognostic tool, often accompanied by low mood, poor appetite, and apparent resignation that could reflect either the patient's considered assessment of their situation or an undertreated depressive or pain syndrome. DECISION: Screen explicitly for depression and inadequately controlled symptoms before finalizing a conservative management recommendation, treating any identified depression or pain aggressively, and revisit the candidacy conversation once those are addressed rather than accepting apparent resignation at face value. Treat depression and uncontrolled symptoms before finalizing a conservative management decision — an apparently settled preference for comfort-focused care should persist once those confounders are addressed, not simply be accepted at the point of maximal distress.

A patient and family express differing preferences during a goals-of-care discussion — The patient states a clear preference — for example, to decline further escalation of care — while family members present express distress and advocate for continued aggressive treatment, sometimes speaking over or for the patient during the encounter. DECISION: Prioritize the documented, directly expressed preference of a patient who retains decision-making capacity, while offering the family a separate, structured meeting to process their distress and understand the reasoning behind the patient's choice, rather than allowing the family's more vocal objection to override a competent patient's stated preference in the moment. A capacitated patient's directly expressed preference governs the plan; family distress is addressed through dedicated support, not by overriding the patient's own stated goals.

An established dialysis patient voices a request to stop treatment — A stated wish to discontinue dialysis, which may arise during a difficult but medically survivable complication, an acute mood disturbance, or as a stable, repeatedly expressed preference consistent with the patient's previously stated values. DECISION: Screen explicitly for depression, uncontrolled pain, and delirium; confirm the request's stability across more than one conversation; and, once confirmed as considered and stable, honor it with the same clinical rigor and proactive symptom-management planning applied to any other major treatment decision in this book. Treat reversible contributors first, confirm stability across repeated conversations, then honor a considered withdrawal request with the same respect given to any other informed patient decision in this book.

Chapter 4: Physiology of Solute and Fluid Removal in Hemodialysis

A patient achieves an adequate small-solute Kt/V but continues to report significant uremic symptom burden — Urea reduction ratio and Kt/V both meet or exceed standard adequacy targets, yet the patient reports persistent fatigue, pruritus, or other uremic symptoms that would typically be expected to improve with adequate clearance. DECISION: Consider that small-solute adequacy does not guarantee comparable clearance of middle molecules or protein-bound toxins, and evaluate whether treatment frequency, duration, or convective strategy adjustment, rather than further escalation of the standard Kt/V target, is the more appropriate response to this symptom pattern. An adequate small-solute Kt/V does not rule out an undertreated middle-molecule or protein-bound toxin burden as a contributor to persistent uremic symptoms.

A patient beginning their first several hemodialysis treatments with severe, longstanding pre-treatment acidosis and uremia develops headache and nausea during or shortly after treatment — New-onset headache, nausea, or mild confusion developing during or within hours of an early hemodialysis session in a patient with a markedly elevated pre-treatment blood urea nitrogen and low bicarbonate, typically on one of the first several treatments rather than an established patient on a stable prescription. DECISION: Recognize this as a disequilibrium-type presentation potentially reflecting both rapid urea-driven osmotic shift and rapid bicarbonate correction, and confirm that initial treatments are being conducted at reduced intensity — shortened duration and reduced blood flow — with gradual escalation over subsequent sessions rather than delivering a full-intensity prescription to a new, severely uremic patient. Severely uremic, acidotic patients begin hemodialysis at reduced intensity with gradual escalation — this is a preventive prescription choice, not merely a response to symptoms once they occur.

Chapter 5: Dialyzers, Membranes, and Water Treatment Systems

A patient develops respiratory and cutaneous symptoms within minutes of starting a hemodialysis treatment using a newly opened dialyzer — Dyspnea, urticaria, and, in severe cases, hypotension developing within the first five to ten minutes of a treatment using a dialyzer the patient has not previously used, particularly if the patient is concurrently taking an ACE inhibitor. DECISION: Stop the treatment immediately, do not return the blood in the extracorporeal circuit to the patient if the reaction is severe, treat as an anaphylactoid reaction, and document the specific dialyzer membrane and sterilization method for future avoidance. Severe symptoms within minutes of a new dialyzer's first use, especially with urticaria, are a dialyzer reaction until proven otherwise — stop the treatment and avoid that membrane and sterilization method going forward.

Multiple patients treated on the same water system develop new, similar symptoms within the same treatment shift — Fatigue, chest or back discomfort, or an unexplained falling hematocrit arising in more than one patient scheduled on the same water loop within the same shift, without an identified source of blood loss in any individual patient. DECISION: Stop treatments on the implicated water system immediately, notify technical staff to inspect water treatment components — chloramine removal and reverse osmosis performance in particular — and arrange alternative water access before resuming any further treatments on that system. Similar new symptoms in multiple patients on the same water system within one shift is a water treatment failure until inspection proves otherwise — stop treatments on that system immediately rather than managing each patient in isolation.

A venous pressure alarm triggers during an otherwise unremarkable treatment — A venous pressure reading outside the expected range for the prescribed blood flow rate, without any accompanying air detection alarm or blood leak alarm, occurring either as an isolated event or with a gradually rising trend over the preceding portion of the treatment. DECISION: Check needle or catheter position and line patency directly rather than simply resetting the alarm; a low pressure warrants checking for dislodgement or disconnection, while a rising or high pressure warrants checking for clot formation in the line or a positional problem with the access itself. A rising venous pressure trend, as opposed to a single isolated spike, warrants a direct patency check of the access and line — not simply an alarm reset.

Chapter 6: The Hemodialysis Prescription: Writing and Adjusting Orders

A patient on a standard dialysate potassium prescription is found to have a persistently elevated predialysis potassium despite reported dietary adherence — Predialysis potassium consistently above target on serial monthly labs, in a patient reporting adherence to dietary potassium restriction, with no recent medication change and no evidence of missed treatments. DECISION: Reassess dialysate potassium prescription and the interdialytic interval and treatment time rather than assuming dietary nonadherence by default; consider a lower dialysate potassium concentration, evaluate whether treatment time or frequency is adequate for this patient's potassium generation rate, and reserve dietary counseling escalation for after the prescription itself has been optimized. Review the dialysate potassium prescription and treatment adequacy before attributing persistent hyperkalemia to dietary nonadherence.

A patient's measured dialysis adequacy falls persistently short of target despite an apparently adequate prescribed blood flow rate and treatment time — A Kt/V or urea reduction ratio below target on repeated measurement, in a patient whose prescribed blood flow rate, dialysate flow rate, and treatment time appear more than sufficient to achieve the target on paper, without an obvious alternative explanation such as missed treatments. DECISION: Evaluate specifically for vascular access recirculation — checking needle placement and spacing, and assessing for access stenosis — rather than responding to the adequacy shortfall by further increasing blood flow rate or treatment time, which will not correct a clearance gap caused by recirculation and may worsen it if the underlying cause is a stenosis limiting available flow. An unexplained adequacy shortfall despite a seemingly sufficient prescription warrants a specific recirculation evaluation before escalating flow rate or treatment time further.

A patient develops new or worsening intradialytic hypotension following a recent hospitalization — Recurrent intradialytic hypotension over several treatments beginning shortly after a hospital admission, particularly one involving a documented weight change, in a patient whose dry weight was not reassessed at the time of discharge. DECISION: Reassess dry weight explicitly in light of the hospitalization, adjusting it sequentially over two or more treatments while monitoring tolerance at each step, rather than treating the hypotension as an isolated hemodynamic problem to be managed with sodium profiling or ultrafiltration adjustment alone without addressing the underlying dry weight change. A recent hospitalization with a documented weight change is a trigger for explicit dry weight reassessment, not simply a background detail to note in the chart.

Chapter 7: Hemodialysis Adequacy: Kt/V, Urea Kinetics, and Their Limits

A patient's measured Kt/V is unexpectedly and persistently low despite an apparently adequate prescription — A calculated Kt/V below target in a patient receiving blood and dialysate flow rates, treatment time, and dialyzer specification that would be expected to achieve an adequate dose, with no other clinical explanation for underdialysis apparent. DECISION: Evaluate for access recirculation using a dedicated recirculation study and review the post-treatment sampling technique used, rather than escalating blood flow rate, treatment time, or dialyzer surface area in response to a Kt/V result that may reflect a measurement artifact rather than a true delivered-dose deficit. An unexpectedly low Kt/V in a prescription that should otherwise be adequate warrants a recirculation and sampling-technique evaluation before the prescription itself is escalated.

A patient with a stable, at-target Kt/V develops new fatigue, declining appetite, or a falling albumin trend — New or worsening constitutional symptoms and a declining nutritional marker in a patient whose Kt/V has remained at or above target throughout, with no change documented in the dialysis prescription itself. DECISION: Pursue a whole-patient adequacy review — residual kidney function, nutritional assessment, volume status — rather than reassuring the patient that a numerically adequate Kt/V excludes a dialysis-related explanation for the new symptoms. New symptoms despite a stable, at-target Kt/V warrant a whole-patient adequacy review, not reassurance based on the Kt/V number alone.

Chapter 8: Anticoagulation in Hemodialysis

A hemodialysis patient develops a substantial, otherwise unexplained decline in platelet count — A platelet count decline of a magnitude and timing — typically five to ten days after heparin exposure, or sooner with recent prior exposure — consistent with an immune-mediated process, in a patient receiving routine heparin anticoagulation for dialysis and, often, heparin locks for catheter maintenance between treatments. DECISION: Evaluate for heparin-induced thrombocytopenia specifically, and if confirmed or strongly suspected, discontinue all heparin exposure across every source — treatment dosing, catheter locks, and coated circuit components — transitioning to a non-heparin anticoagulant, citrate, or anticoagulation-free technique. An unexplained platelet decline in a heparin-exposed dialysis patient is heparin-induced thrombocytopenia until evaluated otherwise — and confirmation requires eliminating heparin from every exposure source, not just the treatment dose.

A patient with an elevated bleeding risk requires hemodialysis anticoagulation — A recent surgical procedure, active gastrointestinal bleeding, or another condition substantially elevating systemic bleeding risk in a patient who otherwise requires standard hemodialysis, with the treating team defaulting toward the unit's standard heparin protocol. DECISION: Select regional citrate anticoagulation or an anticoagulation-free technique rather than standard systemic heparin, matching the anticoagulation approach to the patient's actual bleeding risk rather than applying the unit's default protocol uniformly. An elevated bleeding risk is the trigger to select citrate or an anticoagulation-free approach — not a cue to proceed with the unit's standard heparin protocol by default.

A patient experiences recurrent circuit clotting or prolonged post-treatment bleeding despite an apparently standard anticoagulation protocol — Repeated early circuit clotting requiring dialyzer replacement, or prolonged oozing from needle or catheter sites beyond several minutes of direct pressure, in a patient receiving standard weight-based heparin dosing without individualized clotting time verification. DECISION: Measure clotting time directly to assess whether the standard dose is under- or over-anticoagulating this specific patient, and adjust the dose based on that measurement rather than continuing an unmodified standard protocol or empirically guessing at an adjustment. Recurrent clotting or bleeding on a standard heparin protocol warrants direct clotting time measurement and individualized dose adjustment, not an assumption that the standard dose must be correctly calibrated.

Part III — Vascular Access

Chapter 9: Vascular Access Planning and Creation: Fistula, Graft, and Catheter

A fistula fails to show adequate maturation at the scheduled six-week assessment — A fistula that, at scheduled follow-up assessment approximately six weeks after creation, lacks the expected diameter, depth, or flow characteristics despite an apparently uncomplicated surgical creation and early postoperative course. DECISION: Pursue targeted vascular imaging to identify a correctable cause — juxta-anastomotic stenosis or a diverting accessory branch — and intervene to salvage the fistula, rather than waiting further in the hope that maturation will proceed on its own or proceeding directly to an entirely new access creation without first evaluating for a salvageable cause. Inadequate maturation at the scheduled assessment warrants targeted imaging for a correctable cause before further waiting or before abandoning the fistula for a new access creation.

A patient's Life-Plan trajectory changes after an access type has already been chosen based on the original plan — A patient originally planned for a shorter-duration access, such as a catheter bridging to an anticipated near-term transplant, whose transplant timeline is subsequently delayed substantially beyond what was originally anticipated. DECISION: Reassess access choice against the revised trajectory, considering whether a more durable access — fistula or graft — is now warranted given the extended anticipated duration of dialysis dependence, rather than continuing the original shorter-duration access plan unexamined. A materially changed trajectory is the trigger to reassess access choice, not merely dialysis prescription or goals of care — access decisions require the same active revision discipline established throughout this book.

A patient with bilaterally poor peripheral vessel mapping and a history of prior central venous catheterization is being evaluated for access creation — Inadequate vein caliber on peripheral mapping in both arms, combined with a history of one or more prior central venous catheters, in a patient being considered for graft creation based on the peripheral mapping findings alone. DECISION: Obtain a central venogram before proceeding to graft creation, since central venous stenosis from the prior catheter history could compromise outflow from an otherwise technically adequate graft regardless of peripheral vessel quality. A history of prior central venous catheterization in a patient being evaluated for a new access is the trigger to obtain a central venogram before proceeding — not to rely on peripheral mapping findings alone.

Chapter 10: Cannulation Technique and Vascular Access Physical Examination

Routine pre-treatment physical examination reveals a change in thrill or bruit character from a patient's established baseline — A thrill that has become discontinuous or confined to systole, or a bruit that has become high-pitched and turbulent rather than the patient's usual continuous, low-pitched finding, identified on routine examination before cannulation for that day's treatment. DECISION: Perform the augmentation and elevation tests to localize the suspected stenosis, document the finding and its comparison against the patient's baseline examination, and refer for formal vascular imaging rather than proceeding with cannulation and treatment as though the examination were unremarkable. A change in thrill or bruit character from a patient's own established baseline warrants augmentation testing and imaging referral — not reassurance that the access remains grossly functional.

A patient reports a subjective change in their access's sensation between scheduled treatments — A patient calling on a non-treatment day to report that their fistula or graft feels different than usual, often vaguely described, without other symptoms such as pain, swelling, or fever, and without the patient scheduled to be seen again for a day or more. DECISION: Arrange same-day evaluation rather than deferring assessment to the next scheduled treatment, since a patient's own longstanding familiarity with their access's baseline sensation is a valid clinical signal even when they cannot articulate the change in precise clinical terms. A patient-reported change in access sensation warrants same-day evaluation, not deferral to the next scheduled treatment, regardless of how imprecisely the patient can describe the change.

Chapter 11: Vascular Access Complications: Stenosis, Thrombosis, and Infection

Access flow trend or venous pressure trend shows a gradual decline or rise over several consecutive treatments without a single dramatic threshold-crossing value — A monthly access flow measurement or venous pressure reading that has moved consistently in a concerning direction over three or more consecutive measurements, with each individual value still falling within a technically acceptable range when considered alone. DECISION: Treat the consistent trend itself as the actionable finding and refer for duplex ultrasound evaluation, rather than waiting for any single measurement to cross an absolute numeric threshold before acting. A consistent multi-measurement trend, not any single value, is the actionable surveillance signal — refer for imaging based on the trend rather than waiting for a threshold crossing.

A patient with a vascular access graft develops localized erythema and tenderness at a cannulation site — New warmth, erythema, tenderness, or drainage at a graft cannulation site, with or without accompanying systemic symptoms such as fever, in a patient whose graft has otherwise been functioning normally. DECISION: Obtain blood cultures before initiating empiric antibiotic therapy where clinical stability permits, and monitor closely for response; extensive involvement or failure to respond within the expected timeframe warrants surgical evaluation for possible graft excision rather than continued antibiotic therapy alone. Graft infection that is extensive or fails to respond to appropriate antibiotics within the expected timeframe requires surgical evaluation for excision — not continued antibiotic therapy alone.

A dialysis patient with a large-caliber, proximal fistula develops new or worsening heart failure symptoms — New dyspnea, fatigue, or other heart failure symptoms in a patient with a high-flow, proximal configuration fistula, where the presentation is being attributed solely to volume overload or intrinsic cardiac disease without consideration of the access itself as a contributing factor. DECISION: Consider access-attributable high-output cardiac failure specifically, obtain formal access flow measurement, and involve vascular surgery for possible flow-reduction banding if the access is confirmed as a meaningful contributor, rather than managing the heart failure through volume and cardiac-directed therapy alone. New heart failure in a patient with a large-caliber, high-flow fistula warrants formal access flow measurement to evaluate for an access-attributable contribution, not management directed solely at volume and cardiac causes.

Chapter 12: Central Venous Catheters: Placement, Care, and Catheter-Related Bloodstream Infection

A tunneled catheter shows a gradual decline in aspiration capability while infusion remains relatively preserved — Progressive difficulty achieving adequate blood flow for treatment, developing gradually over days to weeks, with the catheter still able to infuse fluid relatively easily but unable to aspirate blood adequately to support the prescribed blood flow rate. DECISION: Recognize this asymmetric infuse-versus-aspirate pattern as characteristic of a fibrin sheath rather than acute intraluminal thrombus, and proceed toward guidewire exchange or fluoroscopic sheath disruption rather than relying on thrombolytic instillation alone, which is less effective against an external fibrin sheath than against intraluminal clot. An asymmetric infuse-easy, aspirate-poor pattern with gradual onset points to a fibrin sheath — proceed toward guidewire exchange or sheath disruption rather than relying on thrombolytic instillation alone.

A patient with a tunneled catheter and no remaining alternative vascular access develops confirmed catheter-related bloodstream infection — Fever and positive paired blood cultures confirming a catheter source, in a patient whose infecting organism is not Staphylococcus aureus or a fungal species, without tunnel-tract involvement, septic thrombosis, or endocarditis, and who has previously been assessed as having no remaining surgical access option. DECISION: Attempt catheter salvage with systemic antibiotics and antibiotic lock therapy given the organism's favorable salvage prognosis and the patient's lack of alternative access, monitoring closely for treatment response rather than proceeding directly to catheter removal. A favorable-prognosis organism without tunnel-tract involvement or other high-risk features, in a patient with no remaining access alternative, supports a salvage attempt — not reflexive catheter removal as the default first response.

Part IV — Intradialytic Complications and Emergencies

Chapter 13: Intradialytic Hypotension and Hemodynamic Instability

A patient develops nonspecific symptoms such as yawning, restlessness, or mild nausea during the middle-to-later portion of treatment — Vague, nonspecific discomfort, yawning, or restlessness developing during the period of treatment when ultrafiltration rate is typically highest, without yet meeting a formal threshold for measured hypotension on the most recent blood pressure check. DECISION: Treat these nonspecific symptoms as a potential early warning sign of evolving hypotension, obtain an immediate blood pressure check regardless of the scheduled monitoring interval, and consider reducing ultrafiltration rate proactively rather than waiting for the next scheduled check or for more dramatic symptoms to develop. Nonspecific symptoms during the high-ultrafiltration-rate portion of treatment warrant an immediate, unscheduled blood pressure check — not dismissal as unrelated discomfort.

A patient experiences recurrent intradialytic hypotension despite a single, isolated preventive measure already in place — Continued frequent hypotension episodes in a patient already receiving one preventive intervention, such as sodium profiling alone or dialysate temperature reduction alone, without the other complementary measures this chapter describes. DECISION: Implement a multimodal prevention bundle combining several complementary measures — treatment time, sodium and ultrafiltration profiling, temperature, and medication timing — rather than escalating the single measure already in place or concluding that prevention has been fully attempted. Recurrent hypotension despite a single preventive measure warrants a multimodal bundle addressing several mechanisms together — not escalation of the single measure already in place alone.

Chapter 14: Cramps, Dialyzer Reactions, and Other Common Intradialytic Symptoms

A patient develops new intradialytic nausea — New onset of nausea during treatment, without yet having a blood pressure check to correlate the symptom against, in a patient whose nausea could reflect evolving hypotension, disequilibrium syndrome, rapid electrolyte shift, or an unrelated cause. DECISION: Check blood pressure immediately as the first response to any new intradialytic nausea, treating hypotension as the presumptive cause until excluded, before pursuing symptomatic antiemetic treatment or considering the less common alternative causes. New intradialytic nausea warrants an immediate blood pressure check as the first response — not symptomatic antiemetic treatment before hypotension has been assessed.

A patient develops fever and rigors during or shortly after a dialysis treatment — New fever, chills, or rigors developing during or within the hour following a treatment, without yet being characterized as either an isolated event or part of a cluster affecting other patients on the same water system. DECISION: Obtain blood cultures before attributing the episode to a presumed pyrogenic reaction, and simultaneously check whether other patients on the same water system and shift are reporting similar symptoms, since this clustering assessment helps distinguish a water-system-level pyrogenic cause from an individual bacteremic process. Any significant intradialytic fever warrants blood cultures and a clustering check across other patients on the same water system — not an assumption of pyrogenic reaction without this confirmatory evaluation.

Chapter 15: Life-Threatening Intradialytic Emergencies: Air Embolism, Arrhythmia, and Cardiac Arrest

A patient with severe predialysis hyperkalemia shows early electrocardiographic changes during treatment — Peaked T waves or QRS widening on continuous monitoring in a patient with severe predialysis hyperkalemia, developing within the first portion of treatment, without yet progressing to a hemodynamically unstable rhythm. DECISION: Administer calcium gluconate for cardiac membrane stabilization, continue close monitoring, and allow the ongoing dialysis treatment to continue correcting the underlying potassium, escalating to advanced cardiac life support only if progression to an unstable rhythm occurs. Early peaked T waves or QRS widening in a hyperkalemic patient warrant calcium gluconate administration for membrane stabilization — not simply continued observation while awaiting further potassium correction alone.

Blood lines show a distinctive pink or red discoloration of the plasma component during treatment — Visible cherry or burgundy discoloration of the plasma within the blood lines, with or without the patient reporting back or chest pain, raising concern for acute hemolysis. DECISION: Stop the blood pump immediately, do not return the hemolyzed blood to the patient given the severe hyperkalemia risk it carries, and investigate the underlying cause following the water-treatment and machine-malfunction clustering assessment described in Chapter 5. Visible plasma discoloration is acute hemolysis until proven otherwise — stop the pump immediately and do not return the affected blood to the patient.

Part V — Peritoneal Dialysis

Chapter 16: Peritoneal Physiology and Membrane Transport Characteristics

A peritoneal dialysis patient develops declining ultrafiltration despite an unchanged prescription — Progressive difficulty achieving adequate fluid removal, with new or worsening volume overload symptoms, in a patient whose peritoneal dialysis prescription has not been recently modified and who has not had transport category reassessed in some time. DECISION: Obtain a repeat PET to assess for a transport category shift, distinguishing this specific, correctable mechanism from other causes of ultrafiltration failure such as membrane fibrosis or aquaporin dysfunction, and revise the prescription to match whatever transport category the repeat test reveals. Declining ultrafiltration on an unchanged prescription warrants a repeat PET to assess for a transport category shift specifically — not an assumption of generic, unspecified membrane failure.

Chapter 17: Peritoneal Dialysis Catheters and Prescription Design

A peritoneal dialysis patient reports progressively slower or incomplete drainage during exchanges — Gradually worsening drainage time or incomplete drainage volume over days to weeks, without fever, abdominal pain, or cloudy effluent that would instead suggest the peritonitis discussed in Chapter 19. DECISION: Evaluate and address bowel habit and constipation first, since this is the most common and most readily reversible cause, before pursuing an abdominal radiograph to assess for catheter tip migration or considering surgical evaluation for omental wrapping if the drainage problem persists despite an adequate bowel regimen. Impaired peritoneal drainage warrants addressing constipation first — not immediate radiographic or surgical evaluation before this simple, common, and reversible cause has been excluded.

A patient on an incremental peritoneal dialysis prescription has not had residual kidney function reassessed in an extended period — A patient started on a reduced, incremental peritoneal dialysis prescription based on residual function measured at initiation, now well beyond the interval at which reassessment was originally planned, with no repeat measurement yet obtained despite the predictable, expected decline in residual function over time. DECISION: Obtain a repeat residual function measurement and advance the peritoneal prescription proportionally if a meaningful decline is confirmed, rather than allowing the original reduced prescription to continue by default simply because no symptom has yet prompted reconsideration. An overdue residual function reassessment on an incremental prescription warrants proactive repeat measurement and prescription advancement — not continuation of the original reduced dose by default until symptoms eventually appear.

Chapter 18: Peritoneal Dialysis Adequacy and Individualized Prescription

A peritoneal dialysis patient's combined total Kt/V remains stable while their residual function has not been separately reassessed recently — A stable, at-target combined total Kt/V on routine monitoring in a patient whose residual and dialysate components have not been separately reviewed, and whose residual function has not been formally reassessed within the interval this chapter recommends. DECISION: Review the dialysate and residual components of the total Kt/V separately, and obtain a fresh residual function measurement if due, rather than accepting a stable combined total as confirmation that no meaningful change has occurred in either underlying component. A stable combined Kt/V does not confirm stable residual function — review the components separately and reassess residual function on schedule rather than inferring stability from the total alone.

A peritoneal dialysis patient with a stable, at-target total Kt/V develops new fatigue or declining appetite — New constitutional symptoms and a declining nutritional marker in a patient whose combined total Kt/V has remained at target throughout, without an obvious change in the prescription itself. DECISION: Pursue a whole-patient adequacy review, including separate residual and dialysate component tracking, residual urine output trend, and nutritional assessment, rather than reassuring the patient that a numerically adequate total Kt/V excludes a dialysis-related explanation. New symptoms despite a stable total Kt/V warrant a whole-patient adequacy review — not reassurance based on the combined total number alone.

Chapter 19: Peritonitis and Peritoneal Access Infections

A peritoneal dialysis patient's culture returns polymicrobial with enteric organisms identified — More than one organism identified on peritonitis culture, including one or more typically enteric or bowel-flora organisms, in a patient whose clinical presentation may otherwise appear consistent with straightforward peritonitis. DECISION: Pursue surgical evaluation and abdominal imaging to assess for an underlying bowel-related process such as perforation or another intra-abdominal surgical pathology, rather than treating the finding solely as a more complex peritonitis requiring broader antibiotic coverage alone. A polymicrobial culture with enteric organisms is the trigger for surgical evaluation and abdominal imaging — not simply an indication for broader antibiotic coverage alone.

A peritoneal dialysis patient experiences a repeat peritonitis episode with the same organism shortly after completing therapy for a prior episode — A peritonitis episode identifying the same organism as a prior episode, recurring within weeks of that prior episode's treatment completion, in a pattern now established across two or more such episodes rather than a single isolated recurrence. DECISION: Recognize this as a recurrent, relapsing infection pattern suggesting persistent catheter-level colonization, and proceed to catheter removal and replacement rather than a further antibiotic trial with the existing catheter. A recurrent, relapsing pattern with the same organism across multiple episodes is the trigger for catheter removal and replacement — not a further antibiotic trial with the existing catheter retained.

Part VI — Home, Intensive, and Acute Modalities

Chapter 20: Home Hemodialysis and Intensive Dialysis Regimens

A home hemodialysis patient's machine alarm indicates a venous pressure abnormality during an unsupervised treatment — A venous pressure alarm during home treatment, with the patient or care partner needing to determine independently whether this reflects a benign, correctable issue or a genuine access emergency requiring immediate line clamping and emergency response. DECISION: Follow the trained troubleshooting sequence: directly inspect the access site for visible dislodgement or bleeding before resetting the alarm, and if a genuine separation or bleeding is confirmed, immediately clamp lines, apply direct pressure, and contact the unit's emergency protocol rather than simply resetting the alarm and continuing treatment. A venous pressure alarm during home treatment warrants direct access site inspection before any alarm reset — not a reflexive reset without first confirming the access itself is secure.

A patient asks whether intensive home hemodialysis will definitely improve their specific clinical outcomes — A patient considering a transition to short daily or nocturnal home hemodialysis, seeking a clear, confident answer about whether this transition will improve their specific cardiovascular or quality-of-life outcomes. DECISION: Present the genuinely nuanced evidence honestly — generally favorable but not uniformly conclusive, subject to selection-effect limitations in much of the observational data — rather than overstating benefit as more definitively established than the evidence actually supports. Present intensive hemodialysis outcome evidence honestly, including its real limitations — not as a more definitively established benefit than the evidence base actually supports.

Chapter 21: Acute Kidney Injury and Continuous Renal Replacement Therapy

A CRRT filter shows a rising transmembrane pressure trend with declining effluent flow — A gradual rise in transmembrane pressure accompanied by declining effluent or filtrate flow rate over several hours, with blood flow rate unchanged, in a patient on established anticoagulation for continuous renal replacement therapy. DECISION: Recognize this as early filter clotting, review whether the current anticoagulation protocol is properly calibrated for this specific patient, and proceed to a planned, elective filter change before the filter clots outright and interrupts treatment unexpectedly. A rising transmembrane pressure and declining effluent flow trend warrants anticoagulation review and a planned filter change — not simply continued observation until the filter clots outright.

Part VII — Systemic and Metabolic Complications

Chapter 22: Anemia Management in Dialysis Patients

A patient requires progressively escalating ESA doses without the expected hemoglobin response, despite adequate iron studies — A rising ESA dose trend over successive treatments without a corresponding hemoglobin improvement, in a patient whose transferrin saturation and ferritin appear adequate on recent testing. DECISION: Proceed through the structured hyporesponsiveness evaluation sequence — reviewing dialysis adequacy, vascular access for occult infection, and secondary hyperparathyroidism — rather than continuing to escalate ESA dose indefinitely in the absence of an identified explanation. Progressive ESA dose escalation without hemoglobin response, despite adequate iron studies, warrants a structured search for occult inflammation or infection — not continued dose escalation alone.

Chapter 23: Mineral and Bone Disorder in Chronic Kidney Disease

A patient with markedly suppressed PTH develops new bone pain or an unexpected fracture — New bone pain, an unexpected fracture, or a rising alkaline phosphatase inconsistent with a very low PTH, in a patient receiving aggressive calcimimetic or active vitamin D therapy that has suppressed PTH well below the individualized target range. DECISION: Consider adynamic bone disease from PTH over-suppression as the explanation, reduce calcimimetic and vitamin D dosing to allow PTH to rise back into the individualized target range, and monitor for symptomatic improvement rather than assuming the low PTH value is reassuring. New bone pain or fracture with a markedly suppressed PTH warrants considering adynamic bone disease and reducing suppressive therapy — not reassurance that a low PTH value reflects successful treatment.

Chapter 24: Cardiovascular Disease and Fluid Management in Dialysis Patients

A patient's hypertension remains poorly controlled despite escalating antihypertensive medication — Persistently elevated blood pressure despite progressive antihypertensive dose escalation, in a patient whose dry weight has not been formally reassessed recently despite a plausible reason, such as declining muscle mass or weight change, to suspect it may no longer reflect true euvolemic status. DECISION: Reassess dry weight using the structured, multi-method assessment approach this chapter details, and pursue a trial dry weight adjustment if reassessment suggests the current target no longer reflects true euvolemia, rather than continuing to escalate antihypertensive medication alone. Poorly controlled hypertension despite escalating medication warrants dry weight reassessment — not continued antihypertensive escalation alone without first considering a volume-dependent explanation.

Chapter 25: Nutrition, Infection, and Hepatitis C in the Dialysis Population

A dialysis patient develops a new hepatitis C infection after a previously negative screening result — A newly positive hepatitis C test in a patient who had previously tested negative at routine screening, without a clearly identified outside exposure risk on careful history. DECISION: Treat this as a potential sentinel event for a unit-level infection control lapse, immediately reviewing infection control practice and screening other patients treated on the same equipment or in the same area during the relevant period, rather than treating the case as isolated. A new hepatitis C infection in a previously negative patient warrants immediate unit-level investigation and screening of other patients on the same equipment — not treatment as an isolated, unexplained occurrence.

Part VIII — Special Populations and Transitions of Care

Chapter 26: Dialysis in Pediatric, Geriatric, and Pregnant Patients

A dialysis-dependent patient falls into one of this chapter's special populations — pediatric, frail older adult, or pregnant — A patient whose developmental stage, frailty status, or pregnancy status introduces considerations beyond the general adult dialysis framework this book has developed throughout its preceding chapters. DECISION: Adapt the Life-Plan and shared decision-making framework explicitly to this population's specific considerations — growth and transition planning, frailty-adjusted prescription and decision-making, or intensified pregnancy-specific prescription and multidisciplinary monitoring — rather than applying the general adult framework unmodified. A patient in one of this chapter's special populations warrants explicit adaptation of the Life-Plan framework to their specific considerations — not the general adult framework applied unmodified.

Chapter 27: Kidney Transplant Evaluation and Perioperative Dialysis Considerations

A kidney transplant recipient shows a gradually rising creatinine consistent with chronic graft dysfunction — A gradual, sustained rise in creatinine and decline in estimated glomerular filtration rate over successive follow-up visits in a transplant recipient, without an acute, reversible cause identified on evaluation. DECISION: Apply the same trajectory-based Life-Plan reasoning developed in Chapter 1 for native chronic kidney disease progression: initiate proactive vascular access planning and repeat transplant candidacy evaluation well before dialysis becomes urgently necessary, rather than waiting until graft failure is complete. A declining transplant trajectory warrants the same proactive Life-Plan and vascular access planning this book applies to native kidney disease progression — not passive monitoring until dialysis becomes urgently unavoidable.

CONCLUSION

This handbook opened with a single patient's creatinine beginning its final ascent toward kidney failure, and it closes, twenty-seven chapters and a transplant evaluation later, with that same patient's care extending across a lifetime rather than a single decision. That arc was deliberate. Kidney replacement therapy is too often taught and practiced as a series of disconnected technical problems: a prescription to write, a complication to manage, a laboratory value to correct. This book has tried instead to show that these are facets of a single, continuous clinical relationship, one that begins well before dialysis is medically necessary and, for many patients, continues well beyond it.

Three themes have run beneath every chapter of this handbook, regardless of which organ system, modality, or complication was under discussion. The first is that trajectory matters more than any single measurement. A creatinine, a Kt/V, a hemoglobin, a transmembrane pressure, an access flow rate — each of these numbers means something only in relation to where it has been and where it is going. The clinician who reacts to a single value in isolation will, again and again through this book's chapters, arrive at the wrong conclusion; the clinician who tracks the trend arrives at the right one sooner and with greater confidence. The second theme is that escalation is not a strategy. From hemodialysis Kt/V to peritoneal dialysis dosing to CRRT effluent rate to hemoglobin targets, this book has documented the same pattern in trial after trial: pushing a therapeutic target higher once an adequate threshold has been reached rarely helps, and sometimes causes real harm. Adequate, well-individualized treatment, not maximal treatment, is the standard this book has argued for throughout. The third theme is that the earlier a problem is anticipated, the better it resolves. Vein preservation before a fistula is ever needed. Transplant evaluation before dialysis is required. Dry weight reassessment before hypertension becomes entrenched. Transition planning before a graft fails outright. Anticipation, not reaction, is what separates good kidney failure care from adequate kidney failure care, and this book has tried to make that difference concrete rather than aspirational.

The Dialysis Recognition & Response System, built into every chapter's Rhythm Layer and consolidated in the Master Index that follows this conclusion, exists to make that anticipatory instinct teachable. Recognizing a pattern, understanding the decision it calls for, and knowing the trap that catches an inexperienced or hurried clinician are three distinct skills, and this book has tried to build all three together rather than assuming that clinical experience alone will eventually supply them. No index, however thorough, substitutes for judgment developed at the bedside over years of practice. What it can do is compress some of that learning curve, flagging the patterns experienced clinicians already recognize instinctively so that a resident, fellow, or early-career nephrologist recognizes them a little sooner, and a practicing clinician confirms an instinct a little faster.

Kidney replacement therapy will keep changing. Some of what this book documents as current practice will be revised, some of the evidence it cites as settled will be reopened, and some of the technology it describes will be superseded within the working life of anyone reading it now. That is not a weakness particular to this book; it is the ordinary condition of medicine, and it is precisely why this book has emphasized reasoning over memorization wherever the two could be separated. A reader who understands why intensive hemodialysis schedules reduce sudden cardiac death risk, why hepcidin produces functional iron deficiency, or why a transplant evaluation should begin years before dialysis is likely, is better equipped to absorb the next decade's revisions to specific numbers and protocols than a reader who has only memorized this decade's targets.

This book was written for the clinician standing at a patient's bedside at two in the morning, for the fellow reviewing a confusing lab trend before rounds, and for the nephrologist building a Life-Plan with a newly referred patient who is frightened and has a hundred questions. If it has done its job, that reader now has a framework for organizing what they already know, a vocabulary for naming what they are seeing, and the confidence to act on a pattern before it becomes a crisis. The patients on the other side of every one of these chapters are counting on exactly that.

www.ingramcontent.com/pod-product-compliance
Lightning Source LLC
LaVergne TN
LVHW060440061126
851857LV00016B/1679